Strengths-Based Resilience

About the Authors

Tayyab Rashid, PhD, C. Psych., is a licensed school and clinical psychologist and lives in Toronto, Canada. Dr. Rashid has worked with the Toronto District School Board for 5 years as a school psychologist. He has also worked 12 years at the Health and Wellness Centre, University of Toronto Scarborough (UTSC). Dr. Rashid is also a faculty associate with the Human Flourishing Program and a visiting scientist at Chan School of Public Health, Harvard. He completed his doctoral studies at Farleigh Dickinson University and clinical internship and postdoctoral fellowship with Dr. Martin Seligman at the University of Pennsylvania. His expertise includes strength-based clinical psychotherapy focusing on complex mental health challenges, resilience, and posttraumatic growth. He has also worked with individuals experiencing severe trauma, including survivors of the Asian Tsunami of 2004, journalists who have worked in high conflict zones, and survivors of mass shootings. Dr. Rashid has delivered over fifty invited talks and keynotes; trained mental health professionals and educators internationally; and published widely in academic journals. His book *Positive Psychotherapy Clinician Manual* (2018), cowritten with Martin Seligman, is considered one of the most comprehensive clinical resources in the field and has been translated into several languages. Dr. Rashid won the Chancellor Award (2018) from University of Toronto and the Outstanding Practitioner Award (2017) from the International Positive Psychology Association (IPPA).

Jane Gillham, PhD, is a licensed clinical psychologist, educator, and researcher at Swarthmore College in the United States. Dr. Gillham also conducted research at the University of Pennsylvania's Positive Psychology Center for many years. Dr. Gillham's research focuses on promoting resilience and well-being in youth, with a particular focus on how schools, families, and communities can promote children's and adolescents' social and emotional development and help them to thrive. Dr. Gillham completed her BA in psychology at Princeton University, her PhD in psychology at the University of Pennsylvania (under the guidance of Dr. Martin Seligman), and her internship in child clinical psychology at the Yale University Child Study Center. Dr. Gillham is cocreator of the Penn Resilience Program (PRP), a curriculum designed to teach adolescents cognitive and behavioral skills for handling everyday challenges and stressors. PRP has been evaluated in more than 15 randomized controlled studies completed across the world. Dr. Gillham is an author of several other well-being programs for youth, including the Girls' Strengths and Resilience Program and a high school positive psychology curriculum. She has led several large program evaluation studies of these and other curricula designed to promote resilience, strengths, and well-being in youth. Dr. Gillham also serves as a scientific advisor to WorldBeing, a nonprofit organization devoted to promoting resilience and well-being in young people, especially those living in poor communities in low and middle income countries. Dr. Gillham's research has been published in top tier peer-reviewed journals. She previously served as an associate editor for the *Journal of Positive Psychology* (from 2010 to 2020) and has served on editorial boards of several academic journals.

Afroze Anjum, PsyD, C.Psych., is a licensed school psychologist at the Toronto District School Board. Dr. Anjum's expertise includes strengths-based, school-based interventions that incorporate character strengths, resilience, mindfulness, and adaptive problem-solving, to help students cope with challenges such as depression, anxiety, bullying, and lack of motivation. Dr. Anjum obtained her doctoral degree from Fairleigh Dickinson University, New Jersey. She completed her postdoctoral training with Dr. Jane Gillham at Swarthmore College and the University of Pennsylvania where she worked as a researcher and training facilitator for the Penn Resilience Program and the Positive Psychology for Youth Project, a positive psychology curriculum study with high school participants. Dr. Anjum has taught and trained numerous professionals in positive interventions. Her work has been published in peer-reviewed journals and in edited volumes. Dr. Anjum is currently part of the Toronto District School Board's Well-Being Committee in the wake of COVID-19.

Strengths-Based Resilience

A Practitioner's Manual for the SBR Program

Tayyab Rashid
Jane Gillham
Afroze Anjum

hogrefe

Library of Congress of Congress Cataloging in Publication information for the print version of this book is available via the Library of Congress Marc Database under the Library of Congress Control Number 2024931372

Library and Archives Canada Cataloguing in Publication

Title: Strengths-based resilience : a practitioner's manual for the SBR program / Tayyab Rashid, Jane Gillham, Afroze Anjum.
Names: Rashid, Tayyab, author. | Gillham, Jane, author. | Anjum, Afroze, author.
Description: Includes bibliographical references and index.
Identifiers: Canadiana (print) 20240295676 | Canadiana (ebook) 20240295765 | ISBN 9780889375642 (softcover) | ISBN 9781616765644 (PDF) | ISBN 9781613345641 (EPUB)
Subjects: LCSH: Resilience (Personality trait)—Handbooks, manuals, etc. | LCGFT: Handbooks and manuals.
Classification: LCC BF698.35.R47 R37 2024 | DDC 155.2/4—dc23

www.hogrefe.com

Original illustrations *Strengths-Based Resilience Infographic and 7 illustrations in Practice 1: Stretch and Relax section of the Regular Practice: Relaxation and Mindfulness chapter* by Shafik Kamani. Illustration on the cover and illustrations in the following chapters: *Regular Practice: Mindfulness & Relaxation, Module 1: Resilience, Module 2: Fixed & Growth Mindsets, Module 4: Cognitive Flexibility, Module 11: Positive Relationships* modified by Shafik Kamani.

PUBLISHING OFFICES

USA:	Hogrefe Publishing Corporation, 44 Merrimac Street, Newburyport, MA 01950 Phone +1 978 255 3700; E-mail customersupport@hogrefe.com
EUROPE:	Hogrefe Publishing GmbH, Merkelstr. 3, 37085 Göttingen, Germany Phone +49 551 99950 0, Fax +49 551 99950 111; E-mail publishing@hogrefe.com

SALES & DISTRIBUTION

USA:	Hogrefe Publishing, Customer Services Department, 30 Amberwood Parkway, Ashland, OH 44805 Phone (800) 228 3749, Fax (419) 281 6883; E-mail customerservice@hogrefe.com
UK:	Hogrefe Publishing, c/o Marston Book Services Ltd., 160 Eastern Ave., Milton Park, Abingdon, OX14 4SB Phone +44 1235 465577, Fax +44 1235 465556; E-mail direct.orders@marston.co.uk
EUROPE:	Hogrefe Publishing, Merkelstr. 3, 37085 Göttingen, Germany Phone +49 551 99950 0, Fax +49 551 99950 111; E-mail publishing@hogrefe.com

OTHER OFFICES

CANADA:	Hogrefe Publishing, 82 Laird Drive, East York, Ontario M4G 3V1
SWITZERLAND:	Hogrefe Publishing, Länggass-Strasse 76, 3012 Bern

Printed and bound in the Czech Republic

ISBN 978-0-88937-564-2 (print) • ISBN 978-1-61676-564-4 (PDF) • ISBN 978-1-61334-564-1 (EPUB)
http://doi.org/10.1027/00564-000

Dedication

To Diane and Robert Ostermann, who believed in us more than we in ourselves.

T.R. & A.A.

In loving memory of Chris Peterson, who nurtured and celebrated the best in others, and whose work on character strengths inspired this program.

J.G.

Acknowledgments

We are grateful to Martin Seligman whose transformative mentorship inspired us to begin this meaningful work of building resilience through resources without ignoring risks. We thank Chris Peterson for his friendship and foundational work on character strengths, Karen Reivich for her inspiring Penn Resilience Program facilitator training, and Mark Linkins for his deep commitment to promoting students' strengths and his collaboration on previous projects that help set the stage for this program. We owe immense gratitude to Carolyn Lennox and Ruth Baumal at the Toronto District School Board for supporting the initial studies of SBR. We are immensely grateful to Donna and Neal Mayerson, Ryan Niemiec, and Jeffrey Levy for their support with the character strengths assessment. We could not have completed this important work without the Institutional support from our employers – the Toronto District School Board, the University of Toronto Scarborough, and Swarthmore College.

To weave this abstract concept of resilience into measurable, manageable, and teachable skills and strategies required encouragement and support from many individuals across the Toronto District School Board and the University of Toronto Scarborough to whom we are immensely grateful: Michael Alexander, Nabil Ali, Noof Al-Jenebi, Ruth Baumal, James Bowen, Mehmet Buyukcorak, Wenbin Cai, Peter Chang, Lauren Dade, Mehmet Dinc, Avanti and Murtaza Esufally, Lesley Gage, Anushka Fernando Goonetilleke, Milad Hadchiti, Tracy Hale, Dan Halliday, Rick Halpern, Laurie Hambly, Ken Harvey, John Henry, Lucy Horne, Ryan Howes, Khasfia Iqbal, Aaron Jarden, Shafik Kamani, Pomudith Katugampala, Faz Khan, Bruce Kidd, Samantha King, Elsa Kiosses, Calvin Knight, Tom Lazarou, Tim Lomas, Isabel Arias Lopez, Ary Lutchmie-Maharaj, Ed Malabre, Abdullah Mamun, Dessy Marinova, Taaha Muhammad, Ruba Nawaz, Ayesha Nisar, Lindsay Oades, Summayah and Yaseen Poonah, Mahmood Qasim, Denise Quinlan, Joy Reiter, Janine Robb, David Rowen, Marina Schuster, Mariam Shuchman, Laura Sloan, Noman Siddique, Kym Stadnyk, Stuart Snyder, Amanda Uliaszek, Tyler VanderWeele, Dianne Vella-Brodrick, Phil Wall, Sandali Weerakoon, Jennifer Wortham, and Laurie Wright.

We sincerely thank Ruth Louden for her editorial support on the SBR practitioner manual. Ruth is also a coauthor of the *Strengths-Based Resilience Workbook*. Ruth has been working with us on the SBR project for many years and is highly knowledgeable about the program's content, structure, and process. Her editorial insights and attention to detail kept (literally) hundreds of pieces of this project organized and moving. They also improved coherence and clarity throughout the book. We are grateful to Ruth for her expert guidance, diligence, and sincere efforts to make this Manual a good source for those who want to bring out the best in others.

Thank you Lisa Bennett, Robert Dimbleby, and Anne-Lisa Löck at Hogrefe for your enthusiastic support of the SBR program, thoughtful suggestions, advice, and patience through multiple revisions. You helped us to refine and greatly improve the materials while staying true to the lessons, activities, and aesthetic experience that were essential in our earlier unpublished version of the Manual.

To the many participants in our SBR Facilitator Training and students in Flourish and SBR programs, we are immensely grateful for your enthusiastic engagement and helpful feedback.

Contents

Dedication v
Acknowledgments vii
Preface xiii

Section I: Theoretical Background and Development of the Strengths-Based Resilience Program

1 Resilience **3**
Why Resilience Matters 3
Definitions and Descriptions of Resilience 6
Strengths-Based Resilience: Ten Key Considerations 8
Summary 13

2 Theoretical Foundations of Strengths-Based Resilience **21**
Theory of Well-Being: PERMA 21
Classification of Strengths and Virtues 24
Why a Strengths-Based Approach to Resilience? 27
Summary 29

3 SBR Program Development and Validation **35**
Development of the SBR Program 36
Validation of the SBR Program 40
Summary 42

4 SBR Program Content and Delivery **45**
Program Content 45
Program Delivery 51
General Considerations 53
Group Processes 55
Summary 57

Section II: Orientation Session and Regular Practice

Orientation Session **61**
Opening the Session 61
Regular Practices 64

Regular Practice 1: Mindfulness and Relaxation **69**
Core Concepts of Mindfulness and Relaxation 69
General Guidelines for Mindfulness and Relaxation Practice 73
Practice 1: Stretch and Relax 74
Practice 2: Breathe 79
Practice 3: Take a Mindful Minute 80
Practice 4: Use Positive Imagery 81
Practice 5: Visualize Lovingkindness 82
Learning and Cultural Fit 84

Regular Practice 2: Gratitude Journal **93**
Core Concepts of Gratitude 93
Practice: Reflect on Your Gratitude Journal 94
Learning and Cultural Fit 95

Section III: The Modules

Module 1: Resilience **103**
Core Concepts of Resilience 104
Practice: Write Your Own Story of Resilience 105
Learning and Cultural Fit 107
Closing Activities 107

Module 2: Fixed and Growth Mindsets **113**
Core Concepts of Fixed and Growth Mindsets 114
Practice: Identify Your Mindset Reactions 116
Learning and Cultural Fit 118
Closing Activities 119

Module 3: Cognitive Accuracy **125**
Core Concepts of Cognitive Accuracy 126
Practice 1: Unpack Experiences to Understand Challenges 129
Practice 2: Explore Your Thinking Shortcuts 131
Learning and Cultural Fit 133
Closing Activities 134

Module 4: Cognitive Flexibility **139**
Core Concepts of Cognitive Flexibility 140
Practice: Tune in to Your Explanatory Style 142
Learning and Cultural Fit 145
Closing Activities 145

Module 5: Character Strengths **151**
Core Concepts of Character Strengths 152
Practice: Spot Your Character Strengths 154
Learning and Cultural Fit 158
Closing Activities 159

Module 6: Signature Strengths **167**
Core Concepts of Signature Strengths 168
Practice: Compile your Signature Strengths Profile 170
Learning and Cultural Fit 177
Closing Activities 177

Module 7: Problem Solving and Strengths **183**
Core Concepts of Problem Solving and Strengths 184
Practice: Use Strengths to Overcome Challenges 186
Learning and Cultural Fit 189
Closing Activities 193

Module 8: Grudge and Gratitude 199
Core Concepts of Grudge 200
Practice 1: Let Go of the Grudge 201
Core Concepts of Gratitude 204
Practice 2: Express Gratitude 205
Learning and Cultural Fit 208
Closing Activities 208

Module 9: Empathy 215
Core Concepts of Empathy 216
Practice: Build Empathy 217
Learning and Cultural Fit 220
Closing Activities 220

Module 10: Slowness and Savoring 227
Core Concepts of Slowness and Savoring 228
Practice: Slow Down and Savor 230
Learning and Cultural Fit 231
Closing Activities 232

Module 11: Positive Relationships 239
Core Concepts of Positive Relationships 240
Practice: Celebrate Collective Strengths 242
Learning and Cultural Fit 244
Closing Activities 244

Module 12: Positive Communication 251
Core Concepts of Positive Communication 252
Practice: Communicate Actively and Constructively 254
Optional Practice: Active-Constructive Responding (ACR) 256
Learning and Cultural Fit 259
Closing Activities 260

Module 13: Altruism 265
Core Concepts of Altruism 266
Practice: Give the Gift of Time 267
Learning and Cultural Fit 269
Closing Activities 270

Module 14: Meaning and Purpose 275
Core Concepts of Meaning and Purpose 276
Practice: Meaning and Purpose 277
Learning and Cultural Fit 280
Closing Activities 280
Program Wrap-Up 281

Artist's Notes on Illustrations 285

Preface

Stressors and setbacks are inevitable in our contemporary world where we face global pandemics, a climate crisis, racial injustice, and social inequities as well as global unrest. Despite having more money and material goods, living longer, and having more social freedoms, happiness in most Western countries has not increased substantially (Easterlin et al., 2010; Rojas, 2019). On the contrary, rates of mental illness have been increasing steadily (Roth et al., 2020). There is an abundance of self-help books filled with tricks and tips which promise to magically eliminate anger, ambivalence, anxiety, sadness, and other forms of psychological distress. Workshops, courses, and retreats entice individuals to invest a few hours or days and pay a hefty fee to become the best version of themselves and live happily ever after. Though tempting, these untested interventions often overlook the unique needs of living in the 21st century, where people are ambitious, anxious, digitally savvy but increasingly alienated and alone.

Eliminating all risks and vulnerabilities is not feasible. Therefore, we suggest that practicing resilience by tapping into strengths, rather than reducing risks, might be a better approach. Instilling hope, practicing mindfulness, boosting social intelligence, and encouraging citizenship can build confidence and self-efficacy, whereas merely managing stressors cannot. We believe building these skills is essential for everyone, especially for our young people.

Our goal in creating SBR was clear and focused – to explore ways to tap into strengths that build resilience in educational and community settings. The strengths-based resilience (SBR) program described in this manual is informed by positive psychotherapy (PPT; Rashid & Seligman, 2018), the Penn Resilience Program (PRP; Gillham et al., 1995; Jaycox et al., 1994), and the high school positive psychology program (Gillham et al., 2013; Seligman et al., 2009). It was originally developed for youth in secondary school settings but is accessible to a wide range of professionals who work with adolescents and young adults.

The SBR program was created before the worldwide COVID-19 pandemic disrupted life around the world (Rashid et al., 2014). The pandemic caused disruptions in people's learning, work, leisure activities, relationships, and household dynamics that have continued to have an effect. These challenges may have been tougher for some, especially if they were experiencing symptoms of depression, anxiety, or other mental health difficulties. In this postpandemic era that has introduced hybrid work and learning arrangements, people need resilience more than ever to navigate uncertainty and new ways of learning, working, and socializing.

In designing SBR, we integrated knowledge about mindfulness, stressors, and strengths into a holistic program of interventions. We ran implementation studies, mostly in schools, but also some in clinical and community settings (Rashid et al., 2014). Through these studies, we learned ways to strike a balance between mitigating stressors and accentuating strengths and to engage participants through experiential practices. We learned from teachers and facilitators how and where to add more creative room and autonomy for them to deliver the program while keeping the core elements intact. Based on this learning, we included guidelines for facilitators so they can adapt the program to make it culturally relevant, accessible to students with different learning needs, and applicable to everyday life situations that their students are likely to encounter. The result of all this work is this Manual.

SBR is a 14-module program that can be delivered in the form of a life skills or self-development course in a group setting and in one-to-one work with individuals. The program modules can be adapted to various durations (e.g., 60, 75, or 90 minutes). Each module begins and ends with a brief relaxation or mindfulness practice to help participants focus on their experiences in the present moment and settle into a reflective learning journey. Participants are also coached to keep a gratitude journal throughout the program. The aim is to help them spot, reflect on, and write about positive experiences that they may otherwise ignore or minimize.

In addition to the Manual, the Strengths-Based Resilience Workbook (Rashid et al., 2025) is an excellent resource for participants engaged in the SBR program. It can also be utlilized as a standalone book by individuals interested in developing resilience through a strengths-based approach. The Workbook provides ample space for participants to respond to questions and reflect on what they have learnt in the modules. Additionally, extra materials are available to purchasers for download.

After exploring definitions and illustrations of resilience, the first module of the program, *Module 1: Resilience,* encourages participants to recall and write a personalized narrative of resilience. The aim is to define what resilience means to participants and to remind them of times when they used their strengths to overcome significant adversity.

The next three modules, *Module 2: Fixed and Growth Mindsets, Module 3: Cognitive Accuracy*, and *Module 4: Cognitive Flexibility* focus on skills for helping participants appraise and process negative experiences in a realistic and flexible manner. The goal of these modules is to improve their self-awareness about negativity bias – a common human tendency to give negative events and experiences more weight and importance than positive ones.

Modules 5: Character Strengths, 6: Signature Strengths, and *7: Problem-Solving and Strengths* invite participants to acknowledge, assess, and express their core strengths. Participants are encouraged to incorporate multiple perspectives, including those of family members, teachers/colleagues, and friends/peers, resulting in a cohesive understanding of their strengths. Participants also learn to use their strengths in context-specific, goal-directed, and positive ways which are beneficial for them and others.

Modules 8: Grudge and Gratitude, 9: Empathy, and *10: Slowness and Savoring* build essential personal and interpersonal skills, i.e., those that strengthen relationships. The underlying invitation in these modules is to pay closer attention to both positive and negative reactions participants experience when interacting with others. These modules also encourage participants to be mindful of their reactions to their experience in the present and how these might be impacted by the past, especially when associated experiences fuel negative feelings due to unprocessed memories.

Modules 11: Positive Relationships, 12: Positive Communication, and *13: Altruism* focus on cultivating healthy interpersonal and community connections. In the final module, *14: Meaning and Purpose*, participants review their stories of resilience, which they wrote in the first module. They are encouraged to incorporate learning from the program to write a story about their future self.

Culture plays a critical role in individual responses to stress and adversity. Yet, most resilience interventions and programs that have been described in the psychological literature are developed by Western researchers and practitioners. Given today's ethno-culturally diverse, urbanized, polarized, and increasingly anxious world, our program invites facilitators to consider the cultural context from which participants begin their learning journey. For each module, we draw on concepts and skills from positive psychology, cognitive behavioral therapy, and mindfulness and suggest ways to modify program activities so that facilitators consider the unique cultural perspective of participants. Incorporating cultural context can also enable both individuals and communities to become more resilient.

In 2008, we began creating and piloting the SBR program in a variety of high-need educational and clinical settings of the Greater Toronto Area (GTA), Canada, one of the most multicultural cities in the world. Several iterations of the program and extensive consultation after each iteration with educators and healthcare professionals from diverse cultural backgrounds have enhanced its cultural responsiveness.

SBR has been shown to reduce stress and enhance well-being (Rashid & Louden, 2018). However, we do not consider SBR a substitute for evidence-based clinical care. Certain severe psychological conditions may need more focused and specialized interventions. SBR is based on sound theoretical frameworks. These include PERMA (Seligman, 2011) and Classification of Strengths and Virtues (CSV; Peterson & Seligman, 2004), also known as Values in Action (VIA). These frameworks are described in Chapter 2, Theoretical Foundations of Strengths-Based Resilience. However, it is only one of several models of strengths and, like other models, it may not capture all strengths that are important to people in a given community or setting.

In running the SBR program, we recommend that facilitators be mindful of not overlooking stressors, risks, and vulnerabilities in their participants' lives, nor overemphasizing strengths, resources, and assets. In other words, as a facilitator, you help participants to acknowledge their distress while at the same time, use their strengths to build a strong foundation of resilience and well-being.

References

Easterlin, R. A., McVey, L. A., Switek, M., Sawangfa, O., & Zweig, J. S. (2010). The happiness-income paradox revisited. *Proceedings of the National Academy of Sciences – PNAS, 107*(52), 22463–22468. https://doi.org/10.1073/pnas.1015962107

Gillham, J. E., Abenavoli, R. M., Brunwasser, S. M., Linkins, M., Reivich, K. J., & Seligman, M. E. P. (2013). Resilience education. In S. A. David, I. Boniwell, & A. C. Ayers (Eds.), *Handbook of happiness* (pp. 609–630). Oxford University Press.

Gillham, J. E., Reivich, K. J., Jaycox, L. H., & Seligman, M. P. E. (1995). Prevention of depressive symptoms in school children: Two-year followup. *Psychological Science, 6*, 343–351.

Jaycox, L. H., Reivich, K. J., Gillham, J., & Seligman, M. E. P. (1994). Preventing depressive symptoms in school children. *Behaviour Research and Therapy, 32*, 801–816.

Peterson, C., & Seligman, M. E. P. (2004). *Character strengths and virtues: A handbook and classification*. Oxford University Press.

Rashid, T., Anjum, A., Chu, R., Stevanovski, S., Zanjani, A., & Lennex, C. (2014). Strength-based resilience: Integrating risk and resources towards holistic well-being. In G. A. Fava & C. Ruini (Eds.), *Increasing psychological well-being across cultures* (pp. 153–176). Springer.

Rashid, T., Gillham, J., Louden, R., & Anjum, A. (2025). *Strengths-based resilience workbook*. Hogrefe.

Rashid, T., & Louden, R. (2018). *Flourish: A strengths-based resilience (SBR) approach to support students' transition from secondary to post-secondary education*. Ministry of Advanced Education and Skills Development. Toronto, Canada. https://hive.utsc.utoronto.ca/public/iits/flourish/Flourish_Final%20Report_2018.pdf

Rashid, T., & Seligman, M. E. P. (2018). *Positive psychotherapy: Clinician manual*. Oxford University Press. https://doi.org/10.1093/med-psych/9780195325386.001.0001

Rojas, M. (2019). *The economics of happiness how the Easterlin paradox transformed our understanding of well-being and progress*. Springer International Publishing. https://doi.org/10.1007/978-3-030-15835-4

Roth, G. A., Ammirati, E., Barengo, N. C., Beaton, A., Carapetis, J. R., Cooper, L. T., He, F. J., Hu, F., Inker, L., Karthikeyan, G., Misganaw, A. T., Mokdad, A. H., Neal, B., Abedi, A., Abushouk, A. I., Acharya, D., Adair, T., Agarwal, G., Agasthi, P., ... Amini, S. (2020). Global burden of cardiovascular diseases and risk factors, 1990–

2019: Update from the GBD 2019 study. *Journal of the American College of Cardiology, 76*(25), 2982–3021. https://doi.org/10.1016/j.jacc.2020.11.010
Seligman, M. E .P. (2011). *Flourish: A visionary new understanding of happiness and well-being.* Free Press.
Seligman, M. E. P., Ernst, R. M., Gillham, J., Reivich, K., & Linkins, M. (2009). Positive education: Positive psychology and classroom interventions. *Oxford Review of Education, 35*(3), 293–311. https://doi.org/10.1080/03054980902934563

Section I: Theoretical Background and Development of the Strengths-Based Resilience Program

1 Resilience

Resilience is a popular concept both in media and academia, and there are numerous programs which aim to foster it (Calitz, 2018; Joyce et al., 2018; McAvera, 2018). In this chapter, we discuss why we believe another program on resilience is needed. To make our case, we first discuss the increase in mental health difficulties among adolescents and young adults. We then describe various definitions and descriptions of resilience. We conclude with 10 key considerations that we think are important to keep in mind for programs that aim to enhance resilience.

Why Resilience Matters

Stressors are pervasive. Today's young people cope with family dysfunction, academic and social challenges at school, and physical and mental health problems. They face these against a backdrop of sociopolitical conflicts, discrimination, and stress caused by environmental disasters, including wildfires, floods, and extreme temperatures which can jeopardize human development.

According to Carol Dweck (2012), "Debates about human nature often revolve around what is built in. Are people born to be aggressive? Is antipathy toward the outgroup a part of human nature? Is willpower severely limited by biology?" She continues, "To me, however, the hallmark of human nature is how much of who we are – and who we become – is not built in. The hallmark of human nature is each person's great capacity to adapt, to change, and to grow. In fact, perhaps what is built in is this capacity to learn and change according to the world you find yourself in" (Dweck, 2012; p. 614).

We agree, as Dweck suggests, that human beings have the capacity to adapt, change, and grow. By learning about resilience, students learn skills to regulate their emotions, cognition, and behavior, and cope better with stressors.

Immunization from life challenges is neither possible nor desirable. To deal adaptively with challenges, we need resilience. We may not be able to (or want to) eliminate all of the risks and vulnerabilities our children and adolescents will encounter. Still, we can equip them with skills and strengths that promote their resilience by enabling them to cope with challenges more skillfully. Paul Tough, in his book *How Children Succeed* (Tough, 2012), suggests that the qualities that matter most have more to do with character than intelligence alone; these qualities include perseverance, curiosity, conscientiousness, optimism, and self-control.

Our educational systems focus on improving students' academic achievement. Academic and cognitive factors are important, but so are noncognitive characteristics such as leadership, teamwork, adaptability, social responsibility, ethics, and intellectual curiosity (Schmitt et al., 2009). Robert Sternberg and colleagues (Sternberg et al., 2012) have advocated incorporating the broader concept of intelligence in our academic discourse, including creativity, analytical and practical intelligence, and wisdom. This can help us educate all students, including those from diverse cultural backgrounds and academic abilities.

Multiple lines of research indicate that mental health concerns among adolescents and young adults have been increasing steadily. The following are some recent findings:

- To estimate prevalence and changes in adolescent mental health difficulties, a recent meta-analysis by Racine and colleagues (2021), involving 29 studies, including more than 80,000 children and adolescents living in many different areas of the world, showed that, in the first year of the COVID-19 pandemic, 1 in 4 youth globally experienced clinically elevated depression symptoms, while 1 in 5 experienced clinically elevated anxiety symptoms. These rates were double the prepandemic estimates.
- The National Survey on Drug Use and Health (NSDUSH; Twenge et al., 2019; Weinberger et al., 2018) conducted with more than 600,000 American adolescents and young adults found that more American adolescents and young adults in the late 2010s (vs. the mid-2000s) had experienced severe psychological distress, including depression. This group also experienced suicidal ideation more, made more suicide attempts, and had a higher suicide completion rate. These trends were found to be weak or nonexistent among adults aged 26 years and older, suggesting a generational shift in mood disorders and suicide-related outcomes, rather than an overall increase across all ages.
- Cross-sectional surveys of almost half a million students in 8th, 10th, and 12th grades show that depressive symptoms are increasing among the young, especially among girls (Keyes et al., 2019). Likewise, the proportion of college and university students experiencing psychological distress have been increasing steadily. The National College Health Assessment (American College Health Association, 2018), one of the largest of its kind (with more than 30,000 student participants), found that nearly 40% of US college students had reported feeling so depressed during the past 12 months that they could not function. Almost 2% reported attempting suicide and 7.8% reported engaging in self-harming behavior. The World Health Organization Mental Health survey, completed by 1,572 students (aged 18–22 years) from 21 countries, found that 20.3% of students met standardized criteria for a psychiatric disorder (Auerbach et al., 2016).
- From their meta-analysis of 41 studies from 27 countries, Polanczyk and colleagues (2015) estimated that mental health difficulties are experienced by 13.4% of children and adolescents (aged 6–17 years).
- The Ontario Student Drug Use and Health Survey (OSDUHS) is one of the longest ongoing school surveys of adolescents in Canada, and also one of the longest in the world. The 2018 results (Boak et al., 2018), based on a self-report of 11,435 grade 7–12 students, suggested that 39% of students had experienced moderate to severe psychological distress in the past month.
- A meta-analysis of 15 studies with more than 50,000 adolescents found that a considerable proportion of adolescents with mental health concerns (54%) were not receiving needed mental health care (Ghafari et al., 2022).

Mental health difficulties among adolescents and young adults need to be understood within the context of the developmental challenges adolescents typically face, especially their search for identity (Erikson, 1968). This process includes recalibration of relationships with parents, peers, and, perhaps most importantly, with oneself. Often this process is fraught with stressful interactions over culture, creed, and communication. Entangled within the developmental challenges are a myriad of sociocultural, financial, political, climate, and ecological problems.

Could the increase in psychological difficulties reflect an increase in the complexity of challenges faced by this generation? Could the increase in psychological problems reflect a decline in resilience among children and adolescents? In the absence of well-designed, prospective studies, we can only speculate based on broader sociocultural trends, four of which we highlight below: hollow self esteem, helicopter parenting, shrinking imaginative and free playtime, and too much screen time at the expense of in-person social time.

Many psychologists have argued that the self-esteem movement (and its simplistic emphasis on positive feelings about oneself rather than competence) has diverted efforts away from teaching children skills for setting and working toward goals and responding to the challenges and setbacks that are an inevitable part of life (e.g., Baumeister et al., 2003; Seligman et al., 1995). In their book *The Coddling of the American Mind*, Greg Lukianoff and Jonathan Haidt (2018) argue that emphasis, especially in educational settings, on trusting one's feelings as the ultimate lever of truth, without deploying critical thinking and reasoning skills, reinforces cognitive distortions. Similarly, the overinvolvement and overprotectiveness of some parents, also known as helicopter parenting (Padilla-Walker & Nelson, 2012), might be interfering in children's and adolescents' ability to achieve critical developmental milestones, such as self-exploration, self-efficacy, and independent problem-solving (Kouros et al., 2017).

Changes in how children spend time may also be a factor. For example, although research documents the benefits of exercise and recreation on mental health and well-being (e.g., Walsh, 2011), children's opportunities to play have declined significantly from previous generations (Gray, 2011). Through play – free and imaginative – children develop intrinsic interests, social and emotional skills, self-regulation, decision-making and conflict resolution skills, self-confidence, and a variety of character strengths that are related to resilience (Ginsburg, 2007; Gray, 2011).

A major societal shift has been the increase in time spent on social media sites, along with a decrease in time spent interacting with others in person. Tracking the trends of the decade (2010–2019) through its surveys, the Pew Research Center has found that as of 2019, 93% of US millennials (those aged between 23 to 39 in 2019) own a smartphone, and nearly 100% say that they use the Internet (Schaffer, 2019). By age 20, an average young adult in the US will have spent more than 20,000 hours online (Gentina & Chen, 2019). Meta-analytical studies have shown that excessive time spent on social media is associated with poor mental health, including symptoms of depression and anxiety, as well as sleep difficulties (Alimoradi et al., 2019; Marino et al., 2018; Shensa et al., 2020). Children and adolescents who spend less time on social media and more on physical activity, report fewer mental health problems (Aschbrenner et al., 2019; Hrafnkelsdottir et al., 2018). A large study of adolescents found that during COVID-19, the average total daily recreational screen use (excluding hours spent on school-related work) was 7.7 hours per day, representing a doubling of pre-pandemic estimates (3.8 hours) from the same cohort (Nagata et al., 2022).

We cannot say that one or more factors are conclusively associated with an increase in mental health difficulties or with a decline in resilience. Isolating one or more factors from our contemporary lives, which we live mostly housed in the sprawling urban centers around the world, would be a daunting task. In addition to the sociocultural trends mentioned above, we also live amid noise, pollution, traffic, and extreme weather conditions. Compared with people living in rural environments, those in urban settings appear to be at higher risk for psychiatric disorders, including depression (Peen et al., 2010). Many of us also face social adversity such as poverty, racial discrimination, maltreatment, and intergenerational trauma (Gartland et al., 2019). Together, these factors impact us all to varying degrees. It is highly unlikely that we will find a panacea for all of these individual, communal, and societal challenges. Nonetheless, we can attempt to increase individual, interpersonal, and communal resilience through multiple pathways. Programs such as strengths-based resilience (SBR), can offer adolescents pathways to cultivate resilience.

Definitions and Descriptions of Resilience

The concept of resilience has attracted much academic and popular attention in the past two decades. Research on resilience has surged in recent years, offering multiple definitions and descriptions (Luthar, 2003; Métais et al., 2022; Southwick et al., 2014). The following are some selected ones, including resilience as (a) a dynamic process of overcoming challenges, (b) a trait or an attribute, (c) an outcome, and (d) a hybrid of both process and outcome geared explicitly toward growth and transformation. Although these definitions, at times, collide with each other, they also reflect the diversity and complexity of resilience and the numerous ways in which it can be developed.

a. A Dynamic Process

Resilience often refers to a step-by-step process which takes place over time as individuals or communities develop capacities and skills. Resilience can be seen as a dynamic process which involves interactions between both risk and protective processes, internal and external to the individual, that act to modify the effects of an adverse life event (Rutter, 1987, 1999). Dynamic and positive adaptation includes both stress and competence at different levels – individual, family, society – yielding a variety of outcomes which make an individual vulnerable to risks or resilient (Luthar, 1991, 2003). These outcomes or processes include:

- A capacity to adapt to or maintain relatively healthy psychological and physical functioning, in the wake of a significant trauma or setback that threatens the vitality of that system (Bonanno, 2004; Masten, 2014)
- A process to harness resources, especially in challenging settings (e.g., war-ravaged Afghanistan or famine-stricken Niger), to sustain well-being (Panter-Brick et al., 2011)
- The processes that individuals, families, and communities use to cope with, adapt to, and take advantage of assets when facing significant acute or chronic stress or the compounding effect of both together (Ungar & Liebenberg, 2011)
- A dynamic process that enables individuals to actively adapt to challenging situations (Fergus & Zimmerman, 2005)
- The tendency to mobilize a complex repertoire of behavioral resources to deal with a challenge (Agaibi & Wilson, 2005)
- A successful coping mechanism in the face of adversity (Lee & Cranford, 2008)
- The process of adapting well in the face of adversity, trauma, tragedy, threats, or even significant sources of stress (Newman, 2002)

b. A Trait or an Attribute

Resilience can also be used to describe a trait or attribute of an individual or community that we can measure and compare against a standard, such as:

- A person's ability to persevere in the face of challenges, setbacks, and conflicts (Reivich & Shatté, 2002)

- A personal trait that helps individuals to cope with adversity and achieve good adjustment and development (Matson & Gramezy, 1985)
- A combination of personal qualities that enable one to thrive (Conner & Davidson, 2003)
- A psychological ability to overcome the difficulties experienced in the different areas of life with perseverance, as well as a good awareness of one's resources (Sisto et al., 2019)

c. An Outcome

Resilience is often defined as an outcome that emerges from an adverse situation. For example, posttraumatic growth is a resilience outcome. Resilience as an outcome includes:
- A quick recovery under significant adverse conditions (Leipold & Greve, 2009)
- Adaptation to adversity that is influenced by a complex interplay among genetic, environmental, interpersonal, and psychological factors

d. A Hybrid of Process and Outcome

Sometimes resilience is defined as both a process of growth and change and a transformative outcome. Resilience as growth, change, and transformation includes:
- Successful adaptations despite challenging and threatening circumstances (Masten et al., 1990; Rutter, 2006)
- A capacity of any individual to withstand hardship and repair oneself, to transform and change no matter the risks (Bradshaw et al., 2007)
- A class of phenomena characterized by patterns of positive adaptation in the context of significant adversity or risk, which enables individuals to bounce back quickly and effectively from adverse events (Luthans et al., 2010)

e. A Systems Approach

Finally, resilience can be defined from the perspective of a system of dynamic interactions. Ann Masten, a prominent researcher in the area of resilience, has dubbed resilience *ordinary magic* (Masten, 2001), which is a dynamic and evolving process that continues throughout the lifespan, rather than an outcome of adverse experiences. Masten posits that resilience is the ability of a system to adapt successfully to challenges that threaten survival, function, or development. The adaptive process is influenced by personal characteristics and family and social resources. Masten and Barnes (2018, p. 19, Table 1) deem 12 factors to be critical for fostering resilience. An adapted list is below:
1. Nurturing family
2. Close and secure family ties and sense of belonging
3. Effective parenting
4. Agency and willingness to adapt
5. Problem-solving and task management skills
6. Emotion and self regulation

7. Self-efficacy and positive identity
8. Faith, future-mindedness, and hope
9. Sense of meaning and purpose
10. Roles, routines, and rituals
11. Involvement in a well-functioning school
12. Engagement in well-functioning communities

The categories of definitions of resilience described above are not mutually exclusive. Several definitions incorporate elements from more than one category. The concept of resilience in SBR is somewhat consistent with Masten's (2018) notion that resilience is not a singular and stable trait, rather it involves dynamic interactions within and across systems (e.g., families, peers, schools, communities, and cultures).

Strengths-Based Resilience: Ten Key Considerations

Based on our review of the scientific literature on resilience and on our experience developing and implementing the SBR program, we recommend that facilitators keep in mind the 10 considerations below. A central premise across all 10 is that resilience is inherently an interpersonal endeavor. That is, the resilience of adolescents as they grow is influenced by their interactions within and between multiple systems including family, peers, school, community, and culture (Masten, 2018).

1. Make Program Participants Aware of Negativity Bias

Our minds are skewed towards the negative. We perceive negatives as carrying more weight and potency (Ito et al., 1998; Rozin & Royzman, 2001). Stories of deficit, crime, and evil arouse our curiosity more than accounts of virtue, integrity, cooperation, altruism, or modesty. We brood about negative memories for months or even years, while reminiscing less about good things in our past. Negative emotions, bad behavior, and unconstructive feedback exert more impact. Negative impressions and stereotypes are quicker to form and they are more resistant to disconfirmation than are positive ones (Baumeister et al., 2001; Corns, 2018). By focusing on reducing negatives, psychological interventions have done well. They have shown benefits in treating symptoms as well as improving well-being (Houston et al., 2017; Jones, 2020). The effectiveness of psychological interventions, especially those which aim to enhance resilience, can further improve if we recognize our bias towards negativity and give equal attention to positives.

2. Frame Resilience as an Ongoing, Lifelong Process

Resilience is a developmental and ongoing psychosocial process. Each individual's resilience is a complex interplay of genetic, psychological, social, and cultural factors that are domain- and culture-specific. Instead of operationalizing it as a singular construct – trait, outcome, or process – in devising a resilience intervention, it is helpful to consider resilience on a continuum with varying degrees and dimensions. The processes of resilience unfold and change over a lifespan, helping individuals to recover, overcome, withstand, bounce back, adapt positively, survive, and perhaps most importantly thrive while encountering adversity, setbacks, challenges, or trauma. The lifespan approach also implies adverse childhood events do not determine a lifetime of misery and preclude one from enjoying happiness and well-being. Resilience is needed to overcome major life challenges, as well as when dealing with everyday stressors. Ann Masten's concept of ordinary magic (Masten, 2001) can be nurtured through teaching evidence-based skills.

3. Assess Situational Factors

In devising resilience interventions, it is important to assess the acuity or chronicity of stressors. Resilience interventions ought to be informed by the nature, duration, and perceived impact of the stressor. Some stressors are acute or reversible, such as failing an exam, not being selected for a position, or sustaining injuries in an accident from which one can recuperate. Others are more permanent, such as the death of a loved one, accidents which may leave one with permanent disabilities, or permanent displacement due to war, climate disaster, or humanitarian crisis. Acute stressors likely require a different set of interventions and skills than chronic stressors. In assessing the acuity or chronicity of stressors, it is important to consider cultural and situational factors. For example, someone from a collectivist culture may respond to an acute stressor more resiliently because of available social support, whereas someone from an individualistic culture may feel overwhelmed easily by relatively less stressful situations, as they may lack social support.

It is also important to consider individual differences. For example, individuals differ considerably in their temperament, extraversion/introversion, openness to experience, or conscientiousness. That is, an acute stressor will likely yield different responses in two individuals, even among siblings.

4. Teach Resilience Skills

Resilience theory (Zimmerman, 2013) is a strengths-based approach which focuses on positive contextual, social, and individual variables, also known as promotive factors, that contribute to adaption. There are two types of promotive factors: assets and resources. Self-efficacy and self-esteem are considered assets, while resources are factors outside individuals, such as parental support, adult mentors, and youth programs with opportunities to learn and practice. Research has shown that supportive home, community, and peer environments tend to promote adolescent resilience. Furthermore, goal-setting and impulse-control abilities predict resilience (Dias & Cadime, 2017). De Leeuw and Malcolm-Smith (2023) found that social support was a significant protective factor in their review of resilience in children from low- and middle-income countries.

Programs can systematically teach children, adolescents, and adults skills which enhance their resilience. Many resilience promoting programs have been developed and empirically evaluated, although there is great variation in program content and components. As discussed earlier in this chapter, there is also great variability across programs and research in how resilience is conceptualized; that is, whether resilience is conceptualized as an attribute, trait, outcome, process, or system. For example, Penn Resilience Program (PRP) is a group cognitive and behavioral intervention that aims to boost resilience and prevent depression by teaching cognitive and behavioral skills for handling stressors and difficult experiences (Gillham et al., 1995; Gillham et al., 2007). A meta-analysis of 17 controlled PRP evaluations found that PRP significantly reduces depressive symptoms, and these benefits last for at least 12 months following the intervention (Brunwasser et al., 2009). These studies suggest that resilience skills are evidence-based and teachable.

Numerous other programs have attempted to enhance resilience by targeting protective qualities that may buffer against the negative effects of trauma, adversity, and setbacks (Thompson & Dobbins, 2018). Examples of protective factors include positive future orientation, problem-solving skills, self-regulation, family support, safe community, affordable housing, and education (de Leeuw & Malcolm-Smith, 2023). Research indicates that resilience programs that promote protective factors improve mental health and well-being. Examples are interventions for Red Crescent healthcare teams in Iran (Larijani & Garmaroudi, 2018), Chinese medical students (Peng et al., 2014), clergy (Noullet et al., 2018), and nurses (Jackson et al., 2007). Kunzler and colleagues (2022) recently analyzed 24 studies of psychological interventions designed to promote resilience and well-being in nurses. They found that, overall, the interventions improved resilience and well-being. These effects were sustained in the short-term (≤3 months), with additional delayed benefits for anxiety and stress. Delivered mostly as psychoeducational groups, the content of interventions varied. Common strategies included education about stress and self-care, mindfulness and relaxation, cognitive-behavioral skills, identification of personal strengths, and team-building and other activities for strengthening relationships.

Previously, two systematic reviews (Macedo et al., 2014; Robertson et al., 2015) and two meta-analyses (Leppin et al., 2014; Vanhove et al., 2016) found that resilience skills are teachable and that teaching these skills can improve mental health and well-being.

5. Include Evaluation Relevant and Diverse Outcomes in Your Program

We recommend that SBR program administrators and facilitators carefully choose the outcome or evaluative measures to assess the program's effectiveness. SBR facilitators need to familiarize themselves with the overall program goals and the learning outcomes of each module. Identify outcomes that are relevant and important to your setting. Select reliable and valid measures that are related to SBR goals and make sure they are relevant to your context and the demographics of participants, including age, gender, and literacy.

Evaluations of resilience programs rely heavily on self-report outcome measures. Because the SBR program works on multiple dimensions, including feelings, beliefs, cognitions, behaviors, and habits, it might be prudent to incorporate concrete behavioral measures, such as behaviors related to health (hours of sleep, hours spent exercising, number of steps taken, visits to health facilities), interpersonal relationships (number of close friends or positive interactions with others), service to others (hours volunteering), or academic achievement (attendance, academic performance) (Smith et al., 2015).

6. Avoid Denying, Dismissing, or Minimizing Negatives

A common critique about positive psychology interventions is that they tend to minimize, dismiss, or outright ignore risks, vulnerabilities, and adversities (van Zyl et al., 2024). We want to clarify from the onset that our approach to developing SBR does not regard negatives, including setbacks, traumas, adversities, disasters, or challenges, to be any less important than strengths or positives. Negatives in our daily lives – ranging from the death of a loved one; to interpersonal violence, abuse, and discrimination; to traumatic events, including war, famine, climate crises, poverty, accidents, terrorism, industrial disasters, and pandemics – are real challenges and require serious and immediate solutions. Any intervention – however well- or ill-informed by positive psychology – that dismisses or minimizes these issues will likely be ineffective and/or create superficial "feel good" vibes only.

7. Link Resilience to Thriving

Resilience is commonly regarded as an ability to bounce back or adapt to adversities. We invite facilitators to consider resilience a process of not only surviving but also growing and potentially, in the long term, thriving. Early resilience interventions focused on mitigating or managing risk and vulnerability factors (Denny et al., 2004; Werner & Smith, 2001), much like traditional psychological interventions focus on remediating deficits. The contemporary positive psychology and resilience scholarship has expanded the focus to include factors that help invidiudals and communities not only to survive but also to thrive. These include assets such as individual strengths and abilities, as well as interpersonal and environmental resources. Teaching clients about flourishing – a state characterized by positive emotions, a strong sense of personal meaning, good work, and positive relationships – requires far more than simply relieving the symptoms of psychological distress. To foster these outcomes, systematic and sustained effort is essential. In our view, resilience programming is a partnership between participants and practitioners in which the building of positive resources should get as much attention as the reduction of psychological distress. Most individuals tap into their inner resources and/or develop them while dealing with challenges. The seminal works of Tedeschi and Calhoun (1996) and Bonanno (2004) on *posttraumatic growth* show that adversity often also yields growth and helps individuals to foster better relationships, enabling them to put difficult experiences into perspective (meaning making) and to realign their priorities.

8. Promote "Leading with Strengths" as a Catalyst of Resilience

Character strengths are levers or catalysts of change – both in dealing adaptively with stressors as well as in cultivating well-being and resilience. Strengths are catalysts because they not only contribute to individual well-being but also to the well-being of others. For example, when we use humor, we take the edge off a stressful situation. When we express gratitude, even during tough times, we lighten the atmosphere. When we use social intelligence to attune ourselves to someone's needs, that person feels seen and heard.

9. Embed Cultural Context

Resilience is a universal notion. However, survival, recovery, and adaptation are culturally shaped. It is essential to understand resilience within the local context. The bulk of research on resilience interventions has been conducted with samples from WEIRD (Western, Educated, Industrialized, Rich, and Democratic) countries (Henrich et al., 2010). Resilience interventions need to explore cultural context as it may help to examine the coping strategies that adolescents and young adults from marginalized communities use to deal with extreme situations. For example, in one study, the resilience adolescents exposed to trauma and war was related to problem-solving skills and active parental involvement (Fayyad et al., 2017). Therefore, it is important for practitioners to consider how participants' cultural background affects how they deal with distress and how they demonstrate resilience.

Resilience interventions with historically marginalized communities help us to understand not only how these communities survive but also how they thrive. What specific features or processes of their culture facilitate or pose a barrier to resilience (Ungar, 2012)? Unger emphasizes that in an increasingly ethnoracially diverse world, understanding the cultural nuances related to resilience is critical, as it can enrich resilience interventions with local cultural context as well as provide a global perspective. Two examples are noteworthy: first, that of indigenous people. Indigenous people in Canada, Australia, and New Zealand have started social justice initiatives such as truth and reconciliation commissions. Proceedings enable nonindigenous individuals to hear publicly first-hand accounts of how indigenous people have handled cultural genocide and forced placement in residential schools with resilience, despite enduring that horrific abuse. The second example is that of refugee narratives of resilience that show extraordinary courage in the face of extreme hardship. By incorporating the stories and experiences of people who have endured extreme hardships, facilitators can foster an understanding of how resilience unfolds in real-world contexts.

10. Draw on Findings from Other Fields

We find ourselves at an exciting time with regard to resilience interventions, as they intersect with important disciplines including traumatology (adult responses to trauma), developmental psychopathology (children's and adolescents' responses to adversity), positive psychology (emphasis on positive emotions, positive relationships), and humanistic psychology (harnessing one's potential toward self-actualization, meaning and purpose, and growth). In addition, insights from neurobiology and genetics are expanding and consolidating a wholistic understanding of resilience (Graber et al., 2015).

Consistent with this research ethos, SBR integrates findings from traditional clinical psychology, which addresses deficits, vulnerabilities, and stressors, with positive psychology, which amplifies resources, adaptability, and strengths. Resilience reflects an interplay between an individual's skills and attributes (including character strengths) and environmental resources (including caring relationships, social support, and opportunities to contribute). Emerging lines of research are showing that boosting resilience by explicitly enhancing strengths is equally or more efficacious than focusing primarily and exclusively on eliminating deficits (Bird et al., 2010; Brownlee et al., 2013; Larson, 2010; Martínez-Martí & Ruch, 2017; Shoshani & Slone, 2016).

Resilience Interventions: Caveats

In devising resilience interventions, be mindful of some caveats and avoid missteps which can compromise your program's effectiveness and longevity. This includes avoiding simplistic interventions that offer black-and-white solutions to complex stressors, adversities, and challenges. Direct or indirect messages such as *If you work hard, you can overcome any challenge*, *You are the master of your life, take charge*, *It is not your fault*, and *You are stronger than you think* can be true to some extent in some situations, but are not universally true. For most adolescents and young adults, these serve as empty platitudes. These platitudes offer simplistic and clichéd solutions, which may discourage participants from investing effort in practicing, mastering, and applying SBR skills.

Facilitators need to keep in mind that the mental health concerns encountered by adolescents and young adults have numerous causes (e.g., genetic, developmental, environmental, social, financial, and cultural) and numerous consequences (e.g., impacts on academics, social relationships, physical health, recreation, and more). Neither SBR nor any other program can address all the psychological concerns of adolescents and young adults.

We recommend that facilitators also keep in mind that resilience as an adaptation or outcome is not always obvious and may take time to manifest. Facilitators may discover that some participants find the notion of bouncing back or adaptation premature due to their on-going situational challenges. Others may have bounced back and adapted effectively but may not have realized this positive change due to negativity bias. Yet, some others might be fluctuating between adaptation and regression. Remind adolescents and young adults that they are almost always changing. Encourage them to have an open mind and consider numerous ways to be resilient and flexible as they and the circumstances around them change.

Summary

Resilience is a complex and multifaceted construct, encapsulating a dynamic process, a trait or an attribute, an outcome, or a combination of these factors. The aim of this overview is not to reach a consensus about what resilience is and what it is not. Rather, our attempt is to elucidate the ways in which resilience has been conceptualized. Consistent with that diversity of definitions and descriptions, there are myriad interventions to foster it. No one intervention is likely to capture all aspects of resilience. When adversity strikes, it can have a devastating and lifelong impact on the individual. Investing equal attention to building resources, in addition to mitigating risks, will make resilience interventions more effective and accessible.

References

Agaibi, C. E., & Wilson, J. P. (2005). Trauma, PTSD, and resilience: A review of the literature. *Trauma, Violence & Abuse*, 6(3), 195–216. https://doi.org/10.1177/1524838005277438

Alimoradi, Z., Lin, C.-Y., Broström, A., Bülow, P. H., Bajalan, Z., Griffiths, M. D., Ohayon, M. M., & Pakpour, A. H. (2019). Internet addiction and sleep problems: A systematic review and meta-analysis. *Sleep Medicine Reviews, 47,* 51–61. https://doi.org/10.1016/j.smrv.2019.06.004

American College Health Association. (2018). *American College Health Association-National College Health Assessment II: Reference Group Executive Summary Fall 2018.* https://www.acha.org/documents/ncha/NCHA-II_Fall_2018_Reference_Group_Executive_Summary.pdf

Aschbrenner, K. A., Naslund, J. A., Tomlinson, E. F., Kinney, A., Pratt, S. I., & Brunette, M. F. (2019). Adolescents' use of digital technologies and preferences for mobile health coaching in public mental health settings. *Frontiers in Public Health, 7,* Article 178. https://doi.org/10.3389/fpubh.2019.00178

Auerbach, R. P., Alonso, J., Axinn, W. G., Cuijpers, P., Ebert, D. D., Green, J. G., Hwang, I., Kessler, R. C., Liu, H., Mortier, P., Nock, M. K., Pinder-Amaker, S., Sampson, N. A., Aguilar-Gaxiola, S., Al-Hamzawi, A., Andrade, L. H., Benjet, C., Caldas-de-Almeida, J. M., Demyttenaere, K., . . . Bruffaerts, R. (2016). Mental disorders among college students in the world health organization world mental health surveys. *Psychological Medicine, 46*(14), 2955–2970. https://doi.org/10.1017/S0033291716001665

Baumeister, R. F., Bratslavsky, E., Finkenauer, C., & Vohs, K. D. (2001). Bad is stronger than good. *Review of General Psychology, 5*(4), 323–370. https://doi.org/10.1037/1089-2680.5.4.323

Baumeister, R. F., Campbell, J. D., Krueger, J. I., & Vohs, K. D. (2003). Does high self-esteem cause better performance, interpersonal success, happiness, or healthier lifestyles? *Psychological Science in the Public Interest, 4*(1), 1–44. https://doi.org/10.1111/1529-1006.01431

Bird, V., Premkumar, P., Kendall, T., Whittington, C., Mitchell, J., & Kuipers, E. (2010). Early intervention services, cognitive-behavioural therapy and family intervention in early psychosis: Systematic review. *British Journal of Psychiatry, 197*(5), 350–356. https://doi.org/10.1192/bjp.bp.109.074526

Boak, A., Hamilton, H. A., Adlaf, E. M., Henderson, J. L., & Mann, R. E. (2018). *The mental health and well-being of Ontario students, 1991–2017.* CAMH Research Document Series No. 47. https://www.camh.ca/-/media/files/pdf---osduhs/mental-health-and-well-being-of-ontario-students-1991-2017

Bonanno, G. A. (2004). Loss, trauma, and human resilience: Have we underestimated the human capacity to thrive after extremely aversive events? *American Psychologist, 59*(1), 20–28. https://doi.org/10.1037/0003-066X.59.1.20

Bradshaw, B. G., Richardson, G. E., Kumpfer, K., Carlson, J., Stanchfield, J., Overall, J., Brooks, A. M., & Kulkarni, K. (2007). Determining the efficacy of a resiliency training approach in adults with type 2 diabetes. *Diabetes Educator, 33*(4), 650–659. https://doi.org/10.1177/0145721707303809

Brownlee, K., Rawana, J., Franks, J., Harper, J., Bajwa, J., O'Brien, E., & Clarkson, A. (2013). A systematic review of strengths and resilience outcome literature relevant to children and adolescents. *Child and Adolescent Social Work Journal, 30,* 435–459. https://doi.org/10.1007/s10560-013-0301-9

Brunwasser, S. M., Gillham, J. E., & Kim, E. S. (2009). A meta-analytic review of the Penn Resiliency Program's effect on depressive symptoms. *Journal of Consulting and Clinical Psychology, 77*(6), 1042–1054. https://doi.org/10.1037/a0017671

Calitz, C. (2018). Are resilience programs effective? *American Journal of Health Promotion, 32*(3), 822–826. https://doi.org/10.1177/0890117118756180

Connor, K. M., & Davidson J. R. (2003). Development of a new resilience scale: The Connor-Davidson Resilience Scale (CD-RISC). *Depression and Anxiety, 18*(2), 76–82. https://doi.org/10.1002/da.10113

Corns, J. (2018). Rethinking the negativity bias. *Review of Philosophy and Psychology, 9,* 607—625. https://doi.org/10.1007/s13164-018-0382-7

de Leeuw, J. S. H., & Malcolm-Smith, S. (2023). Investigating protective factors that boost resilience in children from low- and middle-income countries: A scoping review. *Vulnerable Children & Youth Studies, 18*(3), 467–500. https://doi.org/10.1080/17450128.2023.2224121

Denny, S., Clark, T. C., Fleming, T., & Wall, M. (2004). Emotional resilience: Risk and protective factors for depression among alternative education participants in New Zealand. *American Journal of Orthopsychiatry, 74*(2), 137–149. https://doi.org/10.1037/0002-9432.74.2.137

Dias, P. C., & Cadime, I. (2017). Protective factors and resilience in adolescents: The mediating role of self-regulation. *Psicología Educativa, 23*(1), 37–43. https://doi.org/10.1016/j.pse.2016.09.003

Dweck, C. S. (2012). Mindsets and human nature: Promoting change in the Middle East, the schoolyard, the racial divide, and willpower. *American Psychologist, 67*(8), 614–622. https://doi.org/10.1037/a0029783

Erikson, E. H. (1968). *Identity: Youth and crisis.* Norton.

Fayyad, J., Cordahi-Tabet, C., Yeretzian, J., Salamoun, M., Najm, C., & Karam, E. G. (2017). Resilience-promoting factors in war-exposed adolescents: An epidemiologic study. *European Child & Adolescent Psychiatry, 26*(2), 191–200. https://doi.org/10.1007/s00787-016-0871-0

Fergus, S., & Zimmerman, M. A. (2005). Adolescent resilience: A framework for understanding healthy development in the face of risk. *Annual Review of Public Health, 6,* 399–419. https://doi.org/10.1146/annurev.publhealth.26.021304.144357

Gartland, D., Riggs, E., Muyeen, S., Giallo, R., Afifi, T. O., MacMillan, H., Hermann, H., Bulford, E., & Brown, S. J. (2019). What factors are associated with resilient outcomes in children exposed to social adversity? A systematic review. *BMJ Open, 9*(4), Article e024870. https://doi.org/10.1136/bmjopen-2018-024870

Gentina, E., & Chen, R. (2019). Digital natives' coping with loneliness: Facebook or face-to-face? *Information & Management, 56*(6), 103138. https://doi.org/10.1016/j.im.2018.12.006

Ghafari, N. T., Bahadivand-Chegini, S., & Doosti-Irani, A. (2022). Global prevalence of unmet need for mental health care among adolescents: A systematic review and meta-analysis. *Archives of Psychiatric Nursing, 36,* 1–6. https://doi.org/10.1016/j.apnu.2021.10.008

Gillham, J. E., Reivich, K. J., Freres, D. R., Chaplin, T. M., Shatté, A. J., Samuels, B., Elkon, A. G., Litzinger, S., Lascher, M., Gallop, R., & Seligman, M. E. (2007). School-based prevention of depressive symptoms: A randomized controlled study of the effectiveness and specificity of the Penn Resiliency Program. *Journal of Consulting and Clinical Psychology, 75*(1), 9–19. https://doi.org/10.1037/0022-006X.75.1.9

Gillham, J. E., Reivich, K. J., Jaycox, L. H., & Seligman, M. E. P. (1995). Prevention of depressive symptoms in schoolchildren: Two-year follow-up. *Psychological Science, 6*(6), 343–351. https://doi.org/10.1111/j.1467-9280.1995.tb00524.x

Ginsburg, K. R. (2007). The importance of play in promoting healthy child development and maintaining strong parent-child bonds. *Pediatrics, 119*(1), 182–191. https://doi.org/10.1542/peds.2006-2697

Graber, R., Pichon, F., & Carabine, E. (2015). *Psychological resilience: State of knowledge and future research agenda.* Overseas Development Institute. https://www.odi.org/publications/9596-psychological-resilience-state-knowledge-future-research-agendas

Gray, P. (2011). The decline of play and the rise of psychopathology in children and adolescents. *American Journal of Play, 3*(4), 443–463.

Henrich, J., Heine, S. J., & Norenzayan, A. (2010). The weirdest people in the world? *The Behavioral and Brain Sciences, 33*(2–3), 61–135. https://doi.org/10.1017/S0140525X0999152X

Houston, J. B., First, J., Spialek, M. L., Sorenson, M. E., Mills-Sandoval, T., Lockett, M., First, N. L., Nitiéma, P., Allen, S. F., & Pfefferbaum, B. (2017). Randomized controlled trial of the resilience and coping intervention (RCI) with undergraduate university students. *Journal of American College Health, 65*(1), 1–9. https://doi.org/10.1080/07448481.2016.1227826

Hrafnkelsdottir, S. M., Brychta, R. J., Rognvaldsdottir, V., Gestsdottir, S., Chen, K. Y., Johannsson, E., Guðmundsdottir, S. L., & Arngrimsson, S. A. (2018). Less screen time and more frequent vigorous physical activity are associated with a lower risk of reporting negative mental health symptoms among Icelandic adolescents. *PLoS ONE, 13*(4), Article e0196286. https://doi.org/10.1371/journal.pone.0196286

Ito, T. A., Larsen, J. T., Smith, N. K., & Cacioppo, J. T. (1998). Negative information weighs more heavily on the brain: The negativity bias in evaluative categorizations. *Journal of Personality and Social Psychology, 75*(4), 887–900. https://doi.org/10.1037//0022-3514.75.4.887

Jackson, D., Firtko, A., & Edenborough, M. (2007). Personal resilience as a strategy for surviving and thriving in the face of workplace adversity: A literature review. *Journal of Advanced Nursing, 60*(1), 1–9. https://doi.org/10.1111/j.1365-2648.2007.04412.x

Jones, C. (2020). *Effectiveness of self-compassion-focused and mindfulness-based interventions in improving the emotional wellbeing of mental health professionals: A systematic review and; The relationships between self-compassion, emotional intelligence, depression, anxiety and carer burden in family caregivers of individuals with a diagnosis of dementia* [Doctoral Dissertation, University of Edinburgh]. Edinburgh Research Archive. https://doi.org/10.7488/era/595

Joyce, S., Shand, F., Tighe, J., Laurent, S. J., Bryant, R. A., & Harvey, S. B. (2018). Road to resilience: A systematic review and meta-analysis of resilience training programmes and interventions. *BMJ Open, 8*(6), Article e017858. https://doi.org/10.1136/bmjopen-2017-017858

Keyes, K. M., Gary, D., O'Malley, P. M., Hamilton, A., & Schulenberg, J. (2019). Recent increases in depressive symptoms among US adolescents: Trends from 1991 to 2018. *Social Psychiatry and Psychiatric Epidemiology, 54*(8), 987–996. https://doi.org/10.1007/s00127-019-01697-8

Kouros, C. D., Pruitt, M. M., Ekas, N. V., Kiriaki, R., & Sunderland, M. (2017). Helicopter parenting, autonomy support, and college students' mental health and well-being: The moderating role of sex and ethnicity. *Journal of Child and Family Studies, 26*(3), 939–949. https://doi.org/10.1007/s10826-016-0614-3

Kunzler, A. M., Chmitorz, A., Röthke, N., Staginnus, M., Schäfer, S. K., Stoffers-Winterling, J., & Lieb, K. (2022). Interventions to foster resilience in nursing staff: A systematic review and meta-analyses of pre-pandemic evidence. *International Journal of Nursing Studies, 134*, Article 104312. https://doi.org/10.1016/j.ijnurstu.2022.104312

Larijani, H. A., & Garmaroudi, G. (2018). Effectiveness of resiliency training in the mental health of the red crescent health care teams. *Romanian Journal for Multidimensional Education/Revista Romaneasca Pentru Educatie Multidimensionala, 10*(1), 1064–1083. https://doi.org/10.18662/rrem/37

Larson, S. (2010). Strength-based discipline that taps into the resilience of youth. *Reclaiming Children and Youth, 18*(4), 22.

Lee, H. H., & Cranford, J. A. (2008). Does resilience moderate the associations between parental problem drinking and adolescents' internalizing and externalizing behaviors? A study of Korean adolescents. *Drug and Alcohol Dependence, 96*(3), 213–221. https://doi.org/10.1016/j.drugalcdep.2008.03.007

Leipold, B., & Greve, W. (2009). Resilience: A conceptual bridge between coping and development. *European Psychologist, 14*(1), 40–50. https://doi.org/10.1027/1016-9040.14.1.40

Leppin, A. L., Bora, P. R., Tilburt, J. C., Gionfriddo, M. R., Zeballos-Palacios, C., Dulohery, M. M., Sood, A., Erwin, P. J., Brito, J. P., Boehmer, K. R., & Montori, V. M. (2014). The efficacy of resiliency training programs: A systematic review and meta-analysis of randomized trials. *PLOS ONE, 9*(10), Article e111420. https://doi.org/10.1371/journal.pone.0111420

Lukianoff, G., & Haidt, J. (2018). *The coddling of the American mind: How good intentions and bad ideas are setting up a generation for failure.* Penguin.

Luthans, F., Avey, J. B., Avolio, B. J., & Peterson, S. J. (2010). The development and resulting performance impact of positive psychological capital. *Human Resource Development Quarterly, 21*(1), 41–67. https://doi.org/10.1002/hrdq.20034

Luthar, S. S. (1991). Vulnerability and resilience: A study of high-risk adolescents. *Child Development, 62*(3), 600–616. https://doi.org/10.2307/1131134

Luthar, S. S. (2003). *Resilience and vulnerability.* Cambridge University Press. https://doi.org/10.1017/CBO9780511615788

Macedo, T., Wilheim, L., Gonçalves, R., Coutinho, E. S. F., Vilete, L., Figueira, I., & Ventura, P. (2014). Building resilience for future adversity: A systematic review of interventions in non-clinical samples of adults. *BMC Psychiatry, 14*(1), 227. https://doi.org/10.1186/s12888-014-0227-6

Marino, C., Gini, G., Vieno, A., & Spada, M. M. (2018). The associations between problematic Facebook use, psychological distress and well-being among adolescents and young adults: A systematic review and meta-analysis. *Journal of Affective Disorders, 226*, 274–281. https://doi.org/10.1016/j.jad.2017.10.007

Martínez-Martí, M. L., & Ruch, W. (2017). Character strengths predict resilience over and above positive affect, self-efficacy, optimism, social support, self-esteem, and life satisfaction. *Journal of Positive Psychology, 12*(2), 110–119. https://doi.org/10.1080/17439760.2016.1163403

Masten, A. S. (2001). Ordinary magic: Resilience processes in development. *American Psychologist, 56*(3), 227–238. https://doi.org/10.1037/0003-066X.56.3.227

Masten, A. S. (2014). *Ordinary magic: Resilience in development.* Guilford Press.
Masten, A. S. (2018). Resilience theory and research on children and families: Past, present, and promise. *Journal of Family Theory and Review, 10*(1), 12–31. https://doi.org/10.1111/jftr.12255
Masten, A. S., & Barnes, A. (2018). Resilience in children: Developmental perspectives. *Children, 5*(7), Article 98. https://doi.org/10.3390/children5070098
Masten, A. S., Best, K., & Garmezy, N. (1990). Resilience and development: Contributions from the study of children who overcome adversity. *Development and Psychopathology, 2*(4), 425–444. https://doi.org/10.1017/S0954579400005812
Masten, A. S., & Garmezy, N. (1985). Risk, vulnerability, and protective factors in developmental psychopathology. In B. B. Lahey, & A. E. Kazdin (Eds.), *Advances in clinical child psychology* (Vol. 8, pp. 1–52). Plenum Press.
McAvera, B. (2018). High bar for resilience programme. *Irish Arts Review, 35*(3), 12.
Métais, C., Burel, N., Gillham, J. E., Tarquinio, C., & Martin-Krumm, C. (2022). Integrative review of the recent literature on human resilience: From concepts, theories, and discussions towards a complex understanding. *Europe's Journal of Psychology, 18*(1), 98–119. https://doi.org/10.5964/ejop.2251
Nagata, J. M., Cortez, C. A., Dooley, E. E., Iyer, P., Ganson, K. T., Bibbins-Domingo, K., Baker, F. C., & Gabriel, K. P. (2022). 10. Screen time and moderate-to-vigorous intensity physical activity among adolescents during the COVID-19 pandemic: Findings from the adolescent brain cognitive development study. *Journal of Adolescent Health, 70*(4), S6–S6. https://doi.org/10.1016/j.jadohealth.2022.01.014
Newman, R. (2002). The road to resilience. *Monitor on Psychology, 33*(9), 62. https://www.apa.org/monitor/oct02/pp
Noullet, C. J., Lating, J. M., Kirkhart, M. W., Dewey, R., & Everly, G. S. (2018). Effect of pastoral crisis intervention training on resilience and compassion fatigue in clergy: A pilot study. *Spirituality in Clinical Practice, 5*(1), 1–7. https://doi.org/10.1037/scp0000158
Padilla-Walker, L. M., & Nelson, L. J. (2012). Black hawk down? Establishing helicopter parenting as a distinct construct from other forms of parental control during emerging adulthood. *Journal of Adolescence, 35*(5), 1177–1190. https://doi.org/10.1016/j.adolescence.2012.03.007
Panter-Brick, C., Goodman, A., Tol, W., & Eggerman, M. (2011). Mental health and childhood adversities: A longitudinal study in Kabul, Afghanistan. *Journal of the American Academy of Child & Adolescent Psychiatry, 50*(4), 349–363. https://doi.org/10.1016/j.jaac.2010.12.001
Peen, J., Schoevers, R. A., Beekman, A. T., & Dekker, J. (2010). The current status of urban-rural differences in psychiatric disorders. *Acta Psychiatrica Scandinavica, 121*(2), 84–93. https://doi.org/10.1111/j.1600-0447.2009.01438.x
Peng, L., Li, M., Zuo, X., Miao, Y., Chen, L., Yu, Y., Liu, B., & Wang, T. (2014). Application of the Pennsylvania resilience training program on medical students. *Personality and Individual Differences, 61*, 47–51. https://doi.org/10.1016/j.paid.2014.01.006
Polanczyk, G. V., Salum, G. A., Sugaya, L. S., Caye, A., & Rohde, L. A. (2015). Annual research review: A meta-analysis of the worldwide prevalence of mental disorders in children and adolescents. *Journal of Child Psychology and Psychiatry, 56*(3), 345–365. https://doi.org/10.1111/jcpp.12381
Racine, N., McArthur, B. A., Cooke, J. E., Eirich, R., Zhu, J., & Madigan, S. (2021). Global prevalence of depressive and anxiety symptoms in children and adolescents during COVID-19: A meta-analysis. *JAMA Pediatrics, 175*(11), 1142–1150. https://doi.org/10.1001/jamapediatrics.2021.2482
Reivich, K., & Shatté, A. (2002). *The resilience factor: Seven essential skills for overcoming life's inevitable obstacles.* Broadway Books.
Robertson, I. T., Cooper, C. L., Sarkar, M., & Curran, T. (2015). Resilience training in the workplace from 2003 to 2014: A systematic review. *Journal of Occupational and Organizational Psychology, 88*(3), 533–562. https://doi.org/10.1111/joop.12120
Rozin, P., & Royzman, E. B. (2001). Negativity bias, negativity dominance, and contagion. *Personality and Social Psychology Review, 5*(4), 296–320. https://doi.org/10.1207/S15327957PSPR0504_2
Rutter, M. (1987). Psychosocial resilience and protective mechanisms. *American Journal of Orthopsychiatry, 57*(3), 316–331. https://doi.org/10.1111/j.1939-0025.1987.tb03541.x
Rutter, M. (1999). Resilience concepts and findings: Implications for family therapy. *Journal of Family Therapy, 21*(2), 119–144. https://doi.org/10.1111/1467-6427.00108

Rutter, M. (2006). The promotion of resilience in the face of adversity. In A. Clarke-Stewart & J. Dunn (Eds.), *Families count: Effects on child and adolescent development* (pp. 26–52). Cambridge University Press. https://doi.org/10.1017/CBO9780511616259.003

Schaffer, K. (2019 December 20). U.S. has changed in key ways in the past decade, from tech use to demographics. *Fact tank: New in the number*. Pew Research Center. https://pewrsr.ch/35HxY2Y

Schmitt, N., Keeney, J., Oswald, F., Pleskac, T. J., Billington, A. Q., Sinha, R., & Zorzie, M. (2009). Prediction of 4-year college student performance using cognitive and noncognitive predictors and the impact on demographic status of admitted participants. *Journal of Applied Psychology, 94*(6), 1479–1497. https://doi.org/10.1037/a0016810

Seligman, M. E. P., Reivich, K. J., Jaycox, L. H., & Gillham, J. E. (1995). *The optimistic child.* Houghton Mifflin.

Shensa, A., Sidani, J. E., Escobar-Viera, C. G., Switzer, G. E., Primack, B. A., & Choukas-Bradley, S. (2020). Emotional support from social media and face-to-face relationships: Associations with depression risk among young adults. *Journal of Affective Disorders, 260,* 38–44. https://doi.org/10.1016/j.jad.2019.08.092

Shoshani, A., & Slone, M. (2016). The resilience function of character strengths in the face of war and protracted conflict. *Frontiers in Psychology, 6,* Article 2006. https://doi.org/10.3389/fpsyg.2015.02006

Sisto, A., Vicinanza, F., Campanozzi, L. L., Ricci, G., Tartaglini, D., & Tambone, V. (2019). Towards a transversal definition of psychological resilience: A literature review. *Medicina, 55*(11), Article 745. https://doi.org/10.3390/medicina55110745

Smith, P. G., Morrow, R. H., & Ross, D. A., (2015). Outcome measures and case definition. In P. Smith, R. H. Morrow, & D. A. Ross (Eds.), *Field trials of health intervention: A toolbox* (3rd ed.; pp. 198–215). Oxford Academic. https://doi.org/10.1093/med/9780198732860.003.0012

Southwick, S. M., Bonanno, G. A., Masten, A. S., Panter-Brick, C., & Yehuda, R. (2014). Resilience definitions, theory, and challenges: Interdisciplinary perspectives. *European Journal of Psychotraumatology, 5*(1), 25338. https://doi.org/10.3402/ejpt.v5.25338

Sternberg, R. J., Bonney, C. R., Gabora, L., & Merrifield, M. (2012). WICS: A model for college and university admissions. *Educational Psychologist, 47*(1), 30–41. https://doi.org/10.1080/00461520.2011.638882

Tedeschi, R. G., & Calhoun, L. G. (1996). The Posttraumatic Growth Inventory: Measuring the positive legacy of trauma. *Journal of Traumatic Stress, 9*(3), 455–472. https://doi.org/10.1002/jts.2490090305

Thompson, S. R., & Dobbins, S. (2018). The applicability of resilience training to the mitigation of trauma-related mental illness in military personnel. *Journal of the American Psychiatric Nurses Association, 24*(1), 23–34. https://doi.org/10.1177/1078390317739957

Tough, P. (2012). *How children succeed: Grit, curiosity, and the hidden power of character.* Houghton Mifflin Harcourt.

Twenge, J. M., Cooper, A. B., Joiner, T. E., Duffy, M. E., & Binau, S. G. (2019). Age, period, and cohort trends in mood disorder indicators and suicide-related outcomes in a nationally representative dataset, 2005–2017. *Journal of Abnormal Psychology, 128*(3), 185–199. https://doi.org/10.1037/abn0000410

Ungar, M. (2012). Researching and theorizing resilience across cultures and contexts. *Preventive Medicine, 55*(5), 387–389. https://doi.org/10.1016/j.ypmed.2012.07.021

Ungar, M., & Liebenberg, L. (2011). Assessing resilience across cultures using mixed methods: Construction of the Child and Youth Resilience Measure. *Journal of Mixed Methods Research, 5*(2), 126–149. https://doi.org/10.1177/1558689811400607

Vanhove, A. J., Herian, M. N., U. Perez, A. L., Harms, P. D., & Lester, P. B. (2016). Can resilience be developed at work? A meta-analytic review of resilience-building programme effectiveness. *Journal of Occupational and Organizational Psychology, 89*(2), 278–307. https://doi.org/10.1111/joop.12123

van Zyl, L. E., Gaffaney, J., van der Vaart, L., Dik, B. J., & Donaldson, S. I. (2024). The critiques and criticisms of positive psychology: A systematic review. *Journal of Positive Psychology, 19*(2), 206–235. https://doi.org/10.1080/17439760.2023.2178956

Walsh, R. (2011). Lifestyle and mental health. *American Psychologist, 66,* 579–592. https://doi.org/10.1037/a0021769

Weinberger, A. H., Gbedemah, M., Martinez, A. M., Nash, D., Galea, S., & Goodwin, R. D. (2018). Trends in depression prevalence in the USA from 2005 to 2015: Widening disparities in vulnerable groups. *Psychological Medicine, 48*(8), 1308–1315. https://doi.org/10.1017/S0033291717002781

Werner, E., & Smith, R. (2001). *Journeys from childhood to midlife: Risk, resilience, and recovery*. Cornell University Press.

Zimmerman, M. A. (2013). Resiliency theory: A strengths-based approach to research and practice for adolescent health. *Health Education & Behavior: The Official Publication of the Society for Public Health Education, 40*(4), 381–383. https://doi.org/10.1177/1090198113493782

2 Theoretical Foundations of Strengths-Based Resilience

The field of positive psychology studies the conditions and processes that enable individuals, families, communities, and institutions to flourish. It explores what works, what is right, and what can be nurtured. Positive psychology does not downplay distress and disorders, nor does it over-emphasize positives. It attempts to strike a balance through its assumption that building positive emotions and strengths can be as essential to well-being as ameliorating stressors and symptoms. In this way, positive psychology compliments, rather than competes with, traditional psychological interventions (Rashid et al., 2023). Strengths-Based Resilience (SBR) is informed by two major concepts in positive psychology. The first one is Martin Seligman's model of well-being (Seligman, 2011), and the second is the classification of strengths and virtues (CSV; Peterson & Seligman, 2004). This chapter provides a brief summary of the foundational concepts of each model and discusses associated research findings relevant to resilience. We conclude this chapter with a discussion of six reasons why a strengths-based approach to building resilience in individuals and communities makes sense.

Theory of Well-Being: PERMA

The PERMA model of well-being was first proposed by Martin Seligman (2011). It describes five ingredients of well-being: *positive emotions, engagement, relationships, meaning,* and *accomplishment* (PERMA; Seligman, 2011). Seligman suggests these five are scientifically measurable and malleable (Seligman, 2011). While the list of elements is neither exhaustive nor exclusive, their fulfillment is associated with higher life satisfaction. There is emerging evidence that fulfillment in these five domains of PERMA is closely linked with resilience (Umucu, 2017). The PERMA framework has shown promise in advancing our understanding of well-being and resilience (e.g., Kovich et al., 2023; van Agteren et al., 2018).

A recent narrative meta-analysis of 64 neuroimaging studies, grouped according to PERMA elements of happiness, showed that happiness as pleasure shows specific and localized neural activity, but so does engagement. Neural activities for pleasure and engagement were active when individuals were doing something. This research suggests that some PERMA elements can be better understood not as just feel-good states but a state of doing something (Tanzer & Weyandt, 2020).

We briefly describe the five domains of well-being and their theoretical and empirical links with resilience.

Positive Emotions

Positive emotions in the PERMA model relate to experiencing positive feelings such as contentment, pride, serenity, hope, optimism, trust, confidence, gratitude, and awe. Research has shown that positive emotions are important for our well-being and carry many benefits (Fredrickson & Joiner, 2018; Terrill et al., 2018).

In the context of resilience, positive emotions build resilience by undoing the adverse, and sometimes lingering, impact of negative emotions. Positive emotions provide a psychological break which is restorative and provides a respite from negative emotions (Folkman & Moskowitz, 2000; Fredrickson et al., 2015). According to Fredrickson's (1998) broaden-and-build theory, whereas negative emotions narrow people's behavioral tendencies toward self-preservation (e.g., fight or flight responses), positive emotions widen the array of thoughts and actions and increase cognitive and behavioral flexibility. In other words, negative emotions constrict people's thought–action repertoires, whereas positive emotions broaden and build these repertoires (Fredrickson, 2001). Positive emotions therefore have the potential of expanding the range of options that one can entertain to cope adaptively with adversity or a challenge.

Engagement

In the PERMA conceptualization, engagement is derived from Csikszentmihalyi's (1990) notion of *flow*. Flow is a profoundly focused and immersive state in which individuals are engaged cognitively, behaviorally, and affectively to produce optimal experience. Engagement generally occurs during a task for which the individual is intrinsically motivated and on which they feel almost compelled to focus, despite distractions.

Many psychological difficulties involve attentional challenges such as lack of interest, boredom, irritability, and restlessness (American Psychiatric Association, 2022; Donaldson et al., 2011; McCormick et al., 2005), which deplete resilience. Engagement promotes resilience by activating and directing inner resources to complete challenging tasks, thereby leaving little room for dwelling on negative thoughts about adversity or setbacks. Although engagement and flow are typically considered individualistic pursuits, research has demonstrated that they can also be fostered in small group settings (Culbertson et al., 2015). Furthermore, a sense of accomplishment after engaged activity can leave one reminiscing about the positive experience and basking in the aftermath (Feldman et al., 2008). Engagement and engagement-related concepts have been studied in business and educational settings (Bakker et al., 2011; Ceja & Navarro, 2011; Grafanaki et al., 2007; Nakamura & Csikszentmihalyi, 2002).

Relationships

The relationship component refers to having positive, secure, and trusting relationships and fulfilling the fundamental human need "to belong." One of the longest studies of adult development, the Harvard Adult Development Study, found that well-being and physical health are strongly associated with the presence of close relationships with others, including those with spouses, family members, and friends (Waldinger & Schulz, 2023). Close relationships are helpful for many reasons. Our loved ones may provide emotional or material support or advice when we encounter difficult times. They may encourage us to care for ourselves and to grow and develop. In addition, social interactions are mentally and emotionally invigorating, whereas social isolation dampens our mood (Waldinger & Schulz, 2023). As Seligman notes (2011), our best moments, such as times we experience joy, meaning, and contentment, often occur with or because of other people.

There is strong evidence that healthy relationships are key to resilience and well-being. For example, in their meta-analysis of 118 studies that focused on more than 100,000 children experiencing violence, Yule and colleagues found that support from family, peers, and school strongly predicted resilience (Yule et al., 2019). A systematic review and meta-analysis of 34 studies, including 2,305 participants, found that stable attachment relationships are critical in building resilience and may reduce the risk of adverse outcomes in adulthood in individuals who experienced adversities in childhood (Darling Rasmussen et al., 2019). Stable attachment relationships also extend beyond primary caregivers and include family members, teachers, and therapists who also can provide protective effects by building secure relationships (Mota & Matos, 2015).

Christopher Peterson, one of the founders of positive psychology, noted that the research on contributors to well-being could be summarized in three words: other people matter (Peterson, 2006). When it comes to resilience, other people matter mightily. Research has consistently shown that having dependable social relationships is associated with greater resilience (Infurna & Luthar, 2018).

Meaning

Meaning entails the extent to which people understand, make sense of, and perceive the significance of their lives. Meaning includes people's perception of having a purpose, mission, or overarching aim in life (Steger, 2012). Meaning has also been conceptualized as belonging to and serving something that is bigger than oneself (Seligman, 2002). Viktor Frankl, who survived the Holocaust, posited that happiness cannot be attained directly (Frankl, 1963). Rather, it must come as the unintended consequence of working for a goal greater than oneself. When meaning is lacking in people's lives, they can experience psychological distress, including symptoms of depression and anxiety, as well as hopelessness and suicidal ideation (Debats, 1996; Frankl, 1963; Mascaro & Rosen, 2006). Meaning provides a sense of coherence and motivation to pursue goals (McNight & Kashdan, 2009).

Meaning helps us to reappraise the significance of adverse or traumatic events and their implications. Making meaning restores harmony within an individual, leading to healing (Park, 2010). Research has shown that meaning making helps people to deal with stressful life situations, including health challenges (Czekierda et al., 2017; Roepke et al., 2013). Finding meaning in life is associated with better physical health, especially when meaning is linked with harmony, peace, and well-being in one's life (Czekierda et al., 2017; Hu et al., 2015).

Meaning contributes to resilience by increasing our motivation and ability to handle challenges. It helps us maintain perspective by placing challenges and setbacks in the larger context of our lives. There are numerous contexts and paths that promote meaning, including close interpersonal relationships; contribution to others' development and well-being; artistic, intellectual, or scientific endeavors; philosophical or religious contemplation; social, political or environmental activism; careers experienced as callings; and spirituality or other potentially solitary pursuits such as meditation (e.g., Stillman & Baumeister, 2009; Wrzesniewski et al., 1997). Regardless of the specific path, achieving a sense of meaningful purpose produces eudaimonic satisfaction, or the sense that one has lived well (Ackerman et al., 2000; Hicks & King, 2009).

Accomplishment

According to the PERMA model, accomplishment (or achievement) involves pursuing success and mastery for their own sake. It involves achieving short- and long-term goals through persistence, engaging in specific behaviors and habits over time, as well as using our strengths optimally. In the psychological literature, accomplishment and achievement are often used interchangeably. Achievement entails mastery, learning a task, and pursuing a goal (Dweck, 2002). Achievement also involves focusing one's skills and abilities toward a specific purpose (Ames, 1992; Pekrun et al., 2002).

In SBR, accomplishment is operationalized throughout the program as framing, pursuing, persisting in, and achieving personally meaningful goals through using our strengths. This is important, because goal setting and goal achievement are associated with well-being and can buffer individuals against future adversities. In other words, when we pursue and accomplish goals despite obstacles, we build resilience. Goal setting is an effective and fundamental component of successful behavior change interventions (Bailey, 2019). Goals which yield accomplishment are future-oriented and intrinsically motivating. They guide our behavior with a commitment to finish (Elliot & Fryer, 2008).

Classification of Strengths and Virtues

Character strengths are central to the SBR program. Whereas resilience, as noted in Chapter 1, has been explored for more than 3 decades (Rutter, 1987), a character-strengths-informed perspective on resilience is relatively new. There are several models of strengths, such as Gallup's Strengths Finder (Rath, 2007); Realise2 (Linley, 2008), behavioral and emotional strengths (Epstein, 2000), the basic human values (Schwartz, 1994), and personal resilience strengths (Benard, 2004).

With the generous support of the Values in Action Institute (https://www.viacharacter.org; now called the VIA Institute on Character), Christopher Peterson and Martin Seligman spearheaded a comprehensive and systematic effort in psychology to classify core human strengths: the *classification of strengths and virtues* (CSV; Peterson & Seligman, 2004). The CSV model has been developed and researched with millions of people from numerous countries. The CSV includes 24 character strengths, broadly parsed into six virtues (Box 1).

Box 1. Classification of character strengths and virtues

1. Wisdom and knowledge – Cognitive strengths that entail the acquisition and use of knowledge

- **Creativity** [originality, ingenuity]: Thinking of novel and productive ways to conceptualize and do things; includes artistic achievement but is not limited to it
- **Curiosity** [interest, novelty seeking, openness to experience]: Taking an interest in ongoing experience for its own sake; finding subjects and topics fascinating; exploring and discovering
- **Judgment** [critical thinking]: Thinking things through and examining them from all sides; not jumping to conclusions; being able to change one's mind in light of evidence; weighing all evidence fairly
- **Love of learning**: Mastering new skills, topics, and bodies of knowledge, whether on one's own or formally; obviously related to the strength of curiosity but goes beyond it to describe the tendency to add systematically to what one knows
- **Perspective** [wisdom]: Being able to provide wise counsel to others; having ways of looking at the world that make sense to oneself and to others

2. Courage – Emotional strengths that involve the exercise of will to accomplish goals in the face of opposition, external or internal

- **Bravery** [valor]: Not shrinking from threat, challenge, difficulty, or pain; speaking up for what is right even against opposition; acting on convictions even if unpopular; includes physical bravery but is not limited to it
- **Perseverance** [persistence, industriousness]: Finishing what one starts; persisting in a course of action in spite of obstacles; "getting it out the door"; taking pleasure in completing tasks
- **Honesty** [authenticity, integrity]: Speaking the truth, but more broadly presenting oneself in a genuine way and acting in a sincere way; being without pretense; taking responsibility for one's feelings and actions
- **Zest** [vitality, enthusiasm, vigor, energy]: Approaching life with excitement and energy; not doing things halfway or halfheartedly; living life as an adventure; feeling alive and activated

3. Humanity – Interpersonal strengths that involve tending to and befriending others

- **Love**: Valuing close relations with others, in particular those in which sharing and caring are reciprocated; being close to people
- **Kindness** [generosity, nurturance, care, compassion, altruistic love, "niceness"]: Doing favors and good deeds for others; helping them; taking care of them
- **Social intelligence** [emotional intelligence, personal intelligence]: Being aware of the motives and feelings of other people and oneself; knowing what to do to fit into different social situations; knowing what makes other people tick

4. Justice – Civic strengths that underlie healthy community life

- **Teamwork** [citizenship, social responsibility, loyalty]: Working well as a member of a group or team; being loyal to the group; doing one's share
- **Fairness**: Treating all people the same according to notions of fairness and justice; not letting personal feelings bias decisions about others; giving everyone a fair chance
- **Leadership**: Encouraging a group of which one is a member to get things done while maintaining good relations within the group; organizing group activities and seeing that they happen

5. Temperance – Strengths that protect against excess
• **Forgiveness**: Forgiving those who have done wrong; accepting the shortcomings of others; giving people a second chance; not being vengeful • **Humility**: Letting one's accomplishments speak for themselves; not regarding oneself as more special than one is • **Prudence**: Being careful about one's choices; not taking undue risks; not saying or doing things that might later be regretted • **Self-regulation** [self-control]: Regulating what one feels and does; being disciplined; controlling one's appetites and emotions
6. Transcendence – Strengths that forge connections to the larger universe and provide meaning
• **Appreciation of beauty and excellence** [awe, wonder, elevation]: Noticing and appreciating beauty, excellence, and/or skilled performance in various domains of life, from nature to art, to mathematics, to science, to everyday experience • **Gratitude**: Being aware of, and thankful for, the good things that happen; taking time to express thanks • **Hope** [optimism, future-mindedness, future orientation]: Expecting the best in the future and working to achieve it; believing that a good future is something that can be brought about • **Humor** [playfulness]: Liking to laugh and tease; bringing smiles to other people; seeing the light side; making (not necessarily telling) jokes • **Spirituality** [faith, purpose]: Having coherent beliefs about the higher purpose and meaning of the universe; knowing where one fits within the larger scheme; having beliefs about the meaning of life that shape conduct and provide comfort

Note. In some cases, the strength name or label is further explained by affiliated concepts that are noted inside square brackets. Adapted from *The VIA Classification of 24 Character Strengths*, by The VIA Institute on Character, 2021. www.viacharacter.org

Peterson and Seligman (2004) note that character strengths are morally desired traits of human existence and, at the same time, are open to empirical examination. Much like psychology has shown that individuals who experience resentment, hostility, vengeance, or vanity are more likely to develop a host of psychological ills, individuals who experience gratitude, forgiveness, humility, love, and kindness are more likely to report being happier and satisfied with life (Emmons & McCullough, 2003; Exline & Hill, 2012; Wood et al., 2010). Character strengths describe various shades and dimensions of human flourishing and well-being.

According to Peterson and Seligman (2004), character strengths are ubiquitous traits and are valued in their own right and do not diminish others; rather, they elevate those who witness the expression of strength, often eliciting admiration, not jealousy. For example, a creative individual may inspire others to be creative through their creative endeavors. Some individuals embody a particular strength extraordinarily, while others may abjectly lack it, at least in specific situations, if not at all times. Societal institutions cultivate character strengths through rituals, ceremonies, and organized events.

Peterson (2006) distinguishes character strengths (e.g., kindness, teamwork, zest) from talents and abilities. Athletic prowess, photographic memory, perfect pitch, excellent dexterity, physical agility, etc. are talents and abilities. Character strengths have a moral undercurrent, whereas talents and abilities are more neutral. Character strengths can help us develop talents. For example, self-regulation and optimism can improve one's athletic performance. To run like Usain Bolt or swim like Michael Phelps, one needs specific muscular agility and physical prowess. These athletes have likely also benefitted from character strengths such as persistence, optimism, and courage to realize their potential. Character strengths can be built on even fragile foundations with enough practice, persistence, good mentoring, and evidence-based interventions (Niemiec, 2018). Character strengths are also distinct from other types of strengths human beings have, including skills (proficiencies one develops such as typing skills, presentation skills, or anger management skills), interests (passions or hobbies for leisure such as sport, art, music, etc.), and resources (external supports such as having many friends or a supportive spiritual community; Peterson, 2006).

Why a Strengths-Based Approach to Resilience?

There are seven reasons why we think that working on strengths to boost resilience is a more effective approach than mitigating deficits alone.

1. **Drawing on their strengths, individuals are better able to adapt to adverse circumstances.** In our view, if resilience entails effective adaptation, the factors that enable this adaptation, such as strengths, abilities, and resources should be an integral part of resilience programming. Adaptive use of character strengths is linked to lower levels of depression and higher levels of well-being (Proctor et al., 2011; Rust et al., 2009; Seligman et al., 2009), greater life satisfaction (Antaramian et al., 2008), and fewer behavior problems (Park & Peterson, 2008). Moreover, eliminating life's challenges is not a desirable goal, as we grow stronger when overcoming challenges and coping successfully with stressful situations. Besides, each of us will face challenging situations, struggles, and suffering as part of life. We will all encounter difficulties. We will all make mistakes. We will all experience loss, including the loss of loved ones.
2. **A strengths-based approach increases individuals' self efficacy and confidence in ways that focusing on their weaknesses cannot.** Being aware of strengths, in addition to vulnerabilities, helps individuals to reinterpret and reframe problems from a strengths-based perspective rather than from a deficit-based approach. Consider the following research findings:
   - Knowing and using one's strengths promotes *valued living* – a style of responding to stressors that involves taking purposeful action – which, in turn, fosters resilience (Ceary et al., 2019).
   - A strengths-based intervention created short-term increases in employees' positive emotions and short- and long-term increases in their psychological capital – self efficacy, optimism, hope, and resilience (Meyers & van Woerkom, 2017).
   - Cultivating personal strengths and resources, such as humor, interpersonal relationships, and daily occupations, may help individuals preserve acceptable levels of well-being despite the presence of symptoms of depression, anxiety, and stress (Bos et al., 2016).
3. **Identifying and nurturing strengths enables individuals to achieve their goals and thrive in their community.** In a globalized knowledge-based educational milieu, a remedial

approach – one that corrects weaknesses of individuals only – gives insufficient preparation for students to accomplish their intellectual, social, and personal goals. From a public health perspective, while fixing weaknesses yields remediation, identifying and nurturing strengths help students to thrive. Empirical research shows that students who report higher levels of strengths tend to be healthier, are more engaged civically, have better physical and mental health, and have healthier interpersonal relationships – factors closely linked with resilience (Cantwell, 2005; Doll et al., 2008; Gillham et al., 2011; Proctor et al., 2011; Waters et al., 2012; Ungar et al., 2014).

4. **A focus on strengths cultivates and cements trust, especially when working with students and young adults from diverse cultural backgrounds, building their sense of belonging and mattering.** Strengths can tap into the communal potential of young adults. Spotting, recognizing, appreciating strengths of students make them feel that they belong and matter to the community. This is crucial for our adolescents and young adults who are reporting increasing levels of loneliness (Gentina & Chen, 2019). By acknowledging students' strengths, educators can demonstrate that students are central to the school community. It is critical in our educational institutions that adolescents and young adults feel that others (e.g., faculty, staff, administrators, peers) are genuinely interested in them and demonstrate that they matter to the institution and larger community in some way (Rayle & Chung, 2007).
5. **Knowledge of one's strengths is essential in nurturing a positive identity.** As noted above, character strengths and not weaknesses or deficits are the most important ingredients for change. However, many adolescents and young adults are often exclusively described by deficit-based labels such as attention-deficit/hyperactivity disorder (ADHD) and conduct disorder. These labels can be stigmatizing and demotivating. Without minimizing the adverse impacts of these conditions, strengths can be a catalyst in overcoming the negative impact of these conditions. We believe that knowledge of one's strengths is essential in nurturing a positive identity.
6. **A strengths-based approach to resilience is supported by emerging lines of research.** The following are examples of recently published studies.
   - Exploring the relationship between resilience and character strengths, Martínez-Martí and Ruch (2017) found that emotional, interpersonal, intellectual, and restraint-oriented strengths were positively related to resilience.
   - In two separate studies involving adults in community settings in China, Duan and Guo (2015) explored the association between character strengths and posttraumatic growth among those who had experienced a natural disaster and a range of traumatic experiences. They found a significant association between virtues (an aggregate of specific strengths) and posttraumatic growth, and between virtues and trait resilience. Resilience also contributed to more posttraumatic growth.
   - Demirci and colleagues (2021) examined the relationship between character strengths and psychological resilience. They found that high levels of wisdom, courage, optimism, and calmness predicted resilience.
   - Strengths-based parenting, which involves noticing and encouraging children's use of their strengths, is associated with greater happiness and life satisfaction and lower levels of depression, anxiety, and stress in youth (Jach et al., 2018; Loton & Waters, 2017; Waters, 2015a; Waters, 2015b).

- In a study of medical students and residents, Hausler and colleagues (2017) found that those who used their signature strengths reported lower levels of emotional exhaustion and better mental health and well-being (Hausler et al., 2017).
- A study of older adults, who described their day-to-day living, found that character strengths were one of the factors that facilitated better coping with challenges and enabled thriving (Russo-Netzer & Littman-Ovadia, 2019).

7. **Strengths-based interventions can promote participants' resilience, well-being, and mental health.**
   - Gillham and colleagues (2013) examined the effects of a high school positive psychology program that focused on helping students to identify and use their personal strengths. They found significant improvements in positive social skills and engagement in school among program participants compared to controls (Gillham et al., 2013; Seligman et al., 2009).
   - Schutte and Malouff (2019) reviewed 14 studies of interventions that focused on helping people to identify and use their personal strengths. They found these interventions significantly increased participants' happiness and satisfaction with life and reduced their feelings of depression. This suggests that understanding and using our best qualities can make a big difference in how we feel.
   - More recently, a meta-analysis of multicomponent positive psychology interventions in school settings found that these interventions enhance psychological well-being and reduce symptoms of depression (Tejada-Gallardo et al., 2020).

Summary

In this chapter, we reviewed two important models in positive psychology that have informed the development of the SBR program. The first one is PERMA, an evidence-based model which posits five components important to well-being: positive emotions, engagement, relationships, meaning, and accomplishment. In addition, SBR is informed by the classification of strengths and virtues (CSV), a model of 24 core human strengths that are valued in every culture. We provided seven reasons why a strengths-based approach can be effective. Research on the PERMA and CSV models provides compelling scientific evidence that we can boost our resilience by amplifying our strengths and abilities while not ignoring or minimizing our deficits and challenges. We review in the next chapter how we developed, piloted, and evaluated the SBR program.

References

Ackerman, S., Zuroff, D. C., & Moskowitz, D. S. (2000). Generativity in midlife and young adults: Links to agency, communion, and subjective well-being. *The International Journal of Aging & Human Development, 50*(1), 17–41. https://doi.org/10.2190/9F51-LR6T-JHRJ-2QW6

American Psychiatric Association. (2022). *Diagnostic and statistical manual of mental disorders* (5th ed., text rev.). https://doi.org/10.1176/appi.books.9780890425787

Ames, C. (1992). Classrooms: Goals, structure, and student motivation. *Journal of Educational Psychology, 84*(3), 261–271. https://doi.org/10.1037/0022-0663.84.3.261

Antaramian, S. P., Huebner, E. S., & Valois, R. F. (2008). Adolescent life satisfaction. *Applied Psychology, 57*(S1), 112–126. https://doi.org/10.1111/j.1464-0597.2008.00357.x

Bailey, R. R. (2019). Goal setting and action planning for health behavior change. *American Journal of Lifestyle Medicine, 13*(6), 615–618. https://doi.org/10.1177/1559827617729634

Bakker, A. B., Oerlemans, W., Demerouti, E., Slot, B. B., & Ali, D. K. (2011). Flow and performance: A study among talented Dutch soccer players. *Psychology of Sport and Exercise, 12*(4), 442–450. https://doi.org/10.1016/j.psychsport.2011.02.003

Benard, B. (2004). *Resiliency: What we have learned*. WestEd.

Bos, E. H., Snippe, E., de Jonge, P., & Jeronimus, B. F. (2016). Preserving subjective wellbeing in the face of psychopathology: Buffering effects of personal strengths and resources. *PLoS ONE, 11*(3), Article e0150867. https://doi.org/10.1371/journal.pone.0150867

Cantwell, L. (2005). A comparative analysis of strengths-based versus traditional teaching methods in a freshman public speaking course: Impacts on student learning and engagement. *Dissertation Abstracts International, 67*(02A), 478–700.

Ceary, C. D., Donahue, J. J., & Shaffer, K. (2019). The strength of pursuing your values: Valued living as a path to resilience among college students. *Stress and Health, 35*(4), 532–541. https://doi.org/10.1002/smi.2886

Ceja, L., & Navarro, J. (2011). Dynamic patterns of flow in the workplace: Characterizing within-individual variability using a complexity science approach. *Journal of Organizational Behavior, 32*(4), 627–651. https://doi.org/10.1002/job.747

Csikszentmihalyi, M. (1990). *Flow: The psychology of optimal experience* (1st ed.). Harper Collins.

Culbertson, S. S., Fullagar, C. J., Simmons, M. J., & Zhu, M. (2015). Contagious flow: Antecedents and consequences of optimal experience in the classroom. *Journal of Management Education, 39*, 319–349. https://doi.org/10.1177/1052562914545336

Czekierda, K., Banik, A., Park, C. L., & Luszczynska, A. (2017). Meaning in life and physical health: Systematic review and meta-analysis. *Health Psychology Review, 11*(4), 387–418. https://doi.org/10.1080/17437199.2017.1327325

Darling Rasmussen, P., Storebø, O. J., Løkkeholt, T., Voss, L. G., Shmueli-Goetz, Y., Bojesen, A. B., Simonsen, E., & Bilenberg, N. (2019). Attachment as a core feature of resilience: A systematic review and meta-analysis. *Psychological Reports, 122*(4), 1259–1296. https://doi.org/10.1177/0033294118785577

Debats, D. L. (1996). Meaning in life: Clinical relevance and predictive power. *British Journal of Clinical Psychology, 35*(4), 503–516. https://doi.org/10.1111/j.2044-8260.1996.tb01207.x

Demirci, İ., Ekşi, H., Ekşi, F., & Kaya, Ç. (2021). Character strengths and psychological vulnerability: The mediating role of resilience. *Current Psychology, 40*(11), 5626–5636. https://doi.org/10.1007/s12144-019-00533-1

Doll, B., Cummings, J. A., & Chapla, B. A. (2008). Best practices in population-based school mental health services. In A. Thomas & J. Grimes, *Best practices in school psychology* (Vol. 5, pp. 1333–1347). National Association of School Psychologists.

Donaldson, S. I., Csikszentmihalyi, M., & Nakamura, J. (Eds.). (2011). *Applied positive psychology: Improving everyday life, health, schools, work, and society*. Routledge Academic. https://doi.org/10.4324/9780203818909

Duan, W., & Guo, P. (2015). Association between virtues and posttraumatic growth: Preliminary evidence from a Chinese community sample after earthquakes. *PeerJ, 3*, Article e883. https://doi.org/10.7717/peerj.883

Dweck, C. (2002). The development of ability conceptions. In A. Wigfield & J. S. Eccles (Eds.), *Development of achievement motivation* (pp. 57–88), Academic Press. https://doi.org/10.1016/B978-012750053-9/50005-X

Elliot, A. J., & Fryer, J. W. (2008). The goal concept in psychology. In J. Shah & W. Gardner (Eds.), *Handbook of motivational science* (pp. 235–250). Guilford Press.

Emmons, R. A., & McCullough, M. E. (2003). Counting blessings versus burdens: An experimental investigation of gratitude and subjective well-being in daily life. *Journal of Personality and Social Psychology, 84*(2), 377–389. https://doi.org/10.1037/0022-3514.84.2.377

Epstein, M. H. (2000). The Behavioral and Emotional Rating Scale: A strength-based approach to assessment. *Diagnostique, 25*(3), 249–256. https://doi.org/10.1177/073724770002500304

Exline, J. J., & Hill, P. C. (2012). Humility: A consistent and robust predictor of generosity. *The Journal of Positive Psychology, 7*(3), 208–218. https://doi.org/10.1080/17439760.2012.671348

Feldman, G. C., Joormann, J., & Johnson, S. L. (2008). Responses to positive affect: A self-report measure of rumination and dampening. *Cognitive Therapy and Research, 32*, 507–525. https://doi.org/10.1007/s10608-006-9083-0

Folkman, S., & Moskowitz, J. T. (2000). Positive affect and the other side of coping. *American Psychologist, 55*(6), 647–654. https://doi.org/10.1037/0003-066X.55.6.647

Frankl, V. E. (1963). *Man's search for meaning: An introduction to logotherapy*. Washington Square Press.

Fredrickson, B. L. (1998). What good are positive emotions? *Review of General Psychology, 2*(3), 300–319. https://doi.org/10.1037/1089-2680.2.3.300

Fredrickson, B. L. (2001). The role of positive emotions in positive psychology: The broaden-and-build theory of positive emotions. *American Psychologist, 56*(3), 218–226. https://doi.org/10.1037/0003-066X.56.3.218

Fredrickson, B. L., Grewen, K. M., Algoe, S. B., Firestine, A. M., Arevalo, J. M. G., Ma, J., & Cole, S. W. (2015). Psychological well-being and the human conserved transcriptional response to adversity. *PLoS ONE, 10*(3), Article e0121839. https://doi.org/10.1371/journal.pone.0121839

Fredrickson, B. L., & Joiner, T. (2018). Reflections on positive emotions and upward spirals. *Perspectives on Psychological Science, 13*(2), 194–199. https://doi.org/10.1177/1745691617692106

Gentina, E., & Chen, R. (2019). Digital natives' coping with loneliness: Facebook or face-to-face? *Information & Management, 56*(6), Article 103138. https://doi.org/https://doi.org/10.1016/j.im.2018.12.006

Gillham, J. E., Abenavoli, R. M., Brunwasser, S. M., Linkins, M., Reivich, K. J., & Seligman, M. E. P. (2013). Resilience education. In S. A. David, I. Boniwell, & A. C. Ayers (Eds.), *Handbook of happiness* (pp. 609–630). Oxford University Press.

Gillham, J., Adams-Deutsch, Z., Werner, J., Reivich, K., Coulter-Heindl, V., Linkins, M., Winder, B., Peterson, C., Park, N., Abenavoli, R., Contero, A., & Seligman, M. E. P. (2011). Character strengths predict subjective well-being during adolescence. *Journal of Positive Psychology, 6*(1), 31–44. https://doi.org/10.1080/17439760.2010.536773

Grafanaki, S., Brennan, M., Holmes, S., Tang, K., & Alvarez, S. (2007). In search of flow in counseling and psychotherapy: Identifying the necessary ingredients of peak moments of therapy interaction. *Person-Centered & Experiential Psychotherapies, 6*(4), 240–255.

Hausler, M., Strecker, C., Huber, A., Brenner, M., Höge, T., & Höfer, S. (2017). Associations between the application of signature character strengths, health and well-being of health professionals. *Frontiers in Psychology, 8*, Article 1307. https://doi.org/10.3389/fpsyg.2017.01307

Hicks, J. A., & King, L. A. (2009). Positive mood and social relatedness as information about meaning in life. *The Journal of Positive Psychology, 4*(6), 471–482. https://psycnet.apa.org/doi/10.1080/17439760903271108

Hu, T., Zhang, D., & Wang, J. (2015). A meta-analysis of the trait resilience and mental health. *Personality and Individual Differences, 76*, 18–27. https://doi.org/10.1016/j.paid.2014.11.039

Infurna, F. J., & Luthar, S. S. (2018). Re-evaluating the notion that resilience is commonplace: A review and distillation of directions for future research, practice, and policy. *Clinical Psychology Review, 65*, 43–56. https://doi.org/10.1016/j.cpr.2018.07.003

Jach, H. K., Sun, J., Loton, D., Chin, T.-C., & Waters, L. E. (2018). Strengths and subjective wellbeing in adolescence: Strength-based parenting and the moderating effect of mindset. *Journal of Happiness Studies, 19*(2), 567–586. https://psycnet.apa.org/doi/10.1007/s10902-016-9841-y

Kovich, M. K., Simpson, V. L., Foli, K. J., Hass, Z., & Phillips, R. G. (2023). Application of the PERMA model of well-being in undergraduate students. *International Journal of Community Well-Being, 6*(1), 1–20. https://doi.org/10.1007/s42413-022-00184-4

Linley, P. A. (2008). *Average to A+: Realising strengths in yourself and others*. CAPP Press.

Loton, D. J., & Waters, L. E. (2017). The mediating effect of self-efficacy in the connections between the strengths-based parenting, happiness, and psychological stress in teens. *Frontiers in Psychology, 8*, Article 1707. https://doi.org/10.3389/fpsyg.2017.01707

Martínez-Martí, M. L., & Ruch, W. (2017). Character strengths predict resilience over and above positive affect, self-efficacy, optimism, social support, self-esteem, and life satisfaction. *Journal of Positive Psychology, 12*(2), 110–119. https://doi.org/10.1080/17439760.2016.1163403

Mascaro, N., & Rosen, D. H. (2006). The role of existential meaning as a buffer against stress. *Journal of Humanistic Psychology, 46*(2), 168–190. https://psycnet.apa.org/doi/10.1177/0022167805283779

McCormick, B. P., Funderburk, J. A., Lee, Y., & Hale-Fought, M. (2005). Activity characteristics and emotional experience: Predicting boredom and anxiety in the daily life of community mental health clients. *Journal of Leisure Research, 37*, 236–253. https://doi.org/10.1080/00222216.2005.11950052

McKnight, P. E., & Kashdan, T. B. (2009). Purpose in life as a system that creates and sustains health and well-being: An integrative, testable theory. *Review of General Psychology, 13*(3), 242–251. https://doi.org/10.1037/a0017152

Meyers, M. C., & van Woerkom, M. (2017). Effects of a strength intervention on general and work-related well-being: The mediating role of positive affect. *Journal of Happiness Studies, 18*(3), 671–689. https://doi.org/10.1007/s10902-016-9745-x

Mota, C. P., & Matos, P. M. (2015). Adolescents in institutional care: Significant adults, resilience and well-being. *Child Youth Care Forum, 44*, 209–224. https://doi.org/10.1007/s10566-014-9278-6

Nakamura, J., & Csikszentmihalyi, M. (2002). The concept of flow. In C. R. Snyder & S. J. Lopez (Eds.), *Handbook of positive psychology* (pp. 89–105). Oxford University Press.

Niemiec, R. M. (2018). *Character strengths interventions: A field guide for practitioners*. Hogrefe.

Park, C. L. (2010). Making sense of the meaning literature: An integrative review of meaning making and its effects on adjustment to stressful life events. *Psychological Bulletin, 136*, 257–301. https://doi.org/10.1037/a0018301

Park, N., & Peterson, C. (2008). Positive psychology and character strengths: Application to strengths-based school counseling. *Professional School Counseling, 12*(2), 85–92. https://doi.org/10.5330/PSC.n.2010-12.85

Pekrun, R., Goetz, T., Titz, W., & Perry, R. P. (2002). Academic emotions in students' self-regulated learning and achievement: A program of qualitative and quantitative research. *Educational Psychologist, 37*(2), 91–105. https://doi.org/10.1207/S15326985EP3702_4

Peterson, C. (2006). *A primer in positive psychology*. Oxford University Press.

Peterson, C., & Seligman, M. E. P. (2004). *Character strengths and virtues: A handbook and classification*. Oxford University Press.

Proctor, C., Tsukayama, E., Wood, A. M., Maltby, J., Eades, J. F., & Linley, P. A. (2011). Strengths Gym: The impact of a character strengths-based intervention on the life satisfaction and well-being of adolescents. *Journal of Positive Psychology, 6*(5), 377–388. https://doi.org/10.1080/17439760.2011.594079

Rashid, T., Summers, R. F., Seligman, M. E. P. (2023). Positive psychology model of mental function and behavior. In A. Tasman, M. B. Riba, R. D. Alarcón, C. A. Alfonso, S. Kanba, D. M. Ndetei, C. H. Ng, T. G. Schulze, & D. Lecic-Tosevski, *Tasman's Psychiatry*. Springer. https://doi.org/10.1007/978-3-030-42825-9_28-1

Rath, T. (2007). *Strengths Finder 2.0 / Tom Rath*. Gallup Press.

Rayle, A. D., & Chung, K.-Y. (2007). Revisiting first-year college students' mattering: Social support, academic stress, and the mattering experience. *Journal of College Student Retention: Research, Theory and Practice, 9*(1), 21–37. https://doi.org/10.2190/X126-5606-4G36-8132

Roepke, A. M., Jayawickreme, E., & Riffle, O. M. (2013). Meaning and health: A systematic review. *Applied Research in Quality of Life, 9*, 1055–1079. https://doi.org/10.1007/s11482-013-9288-9

Russo-Netzer, P., & Littman-Ovadia, H. (2019). 'Something to live for:' Experiences, resources, and personal strengths in late adulthood. *Frontiers in Psychology, 10*, Article 2452. https://doi.org/10.3389/fpsyg.2019.02452

Rust, T., Diessner, R., & Reade, L. (2009). Strengths only or strengths and relative weaknesses? A preliminary study. *Journal of Psychology, 143*(5), 465–476. https://doi.org/10.3200/JRL.143.5.465-476

Rutter, M. (1987). Psychosocial resilience and protective mechanisms. *American Journal of Orthopsychiatry, 57*(3), 316–331. https://doi.org/10.1111/j.1939-0025.1987.tb03541.x

Schutte, N. S., & Malouff, J. M. (2019). The impact of signature character strengths interventions: A meta-analysis. *Journal of Happiness Studies, 20*, 1179–1196. https://doi.org/10.1007/s10902-018-9990-2

Schwartz, S. H. (1994). Are there universal aspects in the structure and contents of human values? *Journal of Social Issues, 50*(4), 19–45. https://doi.org/10.1111/j.1540-4560.1994.tb01196.x

Seligman, M. E. P. (2002). *Authentic happiness: Using the new positive psychology to realize your potential for lasting fulfilment*. Free Press.

Seligman, M. E .P. (2011). *Flourish: A visionary new understanding of happiness and well-being.* Free Press.

Seligman, M. E. P., Ernst, R. M., Gillham, J., Reivich, K., & Linkins, M. (2009). Positive education: Positive psychology and classroom interventions. *Oxford Review of Education, 35*(3), 293–311. https://doi.org/10.1080/03054980902934563

Steger, M. F. (2012). Making meaning in life. *Psychological Inquiry, 23*(4), 381–385. https://doi.org/10.1080/1047840X.2012.720832

Stillman, T. F., & Baumeister, R. F. (2009). Uncertainty, belongingness, and four needs for meaning. *Psychological Inquiry, 20*(4), 249–251. https://doi.org/10.1080/10478400903333544

Tanzer, J. R., & Weyandt, L. (2020). Imaging happiness: Meta analysis and review. *Journal of Happiness Studies, 21*(7), 2693–2734. https://doi.org/10.1007/s10902-019-00195-7

Tejada-Gallardo, C., Blasco-Belled, A., Torrelles-Nadal, C., & Alsinet, C. (2020). Effects of school-based multicomponent positive psychology interventions on well-being and distress in adolescents: A systematic review and meta-analysis. *Journal of Youth and Adolescence, 49*(10), 1943–1960. https://doi.org/10.1007/s10964-020-01289-9

Terrill, A. L., Ellington, L., John, K. K., Latimer, S., Xu, J., Reblin, M., & Clayton, M. F. (2018). Positive emotion communication: Fostering well-being at end of life. *Patient Education and Counseling, 101*(4), 631–638. https://doi.org/10.1016/j.pec.2017.11.018

Umucu, E. (2017). *Evaluating optimism, hope, resilience, coping flexibility, secure attachment, and PERMA as a well-being model for college life adjustment of student veterans: A hierarchical regression analysis* (Publication No. 10608545) [Doctoral dissertation, University of Wisconsin-Medison]. ProQuest Dissertations & Theses Global.

Ungar, M., Russell, P., & Connolly, G. (2014). School-based interventions to enhance the resilience of participants. *Journal of Educational and Developmental Psychology, 4*(1), 66–83. https://doi.org/10.5539/jedp.v4n1p66

Van Agteren, J., Iasiello, M., & Lo, L. (2018). Improving the wellbeing and resilience of health services staff via psychological skills training. *BMC Research Notes, 11*(1), 924. https://doi.org/10.1186/s13104-018-4034-x

Waldinger, R., & Schulz, M. (2023). *The good life: Lessons from the world's longest scientific study of happiness.* Simon Schuster.

Waters, L. (2012). A review of school-based positive psychology interventions. *Australian Educational and Developmental Psychologist, 28*(2), 75–90. https://doi.org/10.1375/aedp.28.2.75

Waters, L. (2015a). Strength-based parenting and life satisfaction in teenagers. *Advances in Social Science Research Journal, 2*(11), 158–173.

Waters, L. (2015b). The relationship between strength-based parenting with children's stress levels and strength-based coping approaches. *Psychology, 6*(6), 689–699. https://doi.org/10.4236/psych.2015.66067

Wood, A. M., Froh, J. J., & Geraghty, A. W. A. (2010). Gratitude and well-being: A review and theoretical integration. *Clinical Psychology Review, 30*(7), 890–905. https://doi.org/10.1016/j.cpr.2010.03.005

Wrzesniewski, A., McCauley, C., Rozin, P., & Schwartz, B. (1997). Jobs, careers, and callings: people's relations to their work. *Journal of Research in Personality, 31*, 21–33. https://doi.org/10.1006/jrpe.1997.2162

Yule, K., Houston, J., & Grych, J. (2019). Resilience in children exposed to violence: A meta-analysis of protective factors across ecological contexts. *Clinical Child and Family Psychology Review*, 22, 406–431. https://doi.org/10.1007/s10567-019-00293-1

3 SBR Program Development and Validation

Resilience interventions have traditionally focused on reducing risk factors (Chmitorz et al., 2018). However, there have been growing calls to also include protective factors in resilience interventions (Fenwick-Smith et al., 2018; Infurna & Luthar, 2018; Masten, 2001). Informed by positive psychotherapy (Rashid & Seligman, 2018), the Penn Resilience Program (Gillham et al., 1995; Jaycox et al., 1994) and the high school positive psychology program (Gillham et al., 2013; Seligman et al., 2009), strengths-based resilience (SBR) addresses mental health and wellness holistically, considering risks and resources, vulnerabilities and assets, and challenges and opportunities. SBR also incorporates techniques from cognitive behavioral therapy (Hofmann et al., 2012; Kreuze et al., 2018) and mindfulness practices, which aim to increase participants' awareness of and perspective on present experiences as well as compassion toward self and others (e.g., Carsley et al., 2018; Kaplan et al., 2017; Luberto et al., 2018).

SBR was created for and tested in a number of settings located in culturally diverse and socio-culturally marginalized neighborhoods since 2010. One of the goals of creating SBR was to offer culturally responsive resilience-building programs to counter-balance resilience scholarship and science dominated by Western theoretical frameworks, concepts, and worldviews (Wyatt, 2021). In the early phases of program validation, SBR went through several iterations, following extensive consultations with educators and healthcare professionals from diverse cultural backgrounds who worked with students and clients from diverse backgrounds. This has enhanced SBR's cultural responsiveness. Each of the 14 modules of the program include a section which offers facilitators strategies to culturally contextualize the SBR modules. For example, while building and strengthening an autonomous self to encounter stressors and adversities is much desired in Western countries, an interdependent self which deals with setbacks by marshalling collective resilience (e.g., of family, clan, group, community) is encouraged by non-Western cultural norms (Raghavan & Sandanapitchai, 2019; Ungar, 2013).

Western cultural norms emphasize individual choice, freedom, and an internal sense of control, relatively free from approval-seeking from others. However, reflections shared in focus groups, and feedback about the cultural relevance of the specific components of each module, made it clear that in many non-Western communities, adversity and resilience are largely understood in relation to other people and contexts, including immediate and extended family and community. From this perspective, resilience is a result of multiple interrelated and interdependent factors which are changeable through collective efforts.

Resilience can also be conceptualized as coping well. To cope well, individuals need assets, abilities, and resources, especially supportive connections with others. Therefore, SBR focuses primarily on helping participants to identify, develop, and use character strengths. Character strengths are valued across cultures and many are essential for developing and sustaining relationships with others.

SBR is appropriate for a variety of educational and clinical settings. In school settings, the program can be delivered as a well-being or psychological well-being curriculum, or as a life skills, health, or personal development course. In postsecondary settings, SBR can be offered either through counseling or clinical services, or in collaboration with various student services, including academic advising, health and wellness services, and athletics. In clinical settings, it can be offered as part of a psychoeducational group of programs to supplement individual therapy. It can also be adapted and offered as a life skills course for adults in a community setting.

Development of the SBR Program

Program Phases

Our original conception of the SBR program involved three phases. We briefly summarize these phases below to provide readers with an overview of the program. The details of each module are described more fully in Chapter 4.

Phase 1

The first phase (Modules 1–4) focuses on resilience, growth, and flexible thinking. This phase begins with building a healthier self-concept by helping participants to recall and reflect on a challenge or setback that they handled adaptively or effectively. Through this activity, participants learn about resilience and the factors that can promote it, including beliefs, skills, behaviors, and internal and external social supports. They learn about negativity bias as well as the skills and strengths they possess that may be helpful in difficult situations in the future.

Next follows an exploration of mindset and thinking habits. Participants learn about specific outcomes associated with a growth or a fixed mindset. For example, if participants perceive their abilities to be largely unchangeable, they are likely to have a fixed mindset, and will be extremely discouraged by challenges and setbacks. They are more likely to lose motivation when tasks become difficult. In contrast, if participants believe that abilities can be nurtured, they are more likely to have a growth mindset, and to view setbacks and challenges as a normal part of the learning process. They are thus more likely to persevere.

Activities in this section are designed to help participants identify their mindset and teach skills that cultivate growth mindset. SBR encourages participants to apply a growth mindset to the development of strengths. Developing strengths (becoming more resilient) is a lifelong process that takes effort and practice. The mindset activity is followed by two practices adapted from cognitive behavioral therapy that help participants learn to think clearly and flexibly in responding to challenges, setbacks, and adversities. Participants learn to unpack challenging experiences into three components: thoughts, feelings, and behavior. They examine the links between these components, especially how our thoughts can influence our feelings and actions. They then identify habitual ways of thinking about negative situations or events, to avoid common thinking errors (e.g., confirmation bias, jumping to conclusions), and to develop more flexible and accurate ways of thinking about problems. These ways include considering alternative interpretations and examining evidence for and against their beliefs.

Skills covered in this first phase are relevant to a variety of character strengths, including optimism, perseverance, open-mindedness, critical thinking, and perspective taking.

Phase 2

SBR's second phase (Modules 5–10) focuses on identifying and cultivating character strengths. This phase begins with a discussion of character strengths, emphasizing the wide variety of strengths that have been valued throughout history and across different cultures. Activities focus on helping participants identify their own actions, behaviors, and habits that are related to strengths. Participants also learn about their signature strengths. Signature strengths refer to a person's central or core strengths. According to Peterson & Seligman (2004), people usually have a few signature strengths and feel more authentic when using them. For example, if someone has a signature strength of playfulness, they easily find ways to use it in their work or personal or family lives. Participants are encouraged to engage in activities designed to help them identify their top strengths and learn practical ways of using strengths in everyday situations. This helps them to translate the abstract notions of strengths, such as gratitude, curiosity, prudence, kindness, and forgiveness, into applicable actions. With the help of scenarios, participants are taught relevant, adaptive, and proportionate use of strengths to address challenges or difficulties they might be experiencing. For example, some challenges may be resolved by a nuanced use of strengths (e.g., playfulness or prudence), while others may themselves be the result of strengths deployed too rigidly or out of context (e.g., being kind to others at the expense of self-care).

Next, participants learn ways to use strengths to solve problems. Later modules in this phase focus on developing and applying specific strengths. For example, in a module on grudge and gratitude, participants explore any stubborn resentments they may have and the adverse and often enduring impact of those resentments. To counterbalance these negative feelings, positive emotions are cultivated through structured practices of gratitude and savoring. Participants also learn about empathy and perspective taking by understanding other's emotions, thoughts, and motives.

Phase 3

The last phase of the SBR program (Modules 11–14) hones the skills that help foster close and supportive relationships. This phase includes modules that focus on spotting and celebrating strengths in family members and friends. Activities emphasize acknowledging others' strengths and engaging in activities with others that allow them to use their strengths. This last phase teaches participants skills for positive communication, helping others, and cultivating a sense of meaning and purpose. After exploring individual and interpersonal strengths, which presumably would have broadened their self-concept and raised their awareness about appreciating and celebrating strengths of loved ones, participants are ready to explore broader themes which encapsulate one of the critical elements of strengths: contributing towards the common good. The last two modules – altruism and meaning and purpose – focus on serving something larger than our individual self to cultivate deeper connections to others. This is in keeping with emerging resilience theory and research that have shifted towards conceptualizing resilience from the individual to the interpersonal and community levels (Infurna & Luthar, 2018; Southwick et al., 2014).

Program Manual Development and Facilitator Training

Program Manual Development

The current manual was developed over a period of 15 years. From its initial rudimentary version in 2009, to its current version, we have conducted validation studies and actively sought feedback from facilitators (teachers, mental health professionals) and students. We have consistently incorporated feedback and recommendations from all stakeholders. In 2014, the manual received a significant uplift with professionally designed, customized illustrations. This was done for a study at a high school. We named that version of the manual *Strong as Me* (Rashid, Anjum, & Gillham, 2014).

During 2015–2017, the SBR program was revised again, incorporating feedback and recommendations from educators and clinicians. Changes included restructuring the format of the lesson delivery, introducing a discussion subsection in every module. As noted earlier, also included in each module was a learning and cultural fit component to raise awareness of the fact that different students have different learning needs and cultural perspectives. No new core content was introduced or removed in this revision. The revised 2016 Manual was used for an intervention with high school students. In that version, we increased the number of lessons from 12 to 14, to cover each lesson within an hour, accommodating requests from educators who preferred to cover content in 60-minute discrete chunks. However, we recommend a 75-minute module to allow ample time for the practice activities, which deepen learning. A suggested breakdown of each session is described in Table 2 in the next chapter.

Facilitator Training: Canadian Settings

In the past 15 years, we have trained hundreds of educators and mental health professionals. These include schoolteachers, administrators, guidance counselors, school psychologists, counselors working in community mental health settings, educators working in school settings in Canadian indigenous communities (Northern Ontario), and counselors working with phone helplines (Kids Phone Help and Nasheeha). We also partnered with a number of community organizations who requested training during the COVID-19 pandemic. Our training is adapted to the needs of settings, with most trainings lasting for three days and some one or two days. At the end of each training, especially three-day long training sessions, we solicited anonymous feedback from trainees.

We asked participants to rate their agreement with each of the following statements on a 5-point Likert scale from strongly disagree (1) to strongly agree (5):

- *The training was well-conducted.*
- *The leaders and facilitators were effective in guiding the training.*
- *It seems that the program will be helpful for my clients/students.*
- *The training video clips and slides were helpful to support my learning.*
- *Having done the activities during the training will help me to better implement the program.*
- *The manual is helpful in reinforcing my learning.*
- *The training sessions increased my understanding of strengths-based resilience.*

A sample of feedback, collected after training more than 127 educators and clinical staff in 2015–17 is presented in Figure 1. Overall, the program received positive feedback. The in-session discussion components, along with the supplementary videos, were among the most frequently cited helpful aspects of the training. Participants also often reported that they gained new perspectives on communication and character strengths. In contrast, a few respondents suggested more concrete instructions for classroom implementation, which we have now incorporated in the manual.

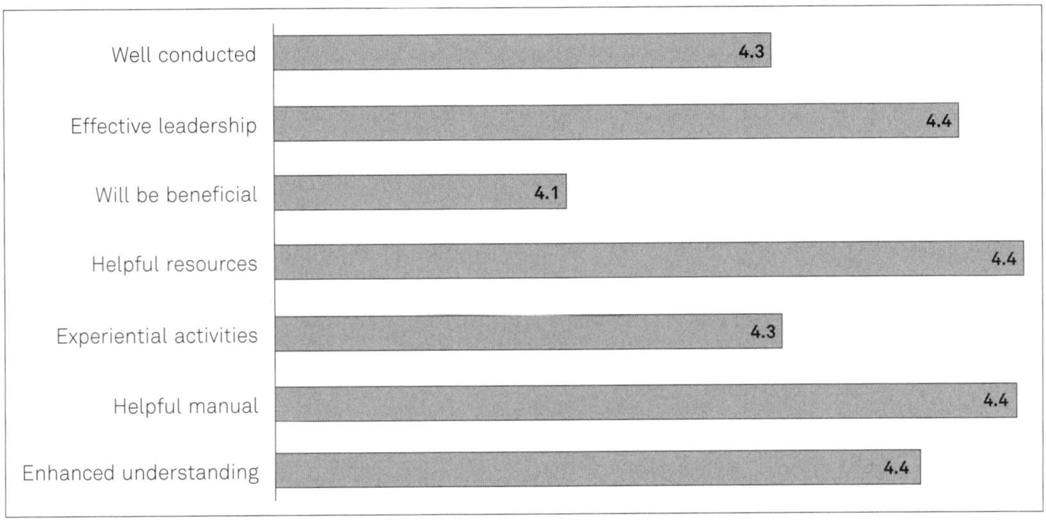

Figure 1. Anonymous feedback regarding 3-day Strengths-Based Resilience (SBR) training completed by 127 professional clinicians and educators in 2015–2017. *Note.* Each item was rated by participants on a 5-point Likert scale from 1 (*strongly disagree*) to 5 (*strongly agree*).

Facilitator Training: International Settings

Cultural responsiveness has been a key feature in attracting the attention of international educators and clinicians for training and collaboration. The program team has been invited to train educators and clinicians in a struggling neighborhood of Karachi, Pakistan (2014), traumatized educators in Kiev, Ukraine (2014), professionals working with adolescents in Graz, Austria (2016), Syrian refugees in Lebanon (2019), traumatized Muslim Community members in New Zealand following the mass shooting in two mosques in Christchurch (2019), teachers and youth workers in disadvantaged communities in Sri Lanka (2022), and transgender community members in Lahore, Pakistan (2022).

SBR is the primary intervention in a large resilience initiative project in Guyana, implemented by the International Development and Relief Foundation (IDRF), a Canadian-based NGO. The project estimates that by its conclusion, more than 67,500 individuals in vulnerable communities in Guyana, including youth in schools and adults in community settings, will be taught resilience and well-being skills. To date, more than 100 educators, mental health professionals, and community leaders have attended three 3-day SBR workshops. A total of 127 participants provided anonymous feedback, rating items on the 1–5 Likert scale described above. On average, participants indicated that the training was informative and engaging (4.8) and that they learned experiential skills (4.7) and skills they can use in their practice (4.8) (Rashid & Ali, 2022).

Validation of the SBR Program

Our team has published several chapters and articles on the theoretical and conceptual framework of SBR (Drvaric et al., 2015; Gillham et al., 2019; Rashid, Anjum, Chu et al., 2014). Our team and other researchers have examined the effectiveness of the SBR program through a number of studies conducted at several schools, an outpatient adolescent unit of a local hospital, the counseling center of a university, and, most recently, at a nursing home in New Zealand (Qureshi, 2022; Rashid & Anjum, 2008; Rashid, Anjum, Chu et al., 2014; Rashid & Louden, 2018). Research indicates that, across these settings, SBR reduces stress and enhances well-being. Furthermore, quantitative and qualitative feedback elicited anonymously from participants as well as from facilitators, shows multiple benefits of a strengths-based approach in the five settings, as discussed below.

First Randomized Trial

The first randomized study of SBR was conducted at a middle school in Toronto, with sixth-grade students who received 8 sessions of SBR in group settings. Tayyab Rashid and Afroze Anjum co-led the group. The class teacher also attended the sessions and often provided illustrations from the classroom curriculum to help students understand SBR concepts. Following the intervention, students in the SBR group reported increased life satisfaction compared with students in the control group, although no statistically significant differences were found in symptoms of depression (Rashid & Anjum, 2008). The second randomized controlled study of SBR evaluated its effects with teachers as participants. Participants in the SBR group, compared to no intervention control, reported a decrease in depressive symptoms and an increase in levels of well-being and life satisfaction.

SBR in Five High Schools

The largest study of SBR was conducted with five Toronto area high schools in 2016–18 (Rashid & Louden, 2018). Teachers were trained to run SBR in classroom settings as part of health or related curriculum or other programming for students. Schools implemented SBR according to their programming needs. For example, one school included SBR in its leadership training program, another incorporated it in its mentorship program, and two schools taught it as a life skills program. Teachers and each school's mental health professionals who also completed the training cofacilitated sessions. In each school, the SBR team also delivered at least one evening workshop called "Resilient Parenting" during school council meetings. This enabled the school administration to introduce the program to parents.

In each school, a regular high school class not receiving the SBR program served as a control group. Seventy-seven high school students completed pre- and post-SBR questionnaires assessing their well-being. Findings indicated that students who completed the SBR program reported a significant reduction in symptoms of psychological distress and in problem behaviors and a significant increase in well-being and resilience compared with students in the control group. At the 6-month follow up, SBR participants continued to report increased resilience, although no differences were found for other outcomes (Rashid & Louden, 2018).

SBR With Young Adults in Clinical Settings

SBR has also been evaluated with university students. In one study, forty-two students seeking counseling services at a university-based counseling center completed 8–10 sessions of SBR group therapy. They were compared with 20 students who participated in an alternative therapy group, offered during the same semester. Students in both study conditions completed questionnaires before the group, shortly after the group, and at 6 and 12 months follow up after the groups ended. Compared with controls, students in the SBR group showed significant reductions in stress and improvements in well-being at the end of the program. These differences in stress and well-being were also significant at the 12-month follow-up, but not at the 6-month follow-up. At the 12-month follow-up, students in SBR group reported less stigma toward mental health concerns than those who received the alternative therapy. Details of the last two studies, with outcome data can found online (Rashid & Louden, 2018).

SBR With Lebanese Journalists

Constant and chronic engagement with traumatic events in any professional field (e.g., healthcare, counseling, trauma work, firefighting) can produce a cumulative effect of internalizing the experiences of clients and survivors. As part of his master's thesis, Milad Hadchiti, who has a background in media, conducted a modified SBR program with Lebanese journalists working in high conflict areas near the Syrian border. The goal was to assess the feasibility of SBR for reducing trauma-related symptoms and as well as enhancing strengths and well-being, which, in turn, could enhance personal and psychological growth. Such growth, especially among a variety of professionals such as counselors, nurses or trauma specialists, could increase their resilience. Hadchiti found that journalists who participated in an SBR intervention showed improvement in their ability to handle traumatic stress compared to journalists who participated in a mindfulness intervention or a no-intervention control group (Hadchiti, 2019).

SBR With Carers of Stroke Survivors

Ayesha Qureshi (2022) adapted the SBR program and conducted a study with 27 participants in New Zealand to examine the feasibility of SBR to support carers of stroke survivors as part of her doctoral thesis. Carers play an important role in the recovery of stroke survivors – from participating in their inpatient rehabilitation to supporting their return home and integration back into the community. In this randomized controlled study, SBR was compared with usual care. Individual interviews with participants in the experimental group explored the benefits and acceptability of the intervention and sought suggestions from the participants for improvements in the program. Quantitative measures were used to compare two groups. Results showed that the SBR intervention was acceptable and potentially beneficial in supporting the resilience of carers of stroke survivors. The intervention appears to be more suitable for carers two years post stroke. The entire study manuscript can be accessed online (https://ourarchive.otago.ac.nz/bitstream/handle/10523/13652/QureshiAyeshaN2022PhD.pdf?sequence=1&isAllowed=y).

Summary

We designed SBR as a well-being program for adolescents and young adults, based on positive psychology, cognitive behavioral therapy, and mindfulness. In our design of the original program and subsequent revisions, we envisioned three broad phases for the program. Phase 1 focuses on understanding resilience, growth mindset, and flexible thinking skills. Phase 2 focuses on identifying and cultivating character strengths. Phase 3 focuses on using strengths and skills to foster positive relationships and to increase meaning and purpose. Over a 15-year period, we adapted the program, accompanying Manual, and pedagogical activities through piloting the program in a variety of settings, from schools and universities to hospitals. Colleagues also used the SBR program with other populations, including reporters in high conflict areas and carers of stroke survivors. All of these activities enabled us to validate the benefits of the SBR program for a wide range of audiences and has led us to the current manual and accompanying workbook.

References

Carsley, D., Khoury, B., & Heath, N. N. (2018). Effectiveness of mindfulness interventions for mental health in schools: A comprehensive meta-analysis. *Mindfulness, 9*(3), 693–707. https://doi.org/10.1007/s12671-017-0839-2

Chmitorz, A., Kunzler, A., Helmreich, I., Tüscher, O., Kalisch, R., Kubiak, T., Wessa, M., & Lieb, K. (2018). Intervention studies to foster resilience: A systematic review and proposal for a resilience framework in future intervention studies. *Clinical Psychology Review, 59*, 78–100. https://doi.org/10.1016/j.cpr.2017.11.002

Drvaric, L., Gerritsen, C., Rashid, T., Bagby, R. M., & Mizrahi, R. (2015). High stress, low resilience in people at clinical high risk for psychosis: Should we consider a strengths-based approach? *Canadian Psychology, 56*(3), 332–347 https://doi.org/10.1037/cap0000035

Fenwick-Smith, A., Dahlberg, E. E., & Thompson, S. C. (2018). Systematic review of resilience-enhancing, universal, primary school-based mental health promotion programs. *BMC Psychology, 6*(1), 30. https://doi.org/10.1186/s40359-018-0242-3

Gillham, J. E., Abenavoli, R. M., Brunwasser, S. M., Linkins, M., Reivich, K. J., & Seligman, M. E. P. (2013). Resilience education. In S. A. David, I. Boniwell, & A. C. Ayers (Eds.), *Handbook of happiness* (pp. 609–630). Oxford University Press.

Gillham, J., Leventhal, K.S., Rashid, T., Anjum, A., & Leventhal, S. (2019). Positive psychology programs for youth in diverse communities. In L. van Zyl & S. I. Rothman (Eds.), *Positive psychological interventions* (pp. 197–226). Springer.

Gillham, J. E., Reivich, K. J., Jaycox, L. H., & Seligman, M. E. P. (1995). Prevention of depressive symptoms in schoolchildren: Two-year follow-up. *Psychological Science, 6*(6), 343–351. https://doi.org/10.1111/j.1467-9280.1995.tb00524.x

Hadchiti, M. (2019). *From vicarious trauma to vicarious resilience: A strength-based resilience intervention* [Unpublished master's thesis]. University of East London, London, UK.

Hofmann, S. G., Asnaani, A., Vonk, I. J., Sawyer, A. T., & Fang, A. (2012). The efficacy of cognitive behavioral therapy: A review of meta-analyses. *Cognitive Therapy and Research, 36*(5), 427–440. https://doi.org/10.1007/s10608-012-9476-1.

Infurna, F. J., & Luthar, S. S. (2018). Re-evaluating the notion that resilience is commonplace: A review and distillation of directions for future research, practice, and policy. *Clinical Psychology Review, 65*, 43–56. https://doi.org/10.1016/j.cpr.2018.07.003

Jaycox, L. H., Reivich, K. J., Gillham, J., & Seligman, M. E. P. (1994). Prevention of depressive symptoms in school children. *Behaviour Research and Therapy, 32*(8), 801–816. https://doi.org/10.1016/0005-7967(94)90160-0

Kaplan, J. B., Bergman, A. L., Christopher, M., Bowen, S., & Hunsinger, M. (2017). Role of resilience in mindfulness training for first responders. *Mindfulness, 8*(5), 1373–1380. https://doi.org/10.1007/s12671-017-0713-2

Kreuze, L. J., Pijnenborg, G. H. M., de Jonge, Y. B., & Nauta, M. H. (2018). Cognitive-behavior therapy for children and adolescents with anxiety disorders: A meta-analysis of secondary outcomes. *Journal of Anxiety Disorders, 60*, 43–57. https://doi.org/10.1016/j.janxdis.2018.10.005

Luberto, C. M., Shinday, N., Song, R., Philpotts, L. L., Park, E. R., Fricchione, G. L., & Yeh, G. Y. (2018). A systematic review and meta-analysis of the effects of meditation on empathy, compassion, and prosocial behaviors. *Mindfulness, 9*(3), 708–724. https://doi.org/10.1007/s12671-017-0841-8

Masten, A. S. (2001). Ordinary magic: Resilience processes in development. *American Psychologist, 56*(3), 227–238. https://doi.org/10.1037/0003-066X.56.3.227

Peterson, C., & Seligman, M. E. P. (2004). *Character strengths and virtues: A handbook and classification.* Oxford University Press; American Psychological Association.

Qureshi, A. (2022). *Strengths-based resilience intervention for informal carers of stroke Survivors* [Doctoral thesis, University of Otago Dunedin, Otago, New Zealand]. http://hdl.handle.net/10523/13652

Raghavan, S. S., & Sandanapitchai, P. (2019). Cultural predictors of resilience in a multinational sample of trauma survivors. *Frontiers in Psychology,* 10. https://www.frontiersin.org/articles/10.3389/fpsyg.2019.00131

Rashid, T., & Ali, N. (2022). Safe guarding human dignity and rights of youth in vulnerable communities in Guyana. Presentation at the Guyana Mental Health & Well-Being Conference, Georgetown, Guyana, November, 15, 2022.

Rashid, T., & Anjum, A. (2008). Positive psychotherapy for young adults and children. In J. R. Z. Abela & B. L. Hankin (Eds.), *Depression in children and adolescents: Causes, treatment and prevention* (pp. 250–287). Guilford Press.

Rashid, T., Anjum, A., Chu, R., Stevanovski, S., Zanjani, A., & Lennex, C. (2014). Strength based resilience: Integrating risk and resources towards holistic well-being. In G. A. Fava & C. Ruini (Eds.), *Increasing psychological well-being in clinical and educational settings: Interventions and cultural contexts* (pp. 153–176). Springer.

Rashid, T., Anjum, A., & Gillham, J. (2014). *Strong as me: A strength based approach to resilience.* Unpublished manuscript.

Rashid, T., & Louden, R. (2018). *Flourish: A strengths-based resilience (SBR) approach to support students' transition from secondary to post-secondary education.* Ministry of Training of College and Universities, Ontario, Canada. https://hive.utsc.utoronto.ca/public/iits/flourish/Flourish_Final%20Report_2018.pdf

Rashid, T., & Seligman, M. E. P. (2018). *Positive psychotherapy: Clinician manual.* Oxford University Press. https://doi.org/10.1093/med-psych/9780195325386.001.0001

Seligman, M. E. P., Ernst, R. M., Gillham, J., Reivich, K., & Linkins, M. (2009). Positive education: Positive psychology and classroom interventions. *Oxford Review of Education, 35*(3), 293–311. https://doi.org/10.1080/03054980902934563

Southwick, S. M., Bonanno, G. A., Masten, A. S., Panter-Brick, C., & Yehuda, R. (2014). Resilience definitions, theory, and challenges: Interdisciplinary perspectives. *European Journal of Psychotraumatology, 5*, 1. https://doi.org/10.3402/ejpt.v5.25338

Ungar, M. (2013). Resilience, trauma, context, and culture. *Trauma, Violence, & Abuse, 14*(3), 255–266. https://doi.org/10.1177/1524838013487805

Wyatt, Z. (2021). Dynamism: Reconceptualising resilience in recovery from trauma. *Asian Journal of Social Science Studies, 6*(4), 28–34. https://doi.org/10.20849/ajsss.v6i4.954

4 SBR Program Content and Delivery

Program Content

The central learning outcomes of SBR are to help participants develop a deep understanding of their strengths and learn how to apply them to better manage everyday stressors and challenges, as well as to increase positive experiences in their everyday lives. Participants learn about their uniqueness in terms of their assets (e.g., signature strengths profile) instead of their deficits (e.g., diagnostic profiles).

The program's 14 modules include in-session experiential activities that teach participants strength-based ways to deal with everyday stressors, challenges, and problems, along with strategies for increasing positive experiences and strengthening relationships. The central feature of the SBR program and each module is the identification and development of participants' internal resources. We believe that it can be effective to engage with strengths rather than focus on symptoms or intervene on deficits. Therefore, the learning goals of the various SBR exercises focus on eliciting, elaborating, and enhancing strengths rather than diagnosing deficits and dysfunctions. However, it is important to underscore that deficits are not dismissed or minimized. Rather, we cultivate an understanding and appreciation of strengths to combat deficits or indeed to co-exist with them, thereby attenuating their impact.

Table 1 provides an overview of the 14 modules as well as the Orientation Session. It lists learning outcomes for each module, provides a brief description of practice activities, and highlights examples of learning and cultural considerations that are further developed in each module. Depending on the setting, these can be referred to as modules, lessons, or sessions.

Table 1. Overview of SBR modules

Module	Learning outcomes	Practice	Learning & cultural considerations
Orientation	Understand goals of the program, introduce the regular practices (gratitude journal and relaxation and mindfulness), and review provisions of confidentiality.	Participants are oriented to program and general protocols and reminded that skills can be practiced within and outside the classroom.	Assuring participants that program skills are applicable to a variety of cultural backgrounds.
Phase 1			
1. Resilience	Define resilience and identify qualities of individual resilience. Develop a coherent and healthier self-narrative. Express an understanding of ways that specific strengths such as persistence, hope, social intelligence, self-regulation, perspective, and spirituality can boost one's resilience.	*Write Your Own Story of Resilience* Participants recall, reflect on, and write a one-page story of resilience, with a beginning, middle, and positive end, describing how they overcame a significant challenge in their lives.	Being mindful that some participants may consider this practice as self-congratulatory and not culturally desirable; others may find it hard to highlight their own role, as the challenge may have been overcome collectively.
2. Fixed & Growth Mindsets	Distinguish between fixed and growth mindsets. Examine and assess their mindset patterns. Explore ways to nurture a growth mindset.	*Identify Your Mindset Reactions* Participants read and reflect on everyday situations and explore whether they tend toward a fixed or growth mindset.	Recognizing limitations as there might be genuine barriers to growth, including specific learning disabilities or systematic socioeconomic barriers; also avoid trite statements such as do your best, you can do anything.

Table 1. Continued

Module	Learning outcomes	Practice	Learning & cultural considerations
3. Cognitive Accuracy	Recognize thinking tendencies, including negativity bias, that can lead to inaccurate interpretations and affect their reactions. Develop more accurate and helpful perceptions about their thoughts, emotions, and reactions.	*Unpack Experiences to Understand Challenges* Participants unpack their negative experiences into three parts: thoughts, emotions, and behaviors. *Explore Your Thinking Shortcuts* Participants apply seven common thinking errors to the situations they unpacked.	Recognizing that some participants might have learned different ways of understanding connections between their thoughts, emotions, and actions.
4. Cognitive Flexibility	Explore habitual patterns of explaining the causes of challenges. Assess the extent to which causes are personal, permanent, and pervasive. Cultivate a flexible thinking style in response to challenging events.	*Tune into Your Explanatory Style* Participants parse their explanations for causes of events into three dimensions: personal, permanent, and pervasive, and learn how these dimensions affect their behaviors.	Increasing cognitive flexibility may not be the most important or relevant intervention for participants facing difficult experiences beyond their control, such as illness, dysfunctional family dynamics, or socioeconomic problems; being careful not to imply that all problems are due to thinking styles.
Phase 2			
5. Character Strengths	Value character strengths as intrinsic attributes which can be used, refined, and developed to boost resilience. Understand that character strengths are as real and impactful in our lives as weaknesses. Hone skills to acknowledge one's own strengths as well as spot strengths in others.	*Spot Your Character Strengths* Participants identify their character strengths from multiple perspectives.	Exploring cultural/religious expressions of strengths with which participants identify, including actions, habits, customs, and rituals; recognizing that there may be additional strengths valued by families and cultures.

Table 1. Continued

Module	Learning outcomes	Practice	Learning & cultural considerations
6. Signature Strengths	Own their cluster of top strengths as sources of energy and learning. Identify opportunities to set personal goals for improvement. Apply strengths adaptively to the unique demands of various situations.	*Compile Your Signature Strengths Profile* Participants compile their signature strengths profile, which includes getting friends, family members and significant others to identify their top strengths. The signature strengths profile helps participants to reflect on how these strengths are an important part of their personality and can be expressed through their actions.	Building awareness of the difference between "leading with one's signature strengths" and "improving weaknesses," so that participants can set personally desirable goals, regardless of whether they scored high or low on a specific strength.
7. Problem Solving & Strengths	Calibrate strengths according to the situational relevance and fit. Recruit strengths optimally to solve everyday problems and setbacks. Learn to use strengths in a balanced and adaptive way.	*Use Strengths to Overcome Challenges* Participants apply strategies for using strengths (considering the specificity, relevance, and potential conflicts between strengths) to solve a personal challenge that needs a solution.	Exploring culturally adaptive use of strengths in solving problems (for example, if cultural norms encourage an individual or collaborative problem-solving approach).
8. Grudge & Gratitude	**Grudge** Gain awareness of the consequences of holding a grudge. Learn the value of forgiveness to enhance well-being and resilience. **Gratitude** Attune awareness toward the goodness of others. Build gratitude skills and positive emotions through concrete actions.	*Let Go of Grudge* Participants reflect on a grudge and are invited to write or draw about consequences of holding onto it. *Express Gratitude* Participants draft a letter of gratitude to someone they have not thanked sufficiently.	Reminding participants who find it hard to recall a grudge, that it is possible to hold a grudge with a valued family member. Recognizing that forgiveness and gratitude are influenced by cultural, spiritual, and family traditions. Recognizing that participants can decide whether it is appropriate or helpful to forgive.

Table 1. Continued

Module	Learning outcomes	Practice	Learning & cultural considerations
9. Empathy	Take the perspective of others who face challenging circumstances. Increase awareness of others' challenging experiences without feeling overwhelmed by negative thoughts and emotions.	*Build Empathy* Participants read a story and discuss in pairs ways to empathize with the painful or emotional experiences of others.	Reinforcing that emotional empathy doesn't necessarily mean participants have to empathize with behavioral consequences, especially if behaviors are valued differently from culture to culture.
10. Slowness & Savoring	Recognize the pressure and cost of doing things faster and frequently. Experience the impact of slowing down to appreciate details. Experience the impact of savoring to amplify positive emotions.	*Slow Down and Savor* Participants learn slowness strategies; participants select at least one object to savor, using different techniques and types of savoring.	Acknowledging it may be difficult for some participants to slow down when they are surrounded by fast-paced culture; not all cultures are time-bound and fast-paced, therefore assess first to ensure cultural relevance.
Phase 3			
11. Positive Relationships	Spot strengths of significant people in their lives. Plan ways to cultivate their relationships by engaging in activities with those who share similar strengths. Explore possibilities to cultivate relationships by learning from those whose strengths are different.	*Celebrate Collective Strengths* Participants create a relationship tree, listing individual strengths of their loved ones who have played significant roles in their lives – could be family or other loved ones.	Being mindful of participants who come from broken, dispersed, deceased, or dysfunctional families, who may find this activity emotionally difficult; for some participants, interpersonal strengths are valued much more than intrapersonal ones.

Table 1. Continued

Module	Learning outcomes	Practice	Learning & cultural considerations
12. Positive Communication	Experience the emotional impact of communication that is active or passive, constructive or destructive. Apply capitalization – a process of being seen, felt, and valued, especially when sharing positive news. Exercise listening skills by asking questions to elaborate on positive events.	*Communicate Actively and Constructively* Participants learn about four different ways of responding to positive news shared by a loved one.	Recognizing that some participants with an introverted disposition or from less expressive or emotive cultures may feel that this exercise is more about celebrating ostentatiously; reminding them that the essence of this practice is being authentic, not elevating oneself.
13. Altruism	Build a sense of connection. Experience positive emotions through helping others. Understand that altruism demands effort by the helper with no obvious benefit in return.	*Give the Gift of Time* Participants plan to give the gift of time doing something that also uses their signature strengths.	Exploring if altruism is part of participants' cultural or religious tradition; adapting the practice within participants' sociocultural context.
14. Meaning & Purpose	Reinterpret their story of resilience for clues to meaning and purpose. Envision a meaningful lifetime accomplishment. Envision a plan of action to achieve the vision within 10 years.	*Reflect on Your Story of Resilience* Participants reinterpret their story of resilience to draw out themes of meaning and purpose in their life. *Envision a Story of Your Future* Participants write a plan of personal actions for how they would like to be remembered and what their positive legacy would be.	Understanding that the pursuit of meaning is highly culturally sensitive and spiritually informed. Recognizing that the pursuit of meaning is deeply influenced by people's cultural and spiritual contexts.

Program Delivery

Each of the 14 SBR modules of the SBR program covers one main topic and follows a consistent structure, beginning with two regular practices (mindfulness and relaxation, gratitude journal) as described in Table 2. Although the full SBR program contains 15 modules, including the Orientation module, facilitators may decide to condense or combine topics, depending on their audience, targeted learning outcomes and time available.

Examples of modules that can be taught together include:
- Modules 3 and 4 (Cognitive Accuracy and Cognitive Flexibility)
- Modules 5 and 6 (Character Strengths and Signature Strengths)
- Modules 13 and 14 (Altruism and Meaning and Purpose)

If you choose to combine topics, you may also need to build in additional time for each session. We have illustrated in Table 2 the difference between a 60- and a 75-minute practice that makes sense for a single module topic. If you choose to combine module topics, we recommend a 90-minute session.

If SBR is being delivered in a counseling/clinical setting, whether in a high school, college, university, hospital, or community organization, we recommend including 8 to 15 participants. When SBR is delivered as a course in high school, college, university, or community settings, we recommend 20 to 30 participants. When conducting training sessions for mental health professionals who would like to facilitate the SBR program, we recommend a size of 20 to 40.

Table 2. Components of a sample module

SBR module components	Description	Example timing	
		60 mins	75 mins
Learning Outcomes	Explain the learning outcomes of the module.	5	5
Opening Activities	Start each session with one of the five mindfulness & relaxation practices, Following the mindfulness & relaxation practice, encourage participants to share a few entries from their gratitude journal.	10	15
Illustration of Core Concepts	Begin with a review of the relevant research related to each module.* Draw on video illustrations to elaborate and deepen knowledge about the topic. Have participants reflect on and discuss their understanding of and reactions to core concepts and video illustrations	15	15
Practice	Invite participants to engage in practice activities relevant to the topic. Have participants debrief their experience with the in-session practice.	20	30
Closing Activities	Discuss practical ways participants can make personalized connections with module learnings to apply them in everyday life to better handle stressors. Refer participants to resources, including relevant published articles, books, websites and multimedia resources, to deepen and consolidate learning. End each session with one of the five mindfulness & relaxation practices	10	10

*Note that Core Concepts in the Workbook are briefer than those in the Practitioner's Manual and generally do not contain references

General Considerations

Facilitators can use this manual in a variety of clinical and educational settings. When delivering the program, facilitators are encouraged to keep in mind the eight considerations below.

1. Adapt the Program to Meet Your Participants' Needs

The present manual provides a framework and structure for facilitators who plan to run an SBR program. However, within each module, the Learning and Cultural Fit section offers you sufficient flexibility to adapt the program to meet your participants' needs.

2. Align Learning Objectives to Stakeholder Goals

Discuss and articulate goals that you want to accomplish by running an SBR program in your setting. Consult Table 1 to assess if your goals align with the learning outcomes listed for each module. Each module of the SBR program offers a Learning and Cultural Fit section. This section can also help you to align your goals with the program.

3. Focus Program Modules on Problems Pertinent to Your Audience

The SBR program modules teach participants to utilize personal strengths to deal with everyday problems and challenges. Each module invites participants to consider the relevance of concepts and skills to their lives. Module 7 specifically outlines 15 common challenges where applying one's strengths can lead to adaptive strengths-based solutions.

4. Anticipate the Resources You Will Need to Deliver an Effective Program

Prepare a list of both tangible and intangible resources you may need to run the program smoothly. These may include training, space, measures, supplies, and staff. Ensure you recruit staff who are genuinely interested in attending training sessions and running a program that incorporates mindfulness, cognitive behavioral interventions, and positive psychology.

5. Know Your Participants

It is important to know who is participating in your program and to tailor the learning outcomes of each module to audience needs. The SBR program is appropriate for a wide range of adolescents and young adults in high school, college, and university settings. It can also be delivered in a community setting as a psychoeducational course or a life skills program. As you tailor your program to your audience, consider cultural context in terms of language proficiency and acculturation, especially if an adolescent has immigrated recently or a young adult is an international student.

The SBR program may not be an appropriate intervention for all, especially individuals who are experiencing severe symptoms related to recent trauma or loss and may need specialized therapeutic support. SBR is not intended to replace therapy. If potential participants have clinical levels of depression, anxiety, or other mental health difficulties, it is important to refer them for appropriate mental health care. Depending on their needs, the SBR program may be helpful as an additional resource.

6. Integrate SBR With Other Programs

The SBR program is but one program. Despite yielding promising results, it is not a panacea. To foster resilience, multiple interventions, from various perspectives, are needed. Establish collaborations whereby activities of the SBR program, such as the Story of Resilience, Cognitive Accuracy and Flexibility, Character Strengths, Gratitude Letter, and Savoring can be incorporated as stand-alone exercises in a variety of programs. For example, the SBR program validation studies at the University of Toronto Scarborough, Canada, included collaborative programming with accessibility and academic advising services, as well as athletics.

7. Know the Outcomes You Want to Evaluate and How Best to Evaluate Them

It is important to include some form of program evaluation. A good evaluation may include valid and reliable measures of resilience and psychological well-being. Include qualitative measures (e.g., open-ended feedback) to ensure participants have an opportunity to share their feedback about the program with minimal cultural or linguistic barriers. Furthermore, ensure that the evaluation aligns with your stated program goals and learning outcomes.

8. Adapt the Experiential Learning Activities to the Size and Needs of Your Group

While our program promotes an experiential approach, one should be mindful that individuals may have different ways of engaging with a concept and practice. Cultural factors play a part. It is important to build sufficient flexibility into each practice so that a maximum number of participants can participate. More importantly, be vigilant that no one in the group is systematically excluded.

Group Processes

In this section, we discuss aspects of the group processes, including establishing group rules and responsibilities and participation-related guidelines.

The SBR program focuses on discovering, building, and using our strengths. The program format emphasizes discussion and application. There will be many opportunities for participants to discuss how concepts they are learning may apply to their own lives, and to apply what they are learning. It is important to create some ground rules to ensure that everyone is comfortable in the group.

At the onset, the facilitator, along with the participants, should discuss creating an inclusive and respectful group environment where everyone is able to participate at their own level of comfort as well as benefit from group processes and practices optimally. To accomplish this, it is important to discuss and establish some guidelines. The following are some important themes about which groups should establish guidelines and rules: respect privacy; respect levels of participation; practice, practice, practice; journal regularly; and begin with mindfulness and relaxation.

Reassure participants about the confidentiality of the information they share. In groups where participants are privy to each other's sensitive information, it is important to emphasize that participants can share concepts and skills covered in the session but must keep confidential information about other participants. Facilitators need to remind participants how they should handle information shared by participants – that is, what remains confidential and what is disclosed to whom and in what circumstances. In discussing the boundaries of confidentiality, facilitators may also discuss the limits of confidentiality.

Also, let participants know that they are in charge of what they share, because some of the practices of the program will invite participants to reflect on personal experiences. They can participate in these exercises at their own level of comfort. Participants have many avenues of learning, from listening to mini lectures and watching video illustrations, to reflecting and writing about their personal experiences.

The SBR program emphasizes practice, both through activities in each module and through the everyday applications section, which is devoted to transferring the lessons in the classroom to everyday experience. Journaling, mindfulness and relaxation, and reflecting in writing in particular are actively practiced. SBR is not simply a group process where participants are likely to foster their resilience by just discussing their problems. It requires an active and ongoing effort which targets a variety of skills that can only be developed by participants when they engage during sessions and practice actively outside of sessions.

To introduce these group process rules, group facilitators or instructors can use the following scripts and modify them according to their group's needs.

Respect Privacy and Confidentiality

The script below is an example of how to introduce to participants the importance of respecting privacy and confidentiality throughout the program.

In this program, participants will learn about specific personal characteristics that build resilience and the specific interpersonal supports that enhance resilience. We often learn about ourselves when we interact with others.

Stories, personal details, and experiences shared in this course must stay in the classroom.

As a member of this class, you will be asked to share your personal stories and opinions. Sharing personal thoughts will make this class more enriching and effective for you. But please only share what you are comfortable sharing. We recognize that your stories may be personal, and we would never wish for you to experience extreme discomfort as a result of anyone unintentionally sharing them. Some participants might not be comfortable sharing if they fear that they will be made fun of by others or if they fear their information will be shared with others.

It is equally important for everyone to respect the privacy of the person who has shared a story and not retell these stories without permission. Sometimes when we retell a story without permission, it becomes gossip and may hurt the person who shared.

One way to respect privacy is to take away the concepts and skills learned from shared stories and experiences, but keep the details of the stories within the group. Treat the personal information of others the way you would like your personal information to be treated. Most importantly, refrain from posting anything about this program or the participants on social media.

If certain situations arise, I may need to disclose your information to relevant professionals, not to get you in trouble, but to ensure that you and others are safe. This is usually information about imminent safety concerns for you or if I learn a minor is being abused. This is my ethical as well as my professional responsibility.

Respect Levels of Participation

This next script invites active yet appropriate group participation and acknowledges that participants' level of participation will vary from meeting to meeting.

We hope that you will all feel comfortable joining in discussions and sharing experiences. This will make the group more interesting and helpful. Sharing experiences also creates a caring group atmosphere. At the same time, we recognize that everyone has different ways of sharing. Everyone has good days and bad days, and this can affect their daily participation. Take your time to gauge your comfort level and trust within the group. The program respects this need and meets you where you are that day. Nothing is imposed on you, and you can decide whether or not to share or participate on a particular day.

Practice, Practice, Practice

The SBR program encourages taking learning outside the classroom. Below is a script to encourage this practice.

To improve at any activity, be it playing the piano, playing soccer, or doing math, one needs practice. Similarly, to boost your resilience, you need to practice some skills which will prepare you to handle unpredictable and tough situations resiliently. You will generally not be asked to do typical academic homework. However, you will be expected to be mindful and find opportunities in your life where you can apply the skills you will learn in this class.

Reflect Regularly in Writing

Our program couples active learning with reflection, a powerful combination that deepens participants, awareness and understanding of resilience. Use the script below to engage them in the process of reflection through writing.

> Most exercises in this program require you to write down your reflections. Writing helps us clarify our thinking and understand jumbled thoughts and emotions. Writing is essential to benefiting from this program. You can choose to reflect in a number of ways, including traditional writing on paper, logging digitally, orally recording on your mobile or smart phone, or drawing pictures or graphics. If you have concerns that someone may read or have access to your writing, we can discuss some practical ways to safeguard your privacy.

Begin With Mindfulness and Relaxation

Fundamental to the SBR program is mind–body awareness. Therefore, each module begins and ends with a mindfulness or relaxation activity. Ensure participants are informed of this feature in your first session using the script below.

> All sessions begin with a brief relaxation or mindfulness exercise. We will practice a number of these exercises during the course of the program. We teach mindfulness and relaxation for many reasons. These exercises can help you to gain a better understanding of your everyday experiences, including how you are feeling and your stress level. You will also learn specific skills to relax yourself to improve your focus and engagement in specific tasks, during and outside this program. By helping you relax and increasing your awareness, some of these activities may help you be kinder and more compassionate to yourself and to others.

Summary

This chapter overviewed the learning outcomes, provided a brief description of practices, and illustrated examples of learning and cultural fit considerations for the SBR program's Orientation Session and 14 Modules. It discussed the common module structure, suggested timing, and recommended optimal group size depending on the setting. In this chapter, we shared eight general considerations for effective delivery and illustrated ground rules to ensure facilitators can run groups effectively.

Section II: Orientation Session and Regular Practice

Orientation Session

This chapter provides facilitators with guidance on introducing the SBR program to participants in an initial orientation session before starting the first module. Facilitators can offer this as a presession, which describes the program, answers participants' questions, covers potential ground rules, and introduces the two regular practices of mindfulness and relaxation and the gratitude journal.

If you require participant, parental, or guardian consent, obtain this prior to the start of this session. Also, share the program schedule in advance, including each module's expected start and end time, and have printed copies available for distribution at the orientation session.

Opening the Session

Welcome participants into the room and invite them to take a seat. You can arrange the seats in a circle or horseshoe to ensure engagement. You can play relaxing music, preferably instrumental, soothing, and somewhat neutral music, at a low volume to create a welcoming atmosphere.

Once everyone has settled in, facilitators can start with an ice-breaker exercise to enable participants to get to know each other better. For example, participants can introduce themselves with a first name and share one strength or positive aspect of themselves or one good thing that happened to them this week.

Introducing the SBR Program

Welcome participants to the strengths-based resilience program, or SBR for short.

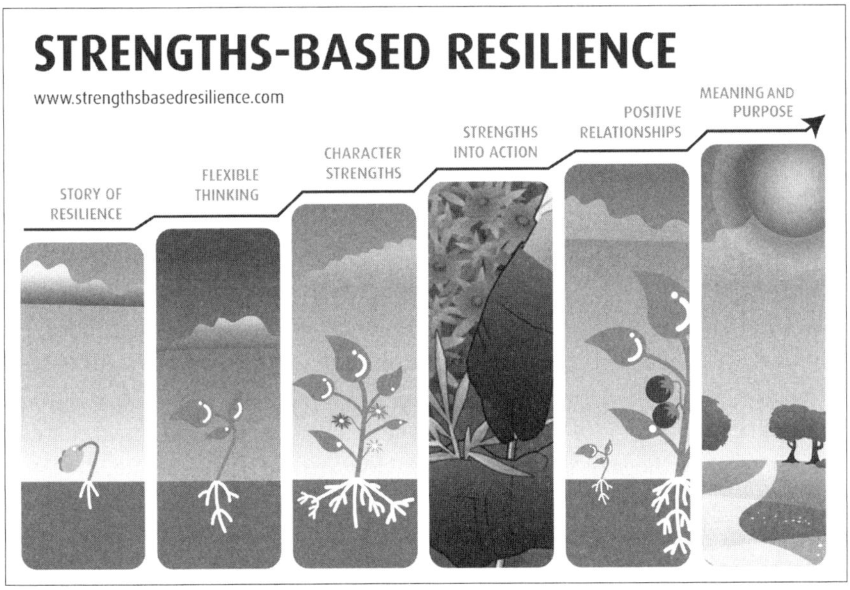

Let participants know that the SBR program of 14 modules is structured around six major content areas, illustrated in the infographic above (also on p. 2 of the participant Workbook), that aim to teach participants concrete strategies to develop their strengths, abilities, and resources.

1. **Story of Resilience.** SBR kicks off with the activity in Module 1 in which participants recall and write a personal narrative centered on overcoming a challenge or a setback.
2. **Flexible Thinking.** In Modules 2, 3, and 4, participants explore their mindsets and learn cognitive skills which foster accurate and flexible thinking.
3. **Character Strengths.** Modules 5 and 6 invite participants to reflect on their character strengths and determine their top strengths.
4. **Strengths into Action.** Modules 7, 8, 9, and 10 provide participants with insights and strategies to translate their character strengths into concrete actions to solve problems, overcome negative experiences, and cultivate positive experiences.
5. **Positive Relationships.** Modules 11 and 12 cultivate skills to foster positive relationships and communication.
6. **Purpose & Meaning.** Modules 13 and 14 explore altruism, purpose, and meaning, inviting participants to envision a future in which they contribute to something larger than themselves.

In addition to these 14 modules, the program has two regular practices that we suggest you describe after discussing the benefits of participation, experiential learning, and ground rules.

Benefits of Participation

SBR was created to enhance people's resilience and well-being. SBR is designed to help counter the mind's negativity bias; that is, our human tendency to attend to negatives (e.g., weaknesses, failures, criticisms, conflicts, and threats) much more than positives (e.g., strengths, triumphs, compliments, solutions, and resources). SBR teaches several specific skills that are designed to help participants to (1) attend to their life experiences in a more balanced way, thus increasing their understanding and appreciation of their lives; (2) understand challenges more fully and think more flexibly about them; (3) use positive qualities, strengths, and experiences to manage difficult experiences and setbacks; and (4) cultivate positive experiences, including greater connection, meaning, and joy.

Experiential Learning

Prepare participants for the experiential nature of SBR sessions. Set the expectation that they will be invited and encouraged to share their ideas and experiences. This program works best when everyone participates.

Provide an overview of how each module will unfold. For example, after learning about key concepts and research findings in the segment called Core Concepts in each module, they will watch one or more videos and be invited to participate in a discussion with group members. (Please note that this section differs a bit between the Manual and Workbook, as the facilitators are provided with more references to the literature.) This is followed by at least one in-session practice activity. After debriefing the practice, they will learn about specific ways this practice can be applied in everyday life and where they can learn more through additional readings, websites, and multimedia resources. See Chapter 4 (p. 56) for a sample script that encourages particpants to practice outside of the sessions.

Participant Goals

Now that participants are prepared for experiential learning, ask them to think about and share their goals with the group. Goals help participants focus on what matters most to them and sustain their motivation throughout the program. Sharing their goals with the group can inspire others who may be uncertain of what they want to accomplish.

Ask participants if they have participated in similar programs or engaged in similar practices. Invite them to share what they hope to gain from attending the program.

Confidentiality and Privacy

Inform participants of expectations regarding their access to other participants' private and confidential information. Request that they treat the personal information of others as they would like their personal information to be treated. Ask them to maintain confidentiality regarding events and experiences within the group's shared space. Differentiate between the insights from the sessions or modules which are shareable, versus the personal details which must remain confidential. See Chapter 4 (p. 55) for a sample script addressing the importance of respecting privacy and confidentiality.

Carefully go through possible limits to confidentiality and your legal and ethical obligations (according to your regional jurisdiction) regarding disclosing personal information to ensure the safety of all those involved.

Emphasize to participants that they are in charge of what they share in the group. Although participation is highly valued, participants are in control of what they decide to share with others. It may help to let participants know that it is natural in a new group to feel hesitant about sharing and that, as the group members continue to meet and get to know each other, they will likely feel more comfortable sharing and discussing their experiences with others. See Chapter 4 (p. 56) for a sample script for inviting respect for each particpant's level of participation.

Establishing the Ground Rules

To maximize the benefits of the group's collective efforts, set the ground rules. This will ensure your and others' safety and foster a welcoming, open, and authentic environment. In this pre-session, facilitators share ground rules consistent with the institution or agency running the SBR program, such as a school, college, university, community health, or mental health setting.

The following are essential topics to cover in your ground rules:

a. **Attendance:** Is there a minimum number of sessions participants are expected to attend?
b. **Joining or leaving a session:** How late can one join a session in progress or how early can one leave if needed?

c. **Dropping out of the program:** What constitutes dropping out of the program, e.g., missing a specific number of sessions continuously or in aggregate? What are the consequences of dropping out, if any? For example, some classes or schools may offer SBR programs as a part of the curriculum with attendance requirements, or attendance could be part of a certificate programming requirement. Likewise, you may state guidelines for when participants face exceptional circumstances beyond their control.
d. **Safeguarding privacy:** What are the expectations regarding safeguarding personal information and managing appropriate boundaries, including when group members share other social or professional activities or roles (e.g., two group members also share a class or a club membership)?
e. **Social media engagement:** Are there expectations regarding interaction on social media or in a shared virtual space with other participants? Examples include commenting about or sharing SBR material on discussion boards, email threads, and social media (e.g., WhatsApp, Facebook, Instagram, Twitter/X, LinkedIn). Be clear about guidelines for recording sessions, i.e., participants can only record sessions (for their personal use only) if they have an accommodation for assistive technology to support their learning and they must delete recordings at the conclusion of the program.
f. **Respect and dignity:** How will you create an open and supportive atmosphere for dialogue? Discuss that differences and disagreements are part of any group process. Underscore the importance of creating and maintaining a respectful group environment which enables every group member to participate, irrespective of their political or religious beliefs and practices. Request that participants treat each other with respect, be supportive of each other, create space for all voices, and approach differences and disagreements with openness, curiosity, and generosity.

After covering the ground rules above, facilitators are encouraged to invite participants to ask questions and share their ideas for additional ground rules. Encourage participants to think about rules to help the group function smoothly and foster an atmosphere of respect, openness, and authenticity.

Downloadable Materials

Inform the participants that there are downloadable materials available for purchasers of the Workbook, and these are highlighted with a download symbol in the modules. They will find details on how to access these in the relevant modules and in the section Notes on Supplementary Materials on p. 171 in the Workbook.

Regular Practices

In addition to the 14 distinct modules that introduce at least one new practice each week, there are two regular practices done weekly: mindfulness and relaxation, and the gratitude journal. Participants need to be aware of these regular practices in advance of the first module. Allow a good half hour in the orientation session to review the core concepts of these practices, to illustrate them through a multi-media resource, and to engage the particpants in discussion and practice. These regular practices help participants consolidate mindfulness and relaxation skills and focus on genuine positives in everyday life.

Inform participants that each program session begins and ends with a brief (3–5 minutes) mindfulness and relaxation practice. The five mindfulness and relaxation practices are rotated throughout the program. See Chapter 4 (p. 57) for a sample script for introducing the regular mindfulness and relaxation practices.

Inform participants that they will be asked to keep a gratitude journal throughout the program. This journal is designed to counter the mind's tendency to attend selectively to negatives while minimizing or ignoring positives. In the gratitude journal practice, participants are encouraged throughout SBR to note three positive experiences every day and write about them in the printable worksheet or a journal. Participants are encouraged to notice a wide range of positive experiences (big or small, strong or subtle, fleeting or lasting). Participants record these positive events, and they are encouraged to share them with the group, if they feel comfortable.

Introduce mindfulness and relaxation and the gratitude journal using the material covered in the next two chapters of this Manual: Mindfulness and Relaxation (pp. 67–90) and Gratitude Journal (pp. 91–99). The Workbook details these two practices in Section I: Regular Practice 1: Mindfulness and Relaxation (pp. 7–25) and Regular Practice 2: Gratitude Journal (pp. 27–31).

Note that the practices from these chapters are intended to be introduced gradually throughout the program, and the main goal of this presession is to introduce these regular practices to participants. The content covered in these chapters does not need to be fully covered in this session (or in any single session). Because these regular practices are part of every session, spread this material throughout multiple sessions. Below are brief pointers to introduce this material in the initial presession meeting.

- Cover the core concepts of mindfulness and relaxation, including playing a selection from the illustrations/videos, facilitating a discussion, and briefly describing the five relaxation exercises (see Regular Practice 1: Mindfulness and Relaxation for information and instructions).
- Lead participants through the first mindfulness and relaxation practice: Stretch and Relax, and then complete the reflection and discussion of that practice. If time permits, end the practice by discussing some of the everyday applications.
- Introduce the gratitude journal, covering core concepts, playing a selection from the illustrations/videos and facilitating a discussion (see Regular Practice 2: Gratitude Journal for information and instructions).
- Introduce the gratitude journal with the help of the workbook sample (Workbook, p. 30.) and instruct participants to start their gratitude journal entries in the coming week. Let participants know that in each meeting, you will invite them to share some of the experiences they wrote about. However, the journal is for their personal use. It will not be collected, and they will not be required to share any particular entry.

Closing the Session

Close the orientation session by reminding participants that resilience is not a trait or quality that we either possess or not. Instead, resilience is a process that unfolds in degrees and requires ongoing effort. It is a process that can be enhanced through life experiences and through learning skills.

It is important that facilitators introduce the program as one based on a unifying framework of hope and optimism. Hope can be a powerful catalyst for behavior change. Participants will learn that cultivating positive emotions and using strengths can enhance their flexible thinking and creative problem-solving skills. SBR is based on the premise that enhancing positives expands participants' array of options in everyday life. Diverse options build stronger and deeper coping mechanisms to manage challenges and stressors. This, in turn, builds resilience.

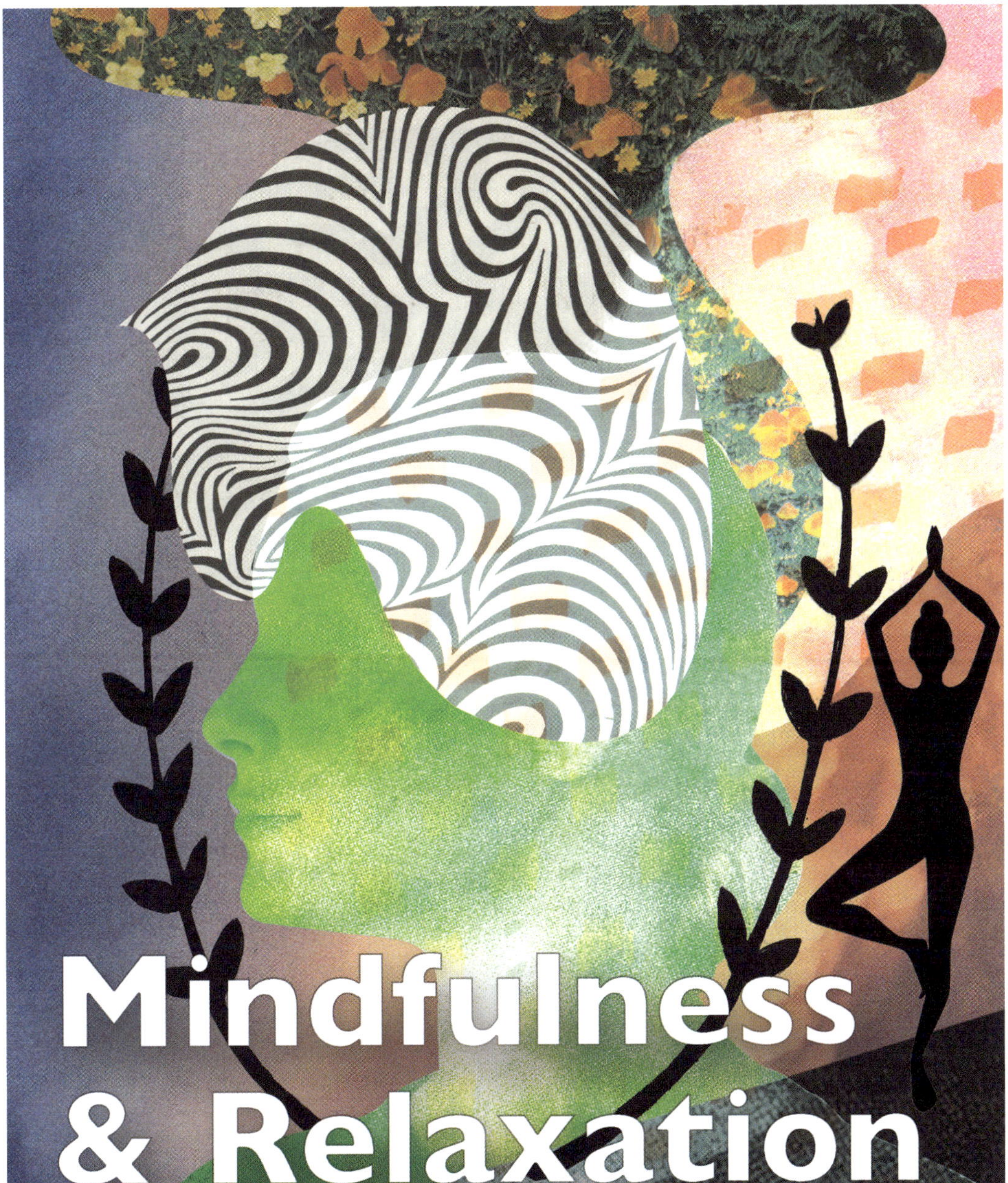
Mindfulness
& Relaxation

Regular Practice 1: Mindfulness and Relaxation

Mindfulness helps us to maintain moment-to-moment awareness of our thoughts, feelings, physical sensations, and our self in the context of our surroundings. Mindfulness enables us to explore how we respond to everyday stressors and challenges. Mindfulness, however, requires regular practice. Each module of the SBR program begins and ends with a brief mindfulness and relaxation practice.

Learning Outcomes for Mindfulness and Relaxation

By starting and ending each session with one of the five mindfulness and relaxation exercises, participants will:

- Increase their awareness of character strengths through specific mindfulness and relaxation exercises
- Increase awareness of their feelings, thoughts, and reactions
- Become more attentive to strengths such as self-regulation, savoring, and personal intelligence
- Incorporate mindfulness and relaxation techniques in their daily life

Core Concepts of Mindfulness and Relaxation

Many of the themes here are also presented in the Core Concepts section of the Workbook (p. 7):

- Mindfulness is a process of regulating attention to explore the quality of one's experiences. Mindfulness entails describing, observing, acting with awareness, and being nonjudging and non-reacting (Baer et al., 2006). These facets of mindfulness help us to make sense of our entangled negative emotions and thoughts. The goal is to widen our perspective to understand and respond to stressors and challenges more adaptively.
- Mindfulness and positive psychology share a common goal – cultivating optimal human functioning (Baer & Lykins, 2011), although both approach this goal in different ways. In mindfulness, the approach is sitting quietly, with closed eyes or with a softened gaze; directing one's attention to the present moment; being aware of sensations, emotions, and thoughts and how one is attached to them. The goal is to develop an inner capacity to enhance our ability to be nonjudgmental and nonreactive to experiences. Positive psychology interventions, on the other hand, involve structured behavioral exercises, such as translating strengths into concrete actions, writing gratitude letters, and undertaking meaningful altruistic actions for others. Mindfulness can help to inform and guide these actions.
- Mindfulness increases our awareness of our thoughts, emotions, and reactions to experiences. Some specific events, experiences, and interactions stick with us. Whenever we think of them, emotions spring up and leave us feeling sad, angry, or unsure. Sometimes we act on these feelings without much awareness. Mindfulness is being aware of this whole process by

observing the flow of our thoughts and emotions, learning about them without judging them or without acting upon them immediately. Understanding this process can help us respond in ways that are more thoughtful and which better reflect our deepest values. The key to this process, however, is creating a psychological space between our self and our thoughts and emotions. This space helps us to develop cognitive flexibility (Gockel, 2010).

- Mindfulness is maintaining moment-by-moment awareness of our thoughts, feelings, bodily sensations, and the surrounding environment without judgment or with less judgment (Kabat-Zinn, 1994). Mindfulness allows us to accept that everything changes. Mindfulness-based interventions (MBIs) in schools may boost resilience (Kuyken et al., 2013); reduce symptoms of anxiety, depression, and physical discomfort (Ding et al., 2023; Linardon et al., 2014); improve sleep (Biegel et al., 2009); decrease levels of impulsivity and aggression (Fuente et al., 2018); reduce mind wandering and improve the ability to ignore distracting and irrelevant stimuli (Sanger & Dorjee, 2016). Research indicates that MBIs can enhance mindfulness and emotional competence, and reduce feelings of depression, anxiety, and stress (Luong et al., 2019).
- Mindfulness also helps us develop awareness of our actions and reactions in specific situations, especially those that bother us. We also learn how our actions impact others. Developing awareness without judgment helps us to be receptive to different perspectives. For example, being mindful about a negative interaction with a friend can help one see the wider perspective. Perhaps the negative interaction was not caused by something you did. Instead, it could be that your friend is upset about something completely unrelated to you. By being mindful, we break down a complex experience into its parts. Mindfulness can strengthen our openness, self-regulation, and social intelligence.

The Role of Mindfulness in SBR

One may think that facilitating mindfulness practices within a strengths-based practice requires specialized training, regular personal practice, and expertise. While prior training in mindfulness may be beneficial, our SBR program offers easy-to-follow, step-by-step instructions to facilitate five brief mindfulness and relaxation practices. In facilitating these exercises, practitioners can keep in mind the following five considerations:

1. **Mindfulness facilitates awareness of character strengths.** Mindfulness and character strengths are closely related. Mindfulness can be a process that directs and supports one's strengths (Niemiec et al., 2012; Niemiec, 2024). It does so when we acknowledge our strengths and those of others, clearly, without biases. The inherent aspects of mindfulness such as self-observation, acceptance, nonjudgment, and detached coping (Sugiura & Sugiura, 2015) can sharpen character strengths (Table 3). Furthermore, integration of character strengths into mindfulness can inform us about the over- and underuse of strengths, and guide us toward a balanced use of our strengths. That said, mindfulness itself is the practice of self-regulation. Almost everyone struggles from time to time to self-regulate to establish a mindfulness practice. Some individuals struggle to manage constant distractions and don't feel they are making sufficient and discernable progress. Progress in mindfulness is often slow and requires sustained effort (Fuente et al., 2018). As a self-regulation process (of increasing attention and observing emotional reactions and attachment patterns),

Table 3. SBR mindfulness and relaxation practices and their relevance to specific character strengths

	Mindfulness and relaxation practice	Relevant modules	Relevant strengths
1	Stretch & Relax	Resilience, Cognitive Accuracy, Cognitive Flexiblity, Fixed & Growth Mindsets	Courage, persistence, open-mindedness, prudence
2	Breathe	Slowness & Savoring	Love of learning, perspective
3	Take a Mindful Minute	Grudge & Gratitude	Curiosity, creativity
4	Use Positive Imagery	Character Strengths, Slowness & Savoring	Appreciation of beauty
5	Visualize Lovingkindness	Positive Relationships	Kindness, love, social intelligence

mindfulness may not be an easy process. Many individuals start a mindfulness practice enthusiastically for a short while but quit for several reasons, including their mind wandering too often, forgetting to practice, or not having sufficient time. Character strengths can offer everyday opportunities to be mindful.

Consider the following illustrations of specific strengths which can be enriched through mindfulness:

- **Appreciation of beauty and excellence**: Being in awe of the beauty in nature, or excellence in arts, sciences, or any human endeavor
- **Creativity**: Letting the mind explore novel and adaptive ways of solving a problem or doing things differently
- **Curiosity**: Exploring aspects of a situation not considered before
- **Gratitude**: Being aware of, and thankful for, the good actions of others
- **Forgiveness**: Consciously abandoning the desire to exact revenge, and letting go of the hurt
- **Kindness**: Feeling love, care, and compassion for self and others
- **Perspective**: Understanding the nature of things, and attending to the most important aspects

Strengths can reinforce our mindfulness. Mindfulness, in turn, can help us to integrate our outer and inner worlds. Almost all psychological programs deal with thinking and feeling – two key parts of our inner world. Our inner world is surrounded and influenced by the outer world: family, friends, colleagues, neighborhoods, cities, states, countries, culture, climate, and technology. Mindfulness is a way to integrate both worlds.

2. **Mindfulness is an evidence-based practice, not a religion.** Mindfulness and relaxation exercises, as presented in SBR, have been adapted from secular evidence-based interventions that have used mindfulness and relaxation skills, either standing alone, such as in lovingkindness meditation (LKM; Salzberg, 1995), mindfulness-based stress reduction (MBSR; Irving et al., 2009; Kabat-Zinn, 2005; Kabat-Zinn et al., 1992), or in conjunction with other established treatments (e.g., dialectical behavior therapy; Linehan, 1993).

3. **Mindfulness and relaxation supplement SBR practices.** In the SBR modules, the brief mindfulness and relaxation exercises are meant to supplement the positive psychology-based interventions. They are not meant to be the primary interventions or to substitute for more comprehensive mindfulness-based interventions such as MBSR or LKM. Furthermore, these exercises are not intended to eliminate negative feelings or experiences, nor are the mindfulness and relaxation exercises alone likely to foster a state of well-being and resilience. Instead, the goal is to facilitate a state of relaxed attention among participants, so they are better prepared to participate in the positive psychology-based interventions in SBR.
4. **Mindfulness broadens attention.** Jon Kabat-Zinn and colleagues (1992, p. 942) hypothesized that "the insight that one is not one's thoughts means that one has a potential range of responses to a given thought if one is able to identify it as such." This increased range of options is associated with a feeling of control. Exploring potential ranges of responses systematically through cognitive behavioral therapy (CBT) focused meditation, Sugiura and Sugiura (2015) outlined five beneficial changes: (1) refraining from catastrophic thinking, (2) logical objectivity, (3) self-observation, (4) acceptance, and (5) detached coping style. SBR exercises aim to broaden the range of options, through promoting flexible thinking and by systematically cultivating positive emotions. Positive emotions make one calm but also expand the scope of attention and cognition.
5. **Mindfulness can enhance motivation.** Like any other intervention, the effectiveness of SBR depends on the motivation of participants. Knowledge of the many benefits of relaxation and mindfulness can increase motivation. For example, by enhancing moment-by-moment awareness, mindfulness can help us to understand which specific emotions bother us. This awareness is nonjudgmental and less reactive. Connecting these benefits with the participants' current stressors can help to enhance their motivation. Furthermore, a deliberate focus on breathing, thoughts, sensations, and specific experiences, in conjunction with their strengths, can help participants establish a connection between mindfulness and the potential for understanding and solving their problems.

Illustrations of Mindfulness and Relaxation

Body Scan Exercise
https://youtu.be/15q-N-_kkrU?si=bGhtUqRI16JY7For
(Duration: 29:02 minutes)
Jon Kabat-Zinn, a distinguished meditation practitioner and researcher, guides you through a nearly half-hour-long comprehensive body scan.

Sharon Salzberg Lovingkindness Meditation
https://www.youtube.com/watch?v=e-TeW9CI0bc
(Duration: 10 minutes)
Sharon Salzberg, a distinguished author and teacher of Buddhist meditation practices, walks you through *lovingkindness meditation.*

Matthieu Ricard Leads a Group Meditation
https://youtu.be/unX4FQqM6vI
(Duration: 39:23 minutes)
Matthieu Ricard, a cellular geneticist who devoted decades to meditation, introduces the concept and practice of meditation.

Reflection and Discussion

Invite participants to complete the Reflection and Discussion section of their Workbook (p. 9) regarding the video(s) they have watched. Discuss the questions:

What are the key messages in the video(s) you just watched?
How might these concepts be relevant in your life?

General Guidelines for Mindfulness and Relaxation Practice

Mindfulness and relaxation can be developed, but they require regular practice. The following pages provide sample scripts and instructions for five practices that you can facilitate in this program (see the Workbook, p. 10–24).

In addition to the mindfulness and relaxation exercises in this module, we have also provided a number of related resources at the end of this module (pp. 89–90). These illustrations offer participants a wider array of options to consolidate their practice. These may be helpful as examples, as you prepare to lead the participants in the mindfulness and relaxation activities. You can share similar online illustrations. We also recommend sharing additional and relevant resources which may help adolescents and young adults to practice together. In facilitating these practices, we recommend the following general guidelines:

- These exercises are designed to be done in a regular seated position. For the initial breathing and relaxation exercise, participants are welcome to gently and slowly close their eyes or select a specific spot nearby to focus on, preferably looking downwards.
- Begin and end each session of the program with one of the five mindfulness and relaxation exercises in this chapter. You may shorten them based on the needs of your participants.
- Use a calm voice, relaxed pace, and if appropriate and available, instrumental background music.
- If you are reading the script, make sure to allow time for participants to breathe and reflect on their breathing.

The five practices that follow can be used in different combinations. It is good to introduce all five practices first and then rotate them, and/or repeat ones that cater better to the group's needs.

Before the first practice, it might help to let participants know that you will be introducing five different practices, which aim to equip participants with a variety of ways to learn applicable skills that they can incorporate into their daily lives. The more frequently participants use them, the more comfortable and beneficial the practices will be for them. Make sure that the space where you will practice SBR skills is quiet, comfortable, and consistent. This will help participants to focus on the subtle aspects of the practice. Invite participants to practice at their level of comfort.

The following five mindfulness and relaxation exercises are kept deliberately simple and easy so that participants can apply them in a variety of ways without requiring any specific apparatus or a significant amount of time.

Practice 1: Stretch and Relax

The Stretch and Relax practice is adapted from two resources:

- *Relaxation: A Comprehensive Manual for Adults, Children and Children With Special Needs* by R. J. Cautela & J. Gorden, 1978, Research Press.
- *Joints and Glands Exercises: As Taught by Sri Swami Rama of the Himalayas*, by R. M. Ballentine, ed., 1977, Himalayan Institute Press.

Invite participants to sit in the *relaxation position* demonstrated below and practice the stretches on the following pages. The full set of stretching exercises takes about 10 minutes. The face massage and remaining postures can be particularly helpful at the end or at times during the middle of the module. For example, the first four postures and face massage can help participants to relax before they participate in the Grudge Exercise in Module 8. Ending the Grudge and Gratitude module with some of the remaining postures (shoulders, arms, stomach, legs) can be helpful for relieving any residual negative emotions.

The Relaxation Position

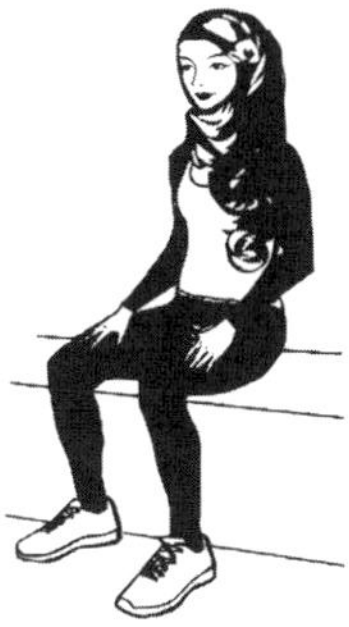

1. Sit in a comfortable position, with your head, neck, and chest aligned. Relax your shoulders.
2. Sit with your back flat against the back of the chair.
3. Uncross your legs and rest your feet flat on the floor.
4. Let your hands rest on your thighs or kneecaps.

Head

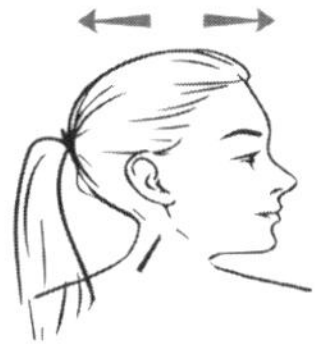

1. Breathe in, move your head slowly to the right.
2. Pause and breathe out, bring your head back to center.
3. Repeat on the left side.
4. Relax your neck, head, and shoulders.

Ear

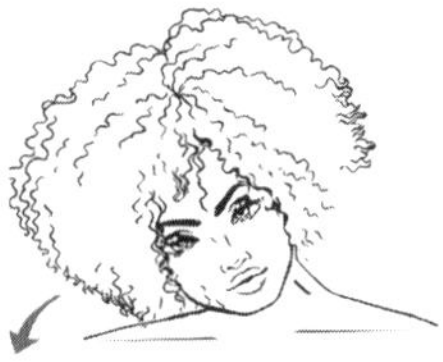

1. Breathe in and slowly bring your ear to your right shoulder, keeping your shoulder down. Feel the stretch as you slowly breathe out.
2. Take one or two additional relaxed breaths in and out.
3. On your final inhalation, bring your head back to center. Slowly exhale.
4. Repeat on the left side.

Neck

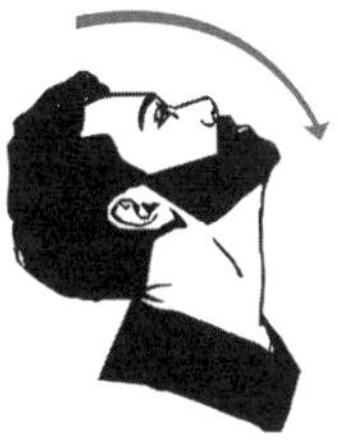

1. Align your head, neck, and chest in a relaxed straight line, keeping your shoulders steady and relaxed.
2. Breathe in, lift your chin up, and slowly tilt your head back.
3. Lift your jaw up, exhale, and feel the stretch. With your jaw extended, take one or two additional relaxed breaths in and out.
4. On your final inhalation, gently bring your head forward, and as you exhale, touch your chin to your chest. With your chin to chest, take one or two additional breaths in and out. Feel the stretch in the muscles at the back of your neck.
5. On your final exhale, bring your head back to a neutral position.

Face Massage

Eyes

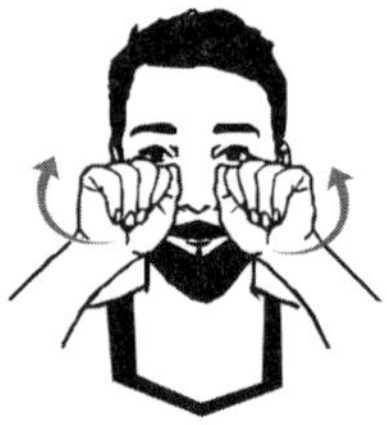

1. Make loose fists and place them under your eye sockets fingers facing forward. Press your fists gently against the bone below your eye sockets, while moving your knuckles across your cheek bones toward your temples.
2. Continue these gentle circular motions against the bony parts of your face, forehead, eyes, cheeks, and mouth, smoothing your muscles and skin.

Face and Forehead Massage

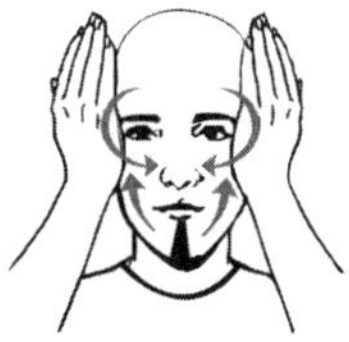

1. Place the lower part of your palms on your cheeks and make circular motions with your palms from cheeks to temple.
2. From your temple, continue to move your palms in a circular motion as you move from your temple to forehead, back to temple, and down to jaw.

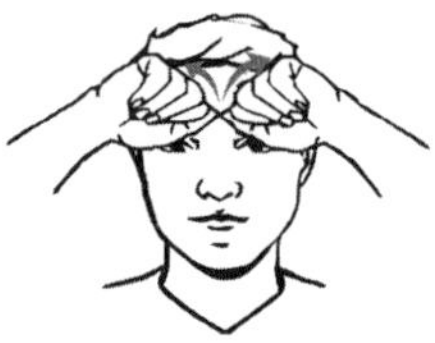

1. Align your head, neck, and chest in a relaxed straight line, keeping your shoulders steady and relaxed.
2. Make loose fists with both of your hands, placing your thumbs between your two eyebrows on your forehead.
3. Massage the forehead with your thumbs using a stroking movement up and out.
4. Follow the bony parts of your face, around the eyes, and moving out toward the temples.

Shoulder Wings

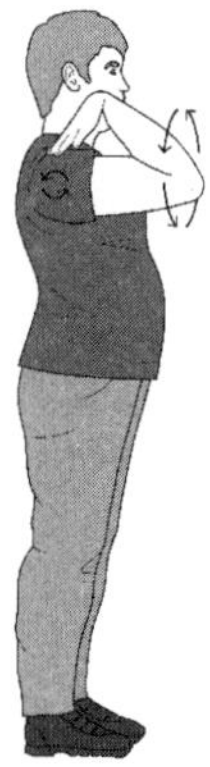

1. As you inhale, fold back your arms, placing your hands on your shoulders.
2. As you exhale, extend the elbows out to the front and bring them together.
3. Move your elbows slowly in a clockwise circular direction, inhaling on the top of the circle and exhaling on the bottom. Make sure to bring your elbows up high and then back with your shoulder blades together and chest extended.
4. Continue the clockwise circular motion a couple of times, repeating an equal number of motions counterclockwise.

Arms

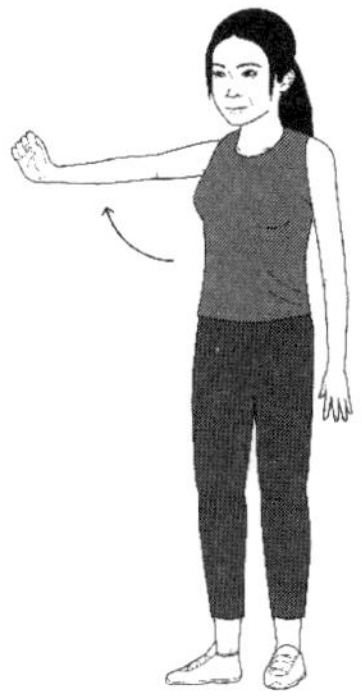

1. As you inhale, stretch out one of your arms in front of you, make a fist, and flex your whole arm.
2. Notice where it feels tense (bicep, forearm, back of arm, wrist, hand, and fingers.)
3. As you exhale, gradually relax your arm, bend it at the elbow, and bring it back to rest at your side.
4. Repeat with the other arm.

Back

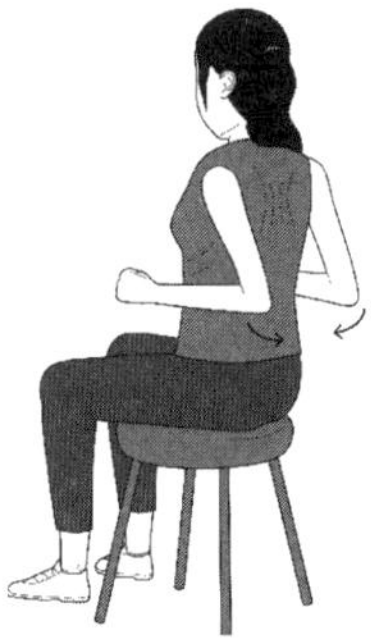

1. Sit up straight, imagining your back against a chair. As you inhale, bring your elbows up. Relax your shoulders. As you exhale, try to get your elbows to touch behind your back.
2. Notice where you feel most tense.
3. Release your arms slowly and place them in a resting position. Repeat two to three times.

Chest

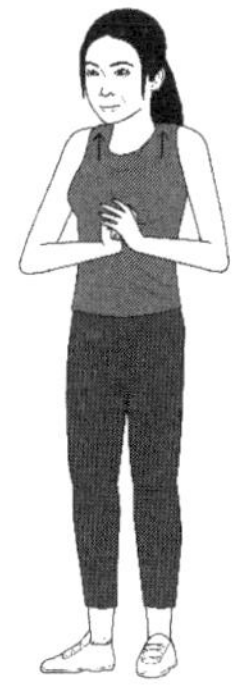

1. As you inhale, raise your shoulders to your ears. Notice the tension.
2. As you exhale, slowly relax your shoulders and chest. Notice how it feels to be relaxed.
3. Feel your heart beating and your lungs expanding with each breath. Repeat two to three times.

Stomach

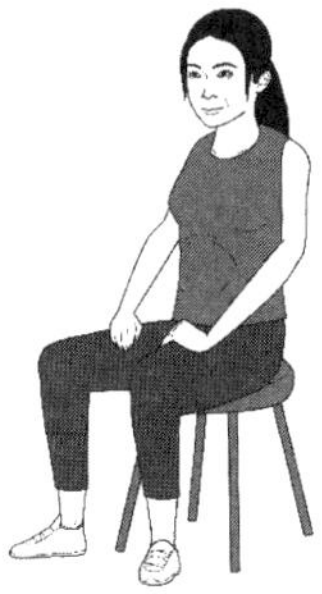

1. Breathe in and tighten your stomach muscles, as tightly as you can. Notice where it feels tense.
2. As you exhale, gradually relax your stomach to its natural position.
3. Notice how it feels to have those muscles loose and relaxed. Repeat two to three times.

Legs

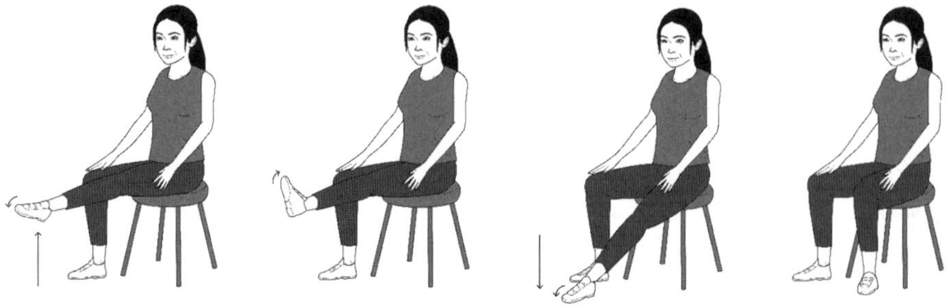

1. Lift your left leg about half a foot from the floor. As you inhale, point your toes away from you. Notice where it feels tense: calf muscles, heel, arch.
2. As you exhale, flex your foot toward you and feel the stretch. Notice where it feels tense: calf muscles, heel, arch.
3. Relax and lower your foot slowly until it rests flat on the floor.
4. Next, bend your knees, hold the posture tight and then relax.
5. Repeat with the other leg.

Below the Waist

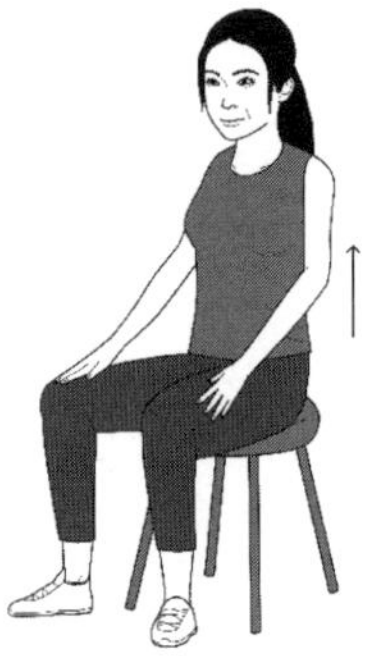

1. Move your concentration to below the waist. On your inhalation, tighten the muscles in your thighs and buttocks, and hold.
2. You may feel slightly elevated on your seat, from the waist up. Notice where you feel particularly tense.
3. As you exhale, release the tension. Relax your muscles.

Breathing Exercise

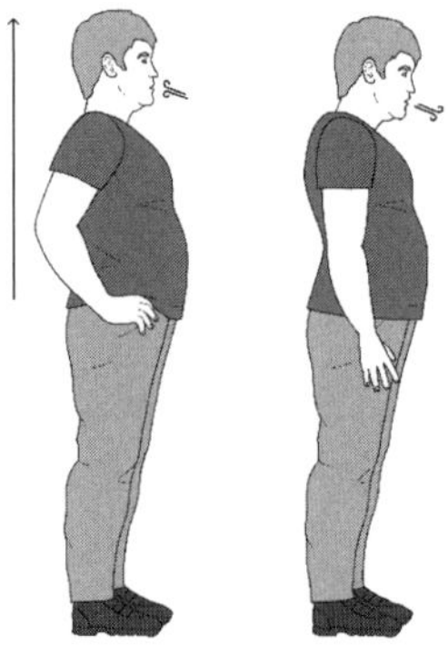

1. Straighten your spine, imagining a string pulling you from your tailbone to the top of your head.
2. Inhale, then hold, and breathe out slowly.
3. As you exhale, feel as if the whole of your body is breathing.
4. Take 10 breaths; inhaling and exhaling, your abdomen expanding with each inhalation and contracting with each exhalation.

Practice Debrief

The first time you lead the group through this activity, invite group members to reflect on and share their experiences. They can complete the practice debrief questions in their Workbook (p. 15):

How was your experience of stretching and then relaxing different muscles? What was it like to stretch and relax different areas of your body? What did you notice?

In your daily life, when and where can you use these practices? How might they be helpful? Note that it can be helpful to stretch and relax specific areas when we notice tension and do not have time to engage in a full body relaxation.

While stretching and relaxing various parts of your body, which exercise did you find most helpful?

Practice 2: Breathe

Before starting this practice, inform participants that they will be participating in a simple breathing exercise (see Workbook, p. 16). Offer participants options to participate at their own level of comfort. Breathing can be improved. A recent meta-analysis has demonstrated that breathwork interventions are associated with lower levels of stress and improve symptoms of depression and anxiety (Fincham et al., 2023).

Facilitate the practice session with the help of the following script:

Sit in a relaxed and comfortable position. Align your head, neck and chest. Feel your back touch the back of the chair.

Bring your shoulders back and relax them away from your ears.

Your hands can rest softly on your kneecaps or wherever you feel comfortable.

Let your eyelids slowly and gently fall, just as the curtain in a theater falls. If you prefer, look at the floor a few feet ahead and gently soften your gaze.

Take a deep breath through your nose, hold it for a few seconds, then exhale slowly and gently.

Repeat two more times, each time trying to deepen the breath, encouraging participants as they breathe in and breathe out, to try to relax their whole body from head to toe.

Encourage the breath to flow without any pauses.

Next, instruct participants to shape their breath; a good breath has three qualities:
1. smooth
2. even (equal duration for inhalation and exhalation)
3. deep

Instruct participants to relax their effort to breathe and let the breath flow naturally, as if their whole body is breathing. Instruct them to focus their attention on the breath as it enters and exits through their nostrils. Ask them to take 10 breaths that are smooth, even, and deep. Once they are done, they can gently open their eyes.

Practice Debrief

The first time you lead the group through this activity, invite group members to reflect on and share their experiences and to complete this Practice Debrief section in their Workbook (p. 16). Some questions you might ask include:

How did you experience this breathing exercise? What was it like to practice attending to your breath? What did you notice?

After completing the breathing exercise, what differences did you feel in your mood (emotions), body, or overall?

In your daily life, when and where can you use this practice? How might it be helpful?

Practice 3: Take a Mindful Minute

In our busy and distracted lives, it may be difficult for some individuals to devote a stretch of time to mindfulness. This practice allows participants to create segments of mindfulness, each lasting only 1 minute (see Workbook, p. 18). Facilitators can use the following script to guide participants through a mindful minute:

Sit in a comfortable position with your hands on your kneecaps. Align your head, neck and chest. Relax your shoulders. Your feet should be touching or resting flat on the floor.

Bring your attention to your breath. Notice how it enters your body and how it leaves your body. Notice that as you inhale, your chest expands. As you exhale, it contracts.

As you inhale, gently bring your breath deep into your belly. Notice your abdomen expanding.

As you exhale, release your breath slowly. Notice your abdomen contracting.

Continue repeating this breathing cycle, expanding your chest and abdomen as you inhale and contracting them as you exhale.

Try to make each inhalation and exhalation last for 10 seconds. Then start over after each count.

Don't worry about doing anything else. To keep your attention focused, count very quietly or in your head. If your attention wanders and you lose count, start again.

When 1 minute is up, I will ring this bell.

Practice Debrief

The first time you lead the group through this activity, invite group members to reflect on and share their experiences and to complete this Practice Debrief section in their Workbook (p. 18). Some questions you might ask include:

How did you experience the mindful minute? What was it like to practice mindfulness for a minute? What did you notice?

After completing the mindful minute, what differences did you feel in your mood (emotions), body, or overall?

In your daily life, when and where can you use this practice? How might it be helpful?

Practice 4: Use Positive Imagery

Guided meditations that use positive imagery can be beneficial in helping participants gain access to their deeper and relaxed selves (see Workbook, p. 20). Positive imagery involves comprehensive involvement of most, if not all of the senses. The practice is built on the image of a positive scene, often of natural beauty, and is based on guided imagery and visualization techniques which have been shown to relieve stress (Lang, 1979; Wilson et al., 2018). The facilitator guides participants through the practice at a leisurely pace. The earlier breathing practice helps participants relax more easily.

Facilitators can use the following script.

Sit comfortably. Bring your back toward the back of your chair.

Sit straight, with your head, neck, and trunk in a straight line – not too rigid, not too soft. Your shoulders should be relaxed, gracefully supporting your head and neck.

With feet flat on the floor, your hands can rest close to your kneecaps. If you feel comfortable doing so, close your eyes. Or look at the floor a few feet ahead, with eyes lowered, and soften your gaze. Inhale and exhale deeply as you complete this visualization.

Imagine a place in your mind, a place where you feel very comfortable. It could be outdoors or indoors. It is a place where you feel calm and peaceful. Take a few deep breaths in and out as you imagine you are in this place.

What does it look like? What objects do you see? Do you hear anything? Can you touch anything? How does it feel? What is the temperature of this place?

Make it comfortable. It is your place, your special spot. If it is indoors, what object can you sit or lie on to relax? If it is outside, feel the ground with your feet, touch something or smell something natural. Relax here. Do what makes you feel relaxed.

Take a few deep breaths, in and out.

In this imagined place, reach out and touch something. Are there pens, pencils, paints, or anything you want to pick up? Is there anything you want to draw, construct, touch, or handle? As you handle these materials, think of a small thing you can do. Select something that feels comfortable. Draw, construct, or paint – whatever feels natural to you. Take your time.

Now take time to savor your expression, your creation.

Enjoy the labor of your hands and of your head. Memorize the details. This is a place where you feel comfortable and can do something that expresses you. Gently prepare and plan to leave this place the same way you arrived.

As you slowly leave, reassure yourself that this is your place to be, your place to do something you like, a place where you can relax.

Practice Debrief

The first time you lead the group through this activity, invite group members to reflect on and share their experiences. Ask the participants to complete the Practice Debrief section in their Workbook (p. 21) and then use the questions to facilitate a discussion:

How did you experience the positive imagery activity? Were you able to imagine being in a comfortable place?

In your daily life, when and where can you use this practice? How might it be helpful?

If participants had trouble with this guided meditation, note that sometimes it can help to have a more specific guided meditation – for example, imagining lying on the beach or sitting in a forest by a stream. Participants may want to try out some of the many guided imagery recordings that are available. Note that many people find guided imagery meditation helpful when they are trying to relax after a stressful experience, to unwind at the end of the day, or to visualize an important upcoming event.

Practice 5: Visualize Lovingkindness

Adapted from Sharon Salzberg's book *Lovingkindness* (Salzberg, 1995), this practice recites specific words and phrases evoking a "boundless warm-hearted feeling." Salzberg describes this practice as compassionate awareness that opens our attention, making it more inclusive. Paying careful and focused attention to our thoughts, feelings, and actions helps us to understand how we treat our loved ones. The positive arc of the practice encourages us to become more loving, forgiving, and accepting of them. The meditation begins with one's self and extends the wish for well-being and happiness to all beings. It is recommended that you read the script a couple of times before using it with participants (see Workbook, p. 22).

You can use the following script to guide this meditation:

Sit comfortably. Bring your spine toward the back of your chair. Sit straight, with your head, neck and trunk in a straight line – not too rigid, not too soft. Your shoulders are relaxed, gracefully supporting your head and neck. With your feet flat on the floor, your hands can rest close to your kneecaps.

If you feel comfortable doing so, close your eyes.

Or focus the floor a few feet in front of you and soften your gaze. Listen to the voice prompts while visualizing.

Begin with the following phrases (adapted from Fronsdal, 2001):

The practice of lovingkindness meditation is usually done by silently repeating the following phrases that show kind wishes first for oneself, followed by kind wishes for others:
May I be happy. May I be well. May I be safe. May I be peaceful and at ease.

As you say these phrases, allow yourself to experience fully the intentions they express. Let feelings of love, kindness, openness, and acceptance embrace you. Let these feelings expand as you repeat these phrases. As you continue the meditation, direct this love and kindness toward yourself.

Lovingkindness meditation helps you to connect your noble intentions with the well-being of others. Continue to direct love and kindness to yourself.

Now, turn your attention to a friend or someone in your life who has deeply cared for you. Then slowly direct phrases of lovingkindness toward them:
May you be happy. May you be well. May you be safe. May you be peaceful and at ease.

As you repeat these phrases, experience fully their intention or heartfelt meaning. And, if any feelings of lovingkindness arise, connect the feelings with the phrases, so that the feelings may become stronger as you repeat the words.

You can also encourage the participants to continue the meditation, enlarging the circle by bringing to mind other friends, neighbors, acquaintances, strangers, and animals. They may also expand the circle to include people with whom they have difficulty.

Practice Debrief

The first time you lead the group through this activity, invite group members to reflect on and share their experiences and to complete this Practice Debrief section in their Workbook (p. 23). Some questions you might ask include:

The lovingkindness meditation aims to harness your attention, thoughts, feelings, and actions toward being kind. Were you able to experience this kindness during the practice? If so, what helped? If you struggled, what were the barriers?
How deeply were you able to feel kindness and compassion for yourself?
How deeply were you able to feel kindness and compassion for others during the practice? Did it change your mood after the practice?
If you could not or had difficulty visualizing a specific person, what made it difficult?

Learning and Cultural Fit

It is important to consider culturally relevant adaptations or refinements that might increase the effectiveness of these mindfulness and relaxation practices.

- Negative emotions such as anger, anxiety, or sadness often keep us stuck in unhealthy states, and stick with us, negatively impacting our emotional well-being. Nonjudgmental mindfulness offers us a relatively simple way to observe these negative emotions and try to untangle emotions, thoughts, and bodily sensations. However, negative emotions provide us with a signal regarding our inner emotional lives. At times, anger, especially when someone is being treated unfairly, can be a justified emotion. Loss of a relationship, an object of significance, or status can make one sad. Fear of the unknown can make one anxious. There are cultural ways to express emotions. Mindfulness should not be used to replace those cultural approaches.
- Mindfulness can help us understand that how we respond to situations (including how we judge, evaluate, and appraise things) is significantly influenced by our cultural background. For instance, people who grow up in cultures or families that emphasize interconnectedness may be more likely to blame themselves in challenging situations (Triandis, 2001). However, within similar cultural settings, experiences related to factors such as gender, age, sibling order, or financial status can lead individuals to handle responsibilities differently, with some possibly avoiding them altogether (Shearman & Dumlao, 2008).
- Most mindfulness practices encourage participants to observe their emotions and thoughts and to reflect upon their actions. This reflection can motivate one to change typical patterns of responding, potentially causing changes and even disruptions to the status quo. Be mindful that change can be difficult and create discomfort, at least initially.
- Relaxation and mindfulness are also about regulation of attention. They are about paying close attention to one's thoughts, emotions, and actions. However, if someone has underlying attentional deficit challenges, they may find it hard to engage in relaxation and mindfulness practices. Offer alternatives such as movement-based practices, practices divided into smaller chunks, or practices supplemented by additional props (e.g., music, artifacts, or customized equipment). That can help individuals to experience benefits of relaxation and mindfulness, according to their abilities.
- Mindfulness is about noticing our feelings, thoughts, and what we do without being hard on ourselves. However, the way we see and understand things is significantly influenced by our socio-cultural context. This means it's important to recognize that being completely nonjudgmental and detached might not always be achievable, or even something we should aim for. It's a reminder that our experiences and who we are can shape how we practice mindfulness.

Everyday Applications

Share with participants ways that mindfulness and relaxation practices can be applied in their daily lives.

- Mindfulness is about enhancing moment-by-moment awareness. With regular practice, it can help you to understand your emotions, especially ones that bother you or preoccupy your thoughts to the point you cannot detach yourself from them. Becoming aware of these bothersome emotions from a less judgmental, less reactive stance can help you understand your attachment to them and generate options to deal with them. SBR modules in the coming pages offer ways to cope with these emotions in a resilient manner.
- Mindfulness and relaxation can be incorporated in everyday life in several informal ways such as walking, sitting, and standing mindfully. By taking long, smooth, and deep breaths during these activities, you can discover a source of relaxation and build a natural buffer against stress. Of course, one may not be able to walk, sit, or stand mindfully all of the time. Nonetheless, the more mindfulness we can incorporate in these everyday activities, the more relaxed and the less stressed we become.
- Eating is one of our most pleasurable activities. However, we often develop mindless eating patterns. We eat to cope with sadness, boredom, or loneliness. We eat with eyes staring at a screen (e.g., a television, computer, tablet, mobile phone). When we are alone, we eat randomly without a schedule. Instead, practice eating mindfully, by slowing down, breathing between bites, and concentrating on the food's flavors, colors, and textures.
- Mindfulness can be incorporated into everyday life in many ways, such as:
  - Begin and/or end each day by spending a few minutes in mindful meditation, using your favorite techniques from visualization to controlled breathing.
  - In conversations, concentrate on listening attentively rather than on planning how you will respond.
  - Be mindful during at least one physical activity, such as walking, climbing up or down stairs, brushing your teeth, or cooking a meal.
  - Bring a lovingkindness orientation to someone who is not in your circle or you do not particularly like. Visualize wishing them well as sincerely as possible and reflect on the impact of this act on your mood.
  - Do at least one interpersonal activity more mindfully. For example, let someone complete their point, even though you think you have more accurate and updated information. Bring someone a cup of coffee or beverage of their choice. Accept the next telemarketing call politely, instead of hanging up.

References

Baer, R. A., & Lykins, E. L. B. (2011). Mindfulness and positive psychological functioning. In K. M. Sheldon, T. B. Kashdan, & M. F. Steger (Eds.) *Designing positive psychology: Taking stock and moving forward* (pp. 335–348). Oxford University Press. https://doi.org/10.1093/acprof:oso/9780195373585.003.0022

Baer, R. A., Smith, G. T., Hopkins, J., Krietemeyer, J., & Toney, L. (2006). Using self-report assessment methods to explore facets of mindfulness. *Assessment, 13,* 27–45. https://doi.org/10.1177/1073191105283504

Biegel, G. M., Brown, K. W., Shapiro, S. L., & Schubert, C. M. (2009). Mindfulness-based stress reduction for the treatment of adolescent psychiatric outpatients: A randomized clinical trial. *Journal of Consulting and Clinical Psychology, 77*(5), 855–866. https://doi.org/10.1037/a0016241

Ding, F., Wu, J., & Zhang, Y. (2023). Can mindfulness-based stress reduction relieve depressive symptoms? A systematic review and meta-analysis. *Journal of Pacific Rim Psychology, 17.* https://doi.org/10.1177/18344909221145814

Fincham, G. W., Strauss, C., & Cavanagh, K. (2023). Effect of breathwork on stress and mental health: A meta-analysis of randomised-controlled trials. *Scientific Reports, 13*(1), 1–14. https://doi.org/10.1038/s41598-022-27247-y

Fronsdal, G. (2001). *The issue at hand: Essays on buddhist mindfulness practice.* Shambala. https://www.insightmeditationcenter.org/books-articles/the-issue-at-hand/

Fuente, J., Mañas, I., Franco, C., Cangas, A. J., & Soriano, E. (2018). Differential effect of level of self-regulation and mindfulness training on coping strategies used by university participants. *International Journal of Environmental Research and Public Health, 15*(10), Article 2230. https://doi.org/10.3390/ijerph15102230

Gockel, A. (2010). The promise of mindfulness for clinical practice education. *Smith College Studies in Social Work, 80*, 248–268. https://doi.org/10.1080/00377311003784184

Irving, J. A., Dobkin, P. L., & Park, J. (2009). Cultivating mindfulness in healthcare professionals: A review of empirical studies of mindfulness-based stress reduction (MBSR). *Complementary Therapies in Clinical Practice, 15*, 61–66. https://doi.org/10.1016/j.ctcp.2009.01.002

Kabat-Zinn, J. (1994). *Wherever you go there you are: Mindfulness meditation in everyday life.* Hyperion.

Kabat-Zinn, J. (2005). *Full catastrophe living: Using the wisdom of your body and mind to face stress, pain, and illness* (15th anniversary ed.). Delta Trade Paperback/Bantam Dell.

Kabat-Zinn, J., Massion, A. O., Kristeller, J., Peterson, L. G., Fletcher, K. E., Pbert, L., Lenderking, W. R., & Santorelli, S. F. (1992). Effectiveness of a meditation-based stress reduction program in the treatment of anxiety disorders. *The American Journal of Psychiatry, 149*(7), 936–943. https://doi.org/10.1176/ajp.149.7.936

Kuyken, W., Weare, K., Ukoumunne, O. C., Vicary, R., Motton, N., Burnett, R., Cullen, C., Hennelly, S., & Huppert, F. (2013). Effectiveness of the mindfulness in schools programme: Non-randomised controlled feasibility study. *British Journal of Psychiatry, 203*(2), 126–131. https://doi.org/10.1192/bjp.bp.113.126649

Lang, P. J. (1979). A bio-informational theory of emotional imagery. *Psychophysiology, 16*, 495–512. https://doi.org/10.1111/j.1469-8986.1979.tb01511.x

Linardon, J., Messer, M., Goldberg, S. B., & Fuller-Tyszkiewicz, M. (2024). The efficacy of mindfulness apps on symptoms of depression and anxiety: An updated meta-analysis of randomized controlled trials. *Clinical Psychology Review, 107*, Article 102370. https://doi.org/10.1016/j.cpr.2023.102370.

Linehan, M. M. (1993). *Cognitive-behavioral treatment of borderline personality disorder.* Guilford Press.

Luong, M. T., Gouda, S., Bauer, J., & Schmidt, S. (2019). Exploring mindfulness benefits for participants and teachers in three German high schools. *Mindfulness, 10*(12), 2682–2702. https://doi.org/10.1007/s12671-019-01231-6

Niemiec, R. M. (2024). *Mindfulness and character strengths: A practical guide to MBSP* (2nd ed.). Hogrefe.

Niemiec, R. M., Rashid, T., & Spinella, M. (2012). Strong mindfulness. *Journal of Mental Health Counseling, 34*(3), 240–253. https://doi.org/10.17744/mehc.34.3.34p6328x2v204v21

Salzberg, S. (1995). *Lovingkindness: The revolutionary art of happiness.* Shambhala.

Sanger, K. L., & Dorjee, D. (2016). Mindfulness training with adolescents enhances metacognition and the inhibition of irrelevant stimuli: Evidence from event-related brain potentials. *Trends in Neuroscience and Education*, 5(1), 1–11. https://doi.org/10.1016/j.tine.2016.01.001

Shearman, S. M., & Dumlao, R. (2008). A cross-cultural comparison of family communication patterns and conflict between young adults and parents. *Journal of Family Communication, 8*(3), 186–211. https://doi.org/10.1080/15267430802182456

Sugiura, T., & Sugiura, Y. (2015). Common factors of meditation, focusing, and cognitive behavioral therapy: Longitudinal relation of self-report measures to worry, depressive, and obsessive-compulsive symptoms among nonclinical participants. *Mindfulness, 6*, 610–623. https://doi.org/10.1007/s12671-014-0296-0

Triandis, H. C. (2001). *Individualism & collectivism.* Westview Press.

Wilson, A. C., Schwannauer, M., McLaughlin, A., Ashworth, F., & Chan, S. W. Y. (2018). Vividness of positive mental imagery predicts positive emotional response to visually presented Project Soothe pictures. *The British Journal of Psychology, 109*(2), 259–276. https://doi.org/10.1111/bjop.12267

Resources

Literature

From classic studies done on a mindfulness-based stress-reduction program to more recent studies on relaxation and meditation in schools and educational settings, please see:

Baer, R. A., & Lykins, E. L. B. (2011). Mindfulness and positive psychological functioning. In K. M. Sheldon, T. B. Kashdan, & M. F. Steger (Eds.), *Designing positive psychology: Taking stock and moving forward* (p. 335–348). Oxford University Press. https://doi.org/10.1093/acprof:oso/9780195373585.003.0022

Biegel, G. M., Brown, K. W., Shapiro, S. L., & Schubert, C. M. (2009). Mindfulness-based stress reduction for the treatment of adolescent psychiatric outpatients: A randomized clinical trial. *Journal of Consulting and Clinical Psychology, 77*(5), 855–866. https://doi.org/10.1037/a0016241

Blanke, E. S., Riediger, M., & Brose, A. (2018). Pathways to happiness are multidirectional: Associations between state mindfulness and everyday affective experience. *Emotion, 18*(2), 202–211. https://doi.org/10.1037/emo0000323

Boroson, M. (2009). *One-moment meditation: Stillness for people on the go.* Winter Road.

Buoncristiani, M., & Buoncristiani, P. (2012). *Developing mindful participants, skillful thinkers, thoughtful schools.* Corwin Press.

Carsley, D., Khoury, B., & Heath, N. (2018). Effectiveness of mindfulness interventions for mental health in schools: A comprehensive meta-analysis. *Mindfulness, 9,* 693–707. https://doi.org/10.1007/s12671-017-0839-2

Evans, S., Ferrando, S., Findler, M., Stowell, C., Smart, C., & Haglin, D. (2008). Mindfulness-based cognitive therapy for generalized anxiety disorder. *Journal of Anxiety Disorders, 22*(4), 716–721. https://doi.org/10.1016/j.janxdis.2007.07.005

Franco, C., Amutio, A., López-González, L., Oriol, X., & Martínez-Taboada, C. (2016). Effect of a mindfulness training program on the impulsivity and aggression levels of adolescents with behavioral problems in the classroom. *Frontiers in Psychology, 7,* Article 1385. https://doi.org/10.3389/fpsyg.2016.01385

Fredrickson, B. L., Arizmendi, C., Van Cappellen, P., Firestine, A. M., Brantley, M. M., Kim, S. L., Brantley, J., & Salzberg, S. (2019). Contemplative moments matter: Effects of informal meditation practice on daily experiences of positive emotions and social integration. *Mindfulness, 10,* 1915–1925. https://doi.org/10.1007/s12671-019-01154-2

Friese, M., & Hofmann, W. (2016). State mindfulness, self-regulation, and emotional experience in everyday life. *Motivation Science, 2*(1), 1–14. https://doi.org/10.1037/mot0000027

Fuente, J., Mañas, I., Franco, C., Cangas, A. J., & Soriano, E. (2018). Differential effect of level of self-regulation and mindfulness training on coping strategies used by university participants. *International Journal of Environmental Research and Public Health, 15*(10), Article 2230. https://doi.org/10.3390/ijerph15102230

Gillham, J., Leventhal, K. S., Rashid, T., Anjum, A., & Leventhal, S. (2019). Positive psychology programs for youth in diverse communities. In L. van Zyl & S. I. Rothman (Eds.), *Positive psychological interventions* (pp. 197–226). Springer. https://doi.org/10.1007/978-3-030-20311-5_9

Gockel, A. (2010). The promise of mindfulness for clinical practice education. *Smith College Studies in Social Work, 80*(2), 248–268. https://doi.org/10.1080/00377311003784184

Grossman, L. M., Mr. Musumeci's 5th Grade Class, Alvarez, A., Kabat-Zinn, J. (2016). *Master of mindfulness: How to be your own superhero in times of stress.* New Harbinger.

Grossman, P., Niemann, L., Schmidt, S., & Walach, H. (2004). Mindfulness-based stress reduction and health benefits: A meta-analysis. *Journal of Psychosomatic Research, 57*(1), 35–43. https://doi.org/10.1016/S0022-3999(03)00573-7

Harvey, J., & Delfabbro, P. H. (2004). Psychological resilience in disadvantaged youth: A critical overview. *Australian Psychologist, 39,* 3–13. https://doi.org/10.1080/00050060410001660281

Hoffman, S.G., Asnaani, A., Vonk, I., Sawyer, A.T., & Fang, A. (2012). The efficacy of cognitive-behavioral therapy: A review of meta-analyses. *Cognitive Therapy and Research, 36,* 427–440. https://doi.org/10.1007/s10608-012-9476-1

Hornich-Lisciandro, T. (2013). Mindfulness in education. *Education Digest, 79*(2), 66–68.

Huppert, F. A., & Johnson, D. M. (2010). A controlled trial of mindfulness training in schools: The importance of practice for an impact on well-being. *Journal of Positive Psychology, 5,* 264–274. https://doi.org/10.1080/17439761003794148

Irving, J. A., Dobkin, P. L., & Park, J. (2009). Cultivating mindfulness in health care professionals: A review of empirical studies of mindfulness-based stress reduction (MBSR). *Complementary Therapies in Clinical Practice, 15*(2), 61–66. https://doi.org/10.1016/j.ctcp.2009.01.002

Ivtzan, I., & Lomas, T. (2016). *Mindfulness in positive psychology.* Routledge. https://doi.org/10.4324/9781315747217

Jennings, P. A., DeMauro, A. A., & Mischenko, P. P. (2019). *The mindful school: Transforming school culture through mindfulness and compassion.* Guilford Press.

Kabat-Zinn, J. (1994). *Wherever you go, there you are: Mindfulness and meditation in everyday life.* Hyperion.

Kabat-Zinn, J., Massion, A. O., Kristeller, J., Peterson, L. G., Fletcher, K. E., Pbert, L., Lenderking, W. R., & Santorelli, S. F. (1992). Effectiveness of a meditation-based stress reduction program in the treatment of anxiety disorders. *American Journal of Psychiatry, 149,* 936–943.

Kuyken, W., Weare, K., Ukoumunne, O. C., Vicary, R., Motton, N., Burnett, R., Cullen, C., Hennelly, S., & Huppert, F. (2013). Effectiveness of the mindfulness in schools programme: Non-randomised controlled feasibility study. *British Journal of Psychiatry, 203*(2), 126–131. https://doi.org/10.1192/bjp.bp.113.126649.

Linehan, M. M. (1993). *Cognitive-behavioral treatment of borderline personality disorder.* Guilford Press.

Luberto, C. M., Shinday, N., Song, R., Philpotts, L. L., Park, E. R., Fricchione, G. L., & Yeh, G. Y. (2018). A systematic review and meta-analysis of the effects of meditation on empathy, compassion, and prosocial behaviors. *Mindfulness, 9,* 708–724. https://doi.org/10.1007/s12671-017-0841-8

Luong, M. T., Gouda, S., Bauer, J., & Schmidt, S. (2019). Exploring mindfulness benefits for participants and teachers in three German high schools. *Mindfulness, 10*(12), 2682–2702. https://doi.org/10.1007/s12671-019-01231-6

Mendelson, T., Dariotis, J. K., Laura, F. G., Ali, S. R., Smith, A. A., Gonzalez, A. A., & Greenberg, M. T. (2013). Implementing mindfulness and yoga in urban schools: A community-academic partnership. *Journal of Children's Services, 8*(4), 276–291. https://doi.org/10.1108/JCS-07-2013-0024

Niemiec, R. M., Rashid, T., & Spinella, M. (2012). Strong mindfulness. *Journal of Mental Health Counseling, 34*(3), 240–253. https://doi.org/10.17744/mehc.34.3.34p6328x2v204v21

Niemiec, R. M. (2024). *Mindfulness and character strengths: A practical guide to MBSP* (2nd ed.). Hogrefe.

Pepping, C. A., Duvenage, M., Cronin, T. J., & Lyons, A. (2016). Adolescent mindfulness and psychopathology: The role of emotion regulation. *Personality and Individual Differences, 99,* 302–307. https://doi.org/10.1016/j.paid.2016.04.089

Rashid, T., Anjum, A., Chu, R., Stevanovski, S., Zanjani, A., & Lennex, C. (2015). Strength based resilience: Integrating risk and resources towards holistic well-being. In G. A. Fava & C. Ruini (Eds.), *Increasing psychological well-being across cultures* (pp. 153–176). Springer. https://doi.org/10.1007/978-94-017-8669-0_10

Rashid, T., & Seligman, M. E. P. (2018). *Positive psychotherapy: Clinician manual.* Oxford University Press.

Salzberg, S. (1995). *Lovingkindness. The revolutionary art of happiness.* Shambhala.

Salzberg, S. (2011). *Real happiness: The power of meditation. A 28-day program.* Workman.

Salzberg, S. (2019, February 7). *Meditation is about recovering and starting again.* Mindful: Healthy Mind, Healthy Life. https://www.mindful.org/meditation-is-about-recovering-and-starting-again/

Sanger, K. L., & Dorjee, D. (2016). Mindfulness training with adolescents enhances metacognition and the inhibition of irrelevant stimuli: Evidence from event-related brain potentials. *Trends in Neuroscience and Education, 5*(1), 1–11. https://doi.org/10.1016/j.tine.2016.01.001

Segal, Z. V., Dimidjian, S., Beck, A., Boggs, J. M., Vanderkruik, R., Metcalf, C. A., Gallop, R., Felder, J. N., & Levy, J. (2020). Outcomes of online mindfulness-based cognitive therapy for patients with residual depressive symptoms: A randomized clinical trial. *JAMA Psychiatry, 77*(6), 563–573. https://doi.org/10.1001/jamapsychiatry.2019.4693

Sugiura, T., & Sugiura, Y. (2015). Common factors of meditation, focusing, and cognitive behavioral therapy: Longitudinal relation of self-report measures to worry, depressive, and obsessive-compulsive symptoms among nonclinical participants. *Mindfulness, 6,* 610–623. https://doi.org/10.1007/s12671-014-0296-0

Wielgosz, J., Goldberg, S. B., Kral, T. R. A., Dunne, J. D., & Davidson, R. J. (2019). Mindfulness meditation and psychopathology. *Annual Review of Clinical Psychology, 15*(1), 285–316. https://doi.org/10.1146/annurev-clinpsy-021815-093423

Willard, C. (2014). *Mindfulness for teen anxiety: A workbook for overcoming anxiety at home, at school, and everywhere else*. Instant Help Books.

Websites

Center for Mindfulness Studies
https://www.mindfulnessstudies.com
A social enterprise, in Toronto, Canada, the Center for Mindfulness Studies provides professional training in mindfulness-based cognitive therapy (MBCT), mindfulness-based stress reduction (MBSR), mindful self-compassion (MSC), and specialized mindfulness training to the general public, healthcare providers, and social service professionals.

Mind & Life Institute
https://www.mindandlife.org
The Mind & Life Institute brings science and contemplative wisdom together to better understand the mind and create positive change in the world. At this critical moment in history, the Institute is expanding our reach beyond individual well-being to focus on societal flourishing and interconnection.

Mindfulness in Schools Project
https://mindfulnessinschools.org/
Mindfulness in Schools Project (MiSP) is a national, not-for-profit charity for young people and schools in the United Kingdom. The organization offers curricula for classroom-based mindfulness.

Action for Happiness
https://www.actionforhappiness.org/
This nonprofit organization offers a variety of resources, including mindfulness exercises, to help people take actions for a happier and kinder world.

Multimedia

The 4-7-8 Breathing Exercise to Alleviate Anxiety and Stress for Teens and Adults
https://youtu.be/PmBYdfv5RSk
This YouTube video introduces 4-7-8 breathing, a method pioneered by Andrew Weill. It is rooted in pranayama and is described as a "natural tranquilizer for the nervous system" helping to quickly reduce tension and allow the body to relax.

How to Stay Calm When You Know You'll Be Stressed
https://youtu.be/8jPQjjsBbIc
One is not at one's best when one is stressed. In fact, our brain has evolved over millennia to release cortisol in stressful situations, inhibiting rational, logical thinking but potentially helping us to survive, for example, being attacked by a lion. Neuroscientist Daniel Levitin thinks there's a way to avoid making critical mistakes in stressful situations, when your thinking becomes clouded: the pre-mortem. "We all are going to fail now and then," he says. "The idea is to think ahead to what those failures might be."

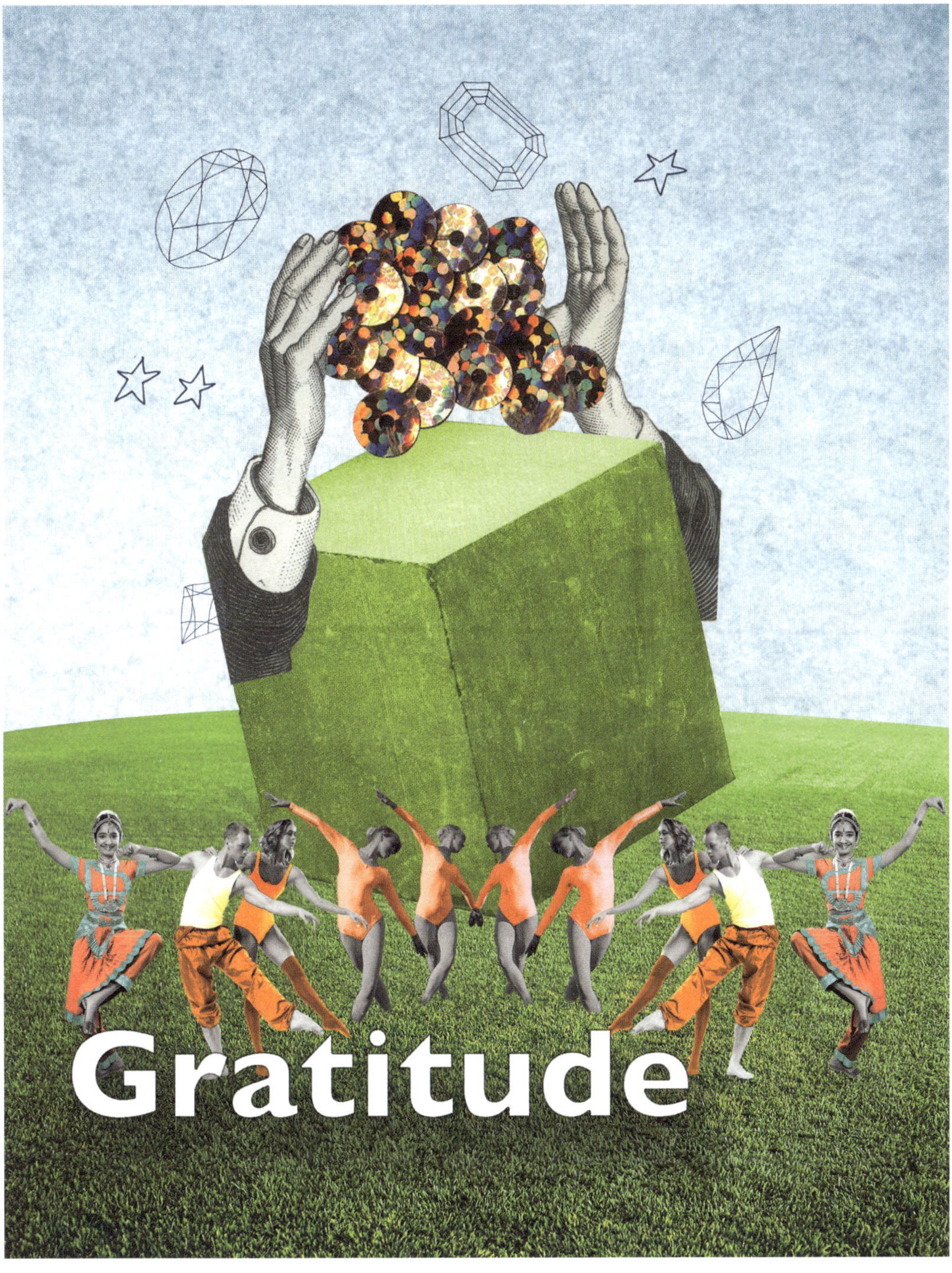
Gratitude

Regular Practice 2: Gratitude Journal

Everyday we face daily stressors, whether they be the number of emails needing a response, traffic gridlock, or sour interactions with family and friends. Daily stresses can have deleterious effects on one's health (Piazza et al., 2013; Seiler et al., 2020). We often notice and remember negative experiences, such as stressors, more readily than positive experiences. To counter this negativity bias and the impact of stressors, the regular practice of gratitude journaling invites participants to note, record, and reflect on positive experiences, big or small, which can uplift them and sustain their positive mood. Each module of the SBR program begins with inviting participants to share a gratitude journal entry.

Learning Outcomes for Gratitude Journal

By writing three positive things in a gratitude journal (big or small) and also recording what made these happen, participants can:

- Sharpen their awareness to notice, acknowledge, and appreciate positive events in daily life
- Counter the human tendency to pay more attention to negatives
- Enhance a sense of enduring thankfulness (gratitude), appreciation of beauty and excellence, savoring, and curiosity

Core Concepts of Gratitude

The themes here are also presented in the Core Concepts section of the Workbook (p. 27):

- The human brain has developed such that we remember failures more readily than successes. Negatives stick with us and often keep us stuck, while positives pass swiftly without staying very long in our attention and memory. We complain and criticize easily, but struggle to compliment and express gratitude (Baumeister et al., 2001).
- One does not need much training to encode, store, and retrieve negative experiences. Our mind has evolved to respond more strongly and frequently to negatives than to positives. No doubt, this built-in tendency helped our ancestors survive and secure shelter, food, and mates in a context of danger (Rozin & Royzman, 2001).
- Though we may live in safer environments today, we require special attention and effort to acknowledge, appreciate, and store positive experiences – that is, it can take effort to cultivate the skills and habits of appreciating these experiences rather than taking them for granted (Renshaw & Olinger Steeves, 2016).
- We can avoid taking positive experiences for granted by deliberately spacing them out. For example, savor autumn colors, spend time with friends, take a warm shower after a long tiring day, or enjoy a greeting from a friend not seen for a while.
- Gratitude is associated with higher levels of life satisfaction and happiness and lower levels of anxiety, stress, depression, and suicidal ideation (Portocarrero et al., 2020). Research indicates that gratitude interventions, such as keeping a gratitude journal, enhance well-being and reduce symptoms of depression and anxiety (Davis et al., 2016; Diniz et al., 2023).

Illustrations of Gratitude

Gateway Public Schools Gratitude Project
https://youtu.be/-m16lKW9ceA
(Duration: 3:42)
This clip shows participants, teachers, and staff at a public school expressing gratitude.

2 Mins Short Gratitude Story for Kids
https://www.youtube.com/watch?v=Y3cpV_dnN_I
(Duration 2:16)
This animated story shows how others appreciate our everyday actions and in turn, how our actions enhance our appreciation and gratitude for others.

Say "Thank You" – A Motivational Video on the Importance of Gratitude
https://youtu.be/7uzynHWxn5Q
(Duration 5:10)
Denzel Washington narrates this motivational video on the importance of gratitude.

Reflection and Discussion

Invite participants to complete the Reflection and Discussion section of their Workbook (p. 28) regarding the video(s) they have watched. Discuss the questions:

What are the key messages in the video(s) you just watched?
How might these concepts be relevant in your life?

Practice: Reflect on Your Gratitude Journal

The gratitude journal is designed to help participants attend to and appreciate positive life experiences.

Introduce the gratitude journal practice by asking group members to think about something they are grateful for and then invite volunteers to share their insights with the group.

Following the group discussion, orient participants to the worksheet on p. 30 in their Workbook and have them complete one entry for yesterday or today. Let participants know that they can copy or adapt the worksheet. You can use the script below (also in the Workbook on p. 29) to facilitate this activity.

> *During the entire program, aim to journal daily, writing three good things about your day, preferably before going to bed. Good things can be big or small as long as they matter to you. Write in the journal each night and recall three good things that happened during your day. Take time to imagine and reexperience each one.*

Let's complete an example right now. Think about three good things that happened either yesterday or today. Describe each good thing briefly, then below it, reflect on one of the following questions:
What made this event happen today?
What have I learned from taking the time to name this good thing?
In what ways did I or others make this good thing happen?

As the program progresses and participants become aware of their character strengths, you can invite them to incorporate new learning into their gratitude journal. In what specific ways did participants express their strengths or spot the strengths of others in their day-to-day routine?

Practice Debrief

Ask the participants to complete the Practice Debrief section in their Workbook (available online as printable PDF and on p. 30) and to address the following:

- *Note on a weekly basis any thoughts you have about completing the gratitude journal or challenges you encounter.*
- *What patterns did you notice about the three things you wrote about?*
- *How did writing about gratitude affect you? Did you notice any changes when writing or at other times of the week?*
- *Did you learn anything from this activity? What did you learn?*
- *How else might you incorporate a practice of gratitude into your daily life?*

Encourage participants to share their gratitude journal entries periodically during the course of the program. Also encourage them to notice and share the impact of this practice on their daily lives.

Learning and Cultural Fit

When introducing concepts of gratitude journaling for the first time, it is important to consider culturally relevant adaptations.

- Be mindful that some participants, especially those with learning challenges related to writing, may find it difficult to write about positive experiences. Offer participants other options to record positive experiences, including taking pictures, making drawings or illustrations of positive experiences, recording voice notes of positive experience, and using artifacts or other tangible objects that manifest positive experiences.
- Participants from Eastern or collectivist cultures may hesitate to focus on individual positive experiences. Encourage them to use collectivist positive experiences, including interactions with siblings, parents, and extended family.
- Since this is a regular practice, some participants might sometimes have difficulty writing about three positive events, especially if they experienced a major setback or encountered a difficulty. Remind participants that positive experiences can be small. Allow participants to skip a week. However, encourage them to review entries from previous weeks, as these might repair their mood or uplift them.

- Participants can become habituated to writing in the gratitude journal. If entries are repeated, the practice can become almost rote, losing its meaning and power. Encourage them to be creative and to alternate the kinds of experiences they focus on. For example, one week a participant can focus on their positive experiences within the family, the next week they can focus on positive experiences at work. Other domains such as nature, art, sport, cuisine, or specific cultural events (e.g., festive seasons, spiritual practices) can be the focus of a gratitude journal.

Everyday Applications

The first time you introduce the regular practice of gratitude journal, share with participants ways that journaling concepts can be applied in their daily lives.

- If you are feeling ungrateful, it is highly likely that you will experience negative emotions at the same time. Instead, cultivate a habit of expressing gratitude, through this practice. It can lead to more positive and genuine experiences on a daily basis.
- Make it a habit to express thanks in daily life. Articulating briefly but specifically how someone's action helped you can infuse mutual respect and affection in our everyday interactions with our loved ones.
- Take a few minutes everyday to feel gratitude in your heart for people whose work benefits you directly or indirectly. For example, nursing and other medical staff do a number of small tasks which make your visit to a doctor effective. Staff at grocery stores do their jobs so you can purchase food which nourishes you. Cleaning staff pick up your garbage to keep your environment clean. Any break in this daily chain of actions can add to your stress. Expressing thanks to others, explicitly, whenever possible and implicitly, in your heart, can maintain or enhance your sense of communal trust and well-being.
- Begin each day by focusing on and listing a few things you are grateful for (e.g., certain people in your life, your pet, beautiful weather outside, a comfortable home, a good cup of coffee or tea).

References

Baumeister, R. F., Bratslavsky, E., Finkenauer, C., & Vohs, K. D. (2001). Bad is stronger than good. *Review of General Psychology*, 5(4), 323–370. https://doi.org/10.1037/1089-2680.5.4.323

Davis, D. E., Choe, E., Meyers, J., Wade, N., Varjas, K., Gifford, A., Quinn, A., Hook, J. N., Van Tongeren, D. R., Griffin, B. J., & Worthington, E. L., Jr. (2016). Thankful for the little things: A meta-analysis of gratitude interventions. *Journal of Counseling Psychology, 63*(1), 20–31. https://doi.org/10.1037/cou0000107

Diniz, G., Korkes, L., Tristão, L. S., Pelegrini, R., Bellodi, P. L., & Bernardo, W. M. (2023). The effects of gratitude interventions: A systematic review and meta-analysis. *Einstein (São Paulo), 21*, Article eRW0371. https://doi.org/10.31744/einstein_journal/2023rw0371

Piazza, J. R., Charles, S. T., Sliwinski, M. J., Mogle, J., & Almeida, D. M. (2013). Affective reactivity to daily stressors and long-term risk of reporting a chronic physical health condition. *Annals of Behavioral Medicine, 45*(1), 110–120. https://doi.org/10.1007/s12160-012-9423-0.

Portocarrero, F. F., Gonzalez, K., & Ekema-Agbaw, M. (2020). A meta-analytic review of the relationship between dispositional gratitude and well-being. *Personality and Individual Differences*, 164, Article 110101. https://doi.org/10.1016/j.paid.2020.110101

Renshaw, T. L., & Olinger Steeves, R. M. (2016). What good is gratitude in youth and schools? A systematic review and meta-analysis of correlates and intervention outcomes. *Psychology in the Schools, 53*(3), 286–305. https://doi.org/10.1002/pits.21903

Rozin, P., & Royzman, E. (2001). Negativity bias, negativity dominance, and contagion. *Personality and Social Psychology Review, 5*, 296–320. https://doi.org/10.1207/S15327957PSPR0504_2

Seiler, A., Fagundes, C. P., & Christian, L. M. (2020). The impact of everyday stressors on the immune system and health. In A. Choukèr (Ed.), *Stress challenges and immunity in space*. Springer. https://doi.org/10.1007/978-3-030-16996-1_6

Resources

Literature

Baumeister, R. F., Bratslavsky, E., Finkenauer, C., & Vohs, K. D. (2001). Bad is stronger than good. *Review of General Psychology, 5*, 323–370. https://doi.org/10.1037/1089-2680.5.4.323

Dziurda, K. (2017). *Gratitude journal: A 52 Week challenge to mastering the art of gratitude and positively transforming your life.* First Publication.

Emmons, R. A. (2007). *Thanks! How the new science of gratitude can make you happier.* Houghton-Mifflin.

Flinchbaugh, C. L., Moore, E. W. G., Chang, Y. K., & May, D. R. (2012). Student well-being interventions: The effects of stress management techniques and gratitude journaling in the management education classroom. *Journal of Management Education, 36*(2), 191–219. https://doi.org/10.1177/1052562911430062

Froh, J. J., Sefick, W. J., & Emmons, R. A. (2008). Counting blessings in early adolescents: An experimental study of gratitude and subjective well-being. *Journal of School Psychology, 46*, 213–233. https://doi.org/10.1016/j.jsp.2007.03.005

Hussong, A. M., Langley, H. A., Thomas, T. E., Coffman, J. L., Halberstadt, A. G., Costanzo, P. R., & Rothenberg, W. A. (2019). Measuring gratitude in children. *Journal of Positive Psychology, 14*(5), 563–575. https://doi.org/10.1080/17439760.2018.1497692

Jiang, H., Sun, P., Liu, Y., & Pan, M. (2016). Gratitude and late adolescents' school well-being: The mediating role of materialism. *Social Indicators Research, 127*(3), 1363–1376. https://doi.org/10.1007/s11205-015-1007-5

Leaf, C. (2019). *Think, learn, succeed: Understanding and using your mind to thrive at school, the workplace, and life.* Baker Books.

Ma, L. K., Tunney, R. J., & Ferguson, E. (2017). Does gratitude enhance prosociality? A meta-analytic review. *Psychological Bulletin, 143*(6), 601–635. https://doi.org/10.1037/bul0000103

Montreuil, T. C., & Tilley, M. A. (Eds.) (2017). *Healthy minds, healthy schools: Strategies and activities for happy and successful learners.* Canadian Scholars' Press.

Sacks, O. (2015). *Gratitude*. Knopf.

Voci, A., Veneziani, C. A., & Fuochi, G. (2019). Relating mindfulness, heartfulness, and psychological well-being: The role of self-compassion and gratitude. *Mindfulness, 10*(2), 339–351. https://doi.org/10.1007/s12671-018-0978-0

Watkins, P. C. (2013). *Gratitude and the good life: Toward a psychology of appreciation.* Springer.

Watkins, P. C., Grimm, D. L., & Kolts, R. (2004). Counting your blessings: Positive memories among grateful persons. *Current Psychology, 23*, 52–67. https://doi.org/10.1007/s12144-004-1008-z

Websites

Grateful Living
https://grateful.org/
Grateful Living is an online nonprofit organization that offers community-based educational programs and practices.

35 Scientific Benefits of Gratitude: Mental Health Research Findings in 2024
https://research.com/education/scientific-benefits-of-gratitude
This website explains what gratitude is, how it works, and what are its major benefits.

Gratitude Works
http://emmons.faculty.ucdavis.edu/
Robert Emmons, one of the most eminent researchers of gratitude, briefly summarizes his research findings, lists his publications, and refers to links to gratitude resources.

Multimedia

Gratitude is Good for You
https://youtu.be/sCV-mEsASLA
This video from John Templeton Foundation describes the benefits of having an attitude of gratitude and how one can practice being more grateful everyday.

Making Gratitude a Part of Everyday Life: Tips From Dr. Robert Emmons
https://www.takingcharge.csh.umn.edu/making-gratitude-part-everyday-life-tips-dr-robert-emmons
Robert Emmons, author of the book *Thanks! How the New Science of Gratitude Can Make You Happier*, shares helpful strategies to integrate gratitude in daily life.

Thanks! By Robert Emmons (Book Summary)
https://www.njlifehacks.com/thanks-robert-emmons-book-summary/
Robert Emmons, an expert in gratitude research, shares some tips for integrating gratitude into daily life.

How to Create a Gratitude Journal
https://blog.mindvalley.com/gratitude-journal/
This blog describes how to create a gratitude journal ritual in five easy steps.

155 Gratitude Journal Prompts
https://www.developgoodhabits.com/gratitude-journal-prompts/
This website provides 155 gratitude journal prompts, including happiest childhood memory, favorite song, and family traditions for which one feels gratitude.

Gratitude: Greater Good Magazine
https://greatergood.berkeley.edu/topic/gratitude
The Greater Good magazine shares scientific research on happiness and well-being, along with related stories, tips, and tools. It aims to make scientific research and evidence-based interventions accessible to a wider audience outside of academia.

How Gratitude Leads to Good Health and Happiness
https://my.happify.com/hd/gratitude-infographic/
This infographic visually describes the evidence-based benefits of gratitude.

Positive Psychology - Gratitude
https://positivepsychology.com/benefits-of-gratitude/
This web article describes 14 evidence-based benefits of gratitude.

The Science Behind Gratitude Journaling
https://wanderersway.com/blogs/wanderers-way/the-science-behind-gratitude-journaling
This blog describes how gratitude journaling improves health from the critical lens of science.

Section III: The Modules

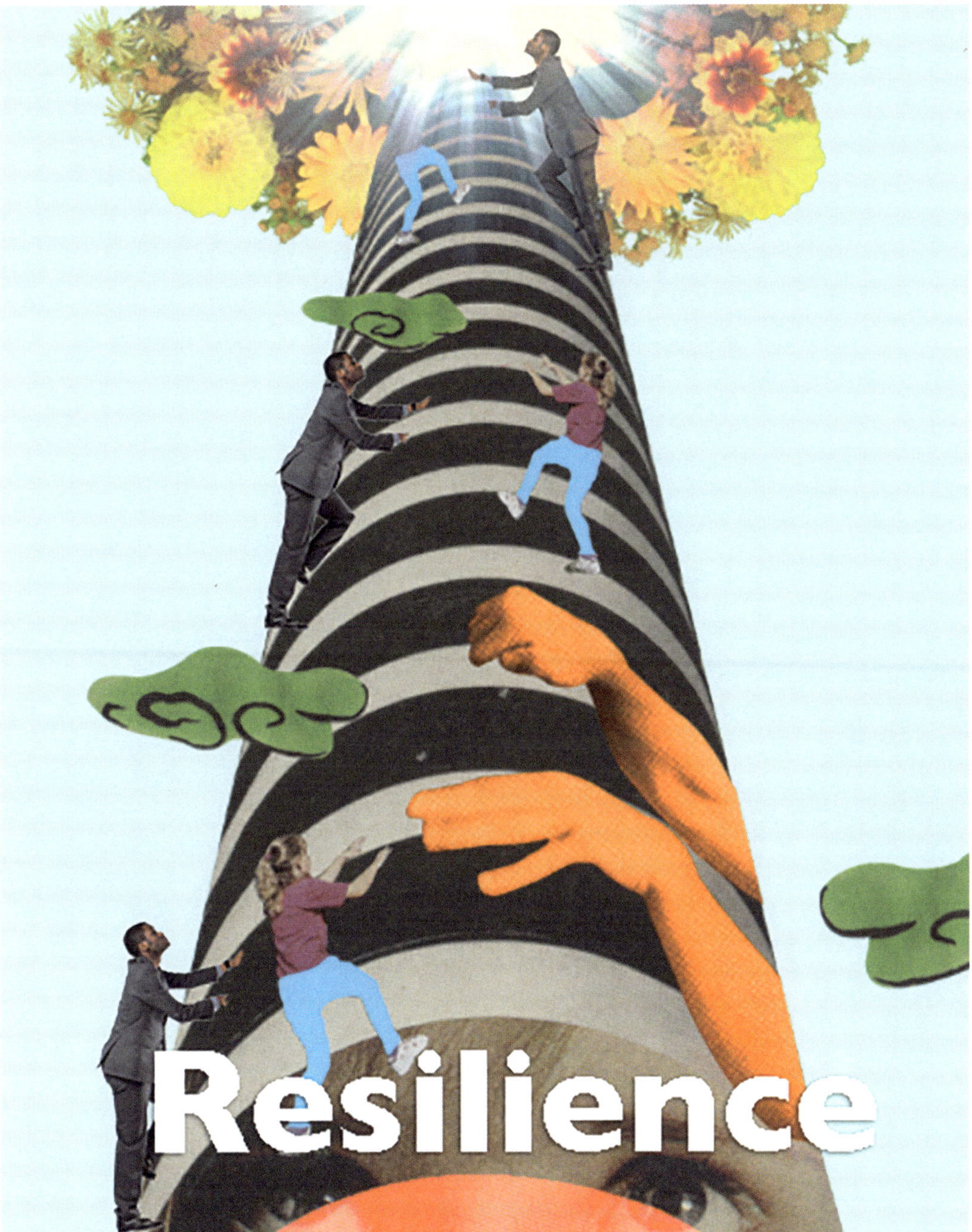
Resilience

Module 1: Resilience

The first module of the SBR program introduces participants to the concept of resilience as it will be used in this 14-module program. A story-telling activity follows in which participants are invited to recall an experience of overcoming a challenge and reappraise it from the perspective of resilience. The module ends by offering ways to enrich everyday life experiences through resilience.

Module Topic	Minutes to Allot	
Learning Outcomes By reflecting and writing about a challenge they overcame effectively, and learning about different ways that resilience can manifest itself, participants: • Define resilience and identify qualities of individual resilience • Develop a coherent and healthier self-narrative • Express an understanding of ways that specific strengths, such as persistence, hope, social intelligence, self-regulation, perspective, and spirituality, can boost one's resilience	5	5
Opening Activities Start the module with a relaxation or mindfulness practice Invite participants to share a few events from their gratitude journal that have occurred since the last session Invite questions about the previous module and practice(s)	10	15
Illustration of Core Concepts Review core concepts and show video illustrations Facilitate reflection and discussion: • *What are the key messages in the video(s) you just watched?* • *Please describe them in relation to resilience and some of its features.*	15	15
Practice: Write Your Own Story of Resilience Introduce Story of Resilience activity and sample Have participants draft their story of resilience Debrief learning from practice(s) using the questions: 1. *How does your own story of resilience represent aspects of resilience discussed earlier?* 2. *What helped you deal with your challenge?* 3. *How did others contribute in your story of resilience? Have you had the opportunity to discuss this specific story with them?*	20	30
Closing Activities Invite discussion of everyday applications Remind participants of relevant resources at the end of the module Guide participants in a 3-minute closing relaxation or mindfulness practice	10	10
Total	60 minutes	75 minutes

Core Concepts of Resilience

Resilience can be understood from a number of perspectives. We will discuss them as part of some broad themes, many of which are also presented in the Core Concepts section of the Workbook (p. 35). Some of these perspectives are:

- Resilience is a dynamic process that involves the interaction between both risk and protective processes, internal and external to the individual, which act to modify the effects of an adverse life event (Rutter, 2012). This involves dynamic and positive adaptation which includes both stress and competence at different levels – individual, family, and society – yielding a variety of outcomes, making an individual vulnerable to risks or resilient (Luthar, 2003).
- Resilience is also a process of adapting well in the face of adversity, trauma, tragedy, threats, or other significant sources of stress (Newman, 2002). It is not a static process, but a dynamic one of maintaining relatively healthier psychological and physical functioning, especially when one faces a significant trauma or setback that jeopardizes one's well-being and survival (Bonanno, 2004; Masten, 2014).
- Resilience can be viewed as an ability that helps individuals to persevere in the face of challenges and setbacks (Reivich & Shatté, 2002). This perseverance is marked by four major components: social competence, problem-solving ability, development of autonomy, and having a sense of purpose and meaning (Songprakun & McCann, 2012). Other factors associated with resilience are altruism, harmony, wisdom, and self-actualization (Gutshall, 2013). It is not about shying away from problems, minimizing them, or avoiding them. We all do this from time to time, but eventually this approach can hurt us and cause us to pick up bad coping habits. It may be tough in the moment, but dealing with our problems head-on helps us to deal with challenges better in the long run.
- Social support has been shown to be exceptionally critical for maintaining good physical and psychological health. Numerous lines of research have shown that high-quality social support can enhance resilience to stress, buffer against developing trauma-related psychiatric disorders, decrease the functional impact of trauma-induced disorders, including posttraumatic stress disorder (PTSD), and can reduce medical mortality and morbidity (Chen et al., 2021; Lee et al., 2021; Ozbay et al., 2007). A number of social factors such as family, school, neighborhood, and community are critical for resilience and are associated with positive outcomes across different contexts and exposures (Joyce et al., 2018).
- Resilience can be enhanced by learning skills and through developing and using strengths.

Illustrations of Resilience

Play at least one of the three videos below to illustrate the core concepts of resilience and encourage discussion.

Disney's Motivational Video
https://youtu.be/m2u9VgKZHDo?si=R3O3vmou-tpKJP99
(Duration: 4:36 minutes)
A collection of clips from Disney movies shows the resilience of the main characters.

Famous Failures
https://youtu.be/zLYECIjmnQs
(Duration: 2:58 minutes)
This inspiring video illustrates through famous role models the importance of persevering no matter how many times you have failed in life.

Brains: Journey to Resilience
https://youtu.be/HJvDrT6N-mw
(Duration: 7:44 minutes)
Learn about the resilience scale in this scientifically rigorous video created by the Alberta Family Wellness Initiative.

Reflection and Discussion

Invite participants to complete the Reflection and Discussion section of their Workbook (p. 36) regarding the video(s) they have watched. Discuss the questions:

What are the key messages in the videos you just watched? Please describe them in relation to resilience and some of its features.

Ask participants what are the qualities and skills that help them to be resilient. Be sure to also ask participants how they understand resilience in their own familial and cultural context. Also ask participants if there are elements of resilience not covered in the concepts discussed or illustrated.

Practice: Write Your Own Story of Resilience

The story of resilience is a powerful activity that creates a starting point for each participant to expand their awareness of their own resilience. By remembering and reflecting on a powerful personal experience of resilience, participants can see ways in which they are already resourceful in times of adversity. Moreover, when they share these experiences in a group setting, they expand their repertoire of resilience resources. Finally, this story from their past that they write in Module 1 becomes the starting point for Module 14, when they are invited to explore a vision for their future self - one that is built on purpose and meaning.

The story of resilience practice is laid out in the participants' Workbook on pp. 37–39. A sample story opens the practice on p. 37 (see below); this follows with a blank page for them to write their own story and three practice debrief questions.

Facilitate the practice by adapting the following steps to your audience and program:

1. Have participants read the sample story of resilience in their Workbook (p. 37).
2. Invite participants to close their eyes and take a couple of deep breaths. You can also use Regular Practice 1: Relaxation and Mindfulness to provide participants with a grounding experience. With eyes closed or fixed at a stationary point, close to the floor, invite them to recall a challenging situation that they handled adaptively and successfully. Remind them that they will each define success in their own way.
3. Ask them to recall an event from the past, remote or recent, but not still ongoing. As instructed on their worksheet (p. 38 of Workbook), participants can recall the story with a clear beginning, middle, and a positive end.
4. After participants have had time to recall, invite them to write their stories of resilience.
5. Encourage them to share stories or parts that they feel comfortable sharing.
6. Ask them how their stories illustrate qualities and features of resilience. You can also choose to get the participants to work in pairs and to take turns sharing their stories.

Keep the stories of resilience shared by participants in mind throughout the program. These stories or highlights from them can be used as powerful motivators in subsequent SBR exercises.

Story of Resilience: An Illustration

In fifth grade, I was a shy girl who always felt as if the eyes of the entire school were on me. I was chubby and uncoordinated. Despite loving and wanting to play sports or participate in events, I never had the courage to ask our sports teacher to join in any competition.

Sitting on the bleachers of the school gym, I watched my friends running, sprinting, and jumping and I did all of these – by imagining them. My best friend, Sabrina, was one of the best sprinters and was on the school's relay team. I cheered for her, at times I envied her, and at times I felt somewhat jealous.

At our annual interschool athletic competition, Sabrina asked me to come with her, as I was supposed to spend the evening at her home to complete our social science project. Just before the final relay race, one of our athletes pulled her muscle and couldn't participate any further. Sabrina came to me and gently asked if I could replace her. I said, "no way, I cannot run.... Our team will lose the race due to me." Sabrina said, "but if you don't participate, we will not be able to even compete in the final." Our sports teacher also urged me to join the team, although I could clearly see he wasn't convinced that I should or even could run.

I felt coerced to compete for the sake of the school, and I agreed reluctantly. I joined the team on the track field, and I was to run first. At the whistle, it took me a while to realize that my competitors had moved on. "Run." Once I put one foot in front of the other, repeating this became easier and easier. I felt lighter, and strangely I did not care who was watching... in fact, for the first time, I felt I wasn't watching myself. I felt lighter, and some strange thing pushed me to run faster and faster. I was not the first to the exchange point but certainly not the last one. Little did I realize that the next runner had taken the baton... our team finished second. I was not the best runner that day, but that was the best I ever ran.

Practice Debrief

Ask the participants to complete the Practice Debrief section in their Workbook (p. 39) and to discuss the following:

1. *How does your own story of resilience represent aspects of resilience discussed earlier?*
2. *What helped you deal with your challenge?*
3. *How did others contribute in your story of resilience? Have you had the opportunity to discuss this specific story with them?*

Learning and Cultural Fit

Adapt this practice to the learning and cultural needs of your participants' and their unique values and demographics. Possible adaptations include:

- Participants can draw pictures or use photographs, artifacts, souvenirs, letters of appreciation, awards, or certificates to describe and share their stories of resilience. Ask participants who are shy or modest what their close family members and best friends might say, if asked to describe a time the participant was resilient. If they still cannot think of a story, have participants ask a close family member or best friend to share a story of resilience about them.
- Participants from cultural backgrounds where modesty is valued may find this exercise challenging initially. They may view it as an expression of self-congratulation and immodesty, and may find it incompatible with their cultural expectations. Emphasize that the exercise is about exploring one's resilience, self-awareness, and growth, and less about showing off to others.
- Participants from collectivist cultures may have stories which involve working, collaborating, and persisting with others. To facilitate cultural appropriateness, a participant can share a story of resilience that involves working with others in overcoming a challenge.
- Participants uncomfortable sharing a personal story for a variety of reasons can share a story of someone they know who overcame a challenge in a resilient way.

Closing Activities

The goal of closing this module is to help participants integrate their understanding of resilience and to take their new learning into everyday life.

Discuss with participants the Everyday Applications section, also found on p. 40 in their Workbook. Invite participants to be mindful in their day-to-day lives by noticing actions and habits which show their resilience or that of others. Encourage them to use relevant resources found at the end of this module, some of which are included in their workbooks starting on p. 40.

Choose an activity from Regular Practice 1: Mindfulness and Relaxation to close the module.

Everyday Applications

- We experience hassles, stressors, and setbacks in everyday life. Remember, resilience is bouncing back from these challenges. Next time you experience a challenge in everyday life, recall the story you wrote in this module. Remembering times when we overcame past challenges reinforces how capable we are of overcoming future ones.
- Reflect on everyday hassles, stressors, and setbacks to better understand aspects of your resilience. Do you apply the same strategies over and over to solve a problem and discover they are not working? By being more observant, can you notice what strategies work better? In your upcoming challenges, are there new strategies you can apply from your story of resilience?
- Failures, setbacks, challenges, and adversities are unfortunately the best times to test your resilience. Remind yourself that setbacks and challenges tend to be temporary, and everyone experiences them. Setbacks do not need to define you or determine everything in your life, and are not caused by you alone.
- Setbacks and challenges provide us with the opportunity to use our resilience skills and to develop new skills. Though usually unwelcome, they provide us with important opportunities to learn and to grow. We see situations as setbacks when our expectations are not met, but it is possible that our expectations are not always realistic.
- When dealing with everyday challenges, think how you use various aspects of resilience discussed in the module. This reflection will help you to estimate which specific aspects of resilience you have, and which ones you may need to develop. Remember too that you can draw on friends and family to support your ability to bounce back, when your inner resources are not up to the task.

References

Bonanno, G. A. (2004). Loss, trauma, and human resilience: Have we underestimated the human capacity to thrive after extremely aversive events? *American Psychologist, 59*(1), 20–28. https://doi.org/10.1037/0003-066X.59.1.20

Chen, J.-J., Wang, Q.-L., Li, H.-P., Zhang, T., Zhang, S.-S., & Zhou, M.-K. (2021). Family resilience, perceived social support, and individual resilience in cancer couples: Analysis using the actor-partner interdependence mediation model. *European Journal of Oncology Nursing, 52*, Article 101932. https://doi.org/https://doi.org/10.1016/j.ejon.2021.101932

Gutshall, C. A. (2013). Teachers' mindsets for participants with and without disabilities. *Psychology in the Schools, 50*(10), 1073–1083. https://doi.org/10.1002/pits.21725

Joyce, S., Shand, F., Tighe, J., Laurent, S. J., Bryant, R. A., & Harvey, S. B. (2018). Road to resilience: A systematic review and meta-analysis of resilience training programmes and interventions. *BMJ Open, 8*(6), e017858. https://doi.org/10.1136/bmjopen-2017-017858

Lee, T. S.-H., Wu, Y.-J., Chao, E., Chang, C.-W., Hwang, K.-S., & Wu, W.-C. (2021). Resilience as a mediator of interpersonal relationships and depressive symptoms amongst 10th to 12th grade students. *Journal of Affective Disorders, 278*, 107–113. https://doi.org/10.1016/j.jad.2020.09.033

Luthar, S. S. (2003). *Resilience and vulnerability*. Cambridge University Press. https://doi.org/10.1017/CBO9780511615788

Masten, A. S. (2014). *Ordinary magic: Resilience in development*. Guilford Press.

Newman, R. (2002). The road to resilience. *Monitor on Psychology, 33*(9), 62. https://www.apa.org/monitor/oct02/pp

Ozbay, F., Johnson, D. C., Dimoulas, E., Morgan, C. A., Charney, D., & Southwick, S. (2007). Social support and resilience to stress: From neurobiology to clinical practice. *Psychiatry (Edgmont), 4*(5), 35–40.

Reivich, K., & Shatté, A. (2002). *The resilience factor: 7 keys to finding your inner strength and overcoming life's hurdles*. Broadway Books.
Rutter, M. (2012). Resilience as a dynamic concept. *Development and Psychopathology, 24*(2), 335–344. https://doi.org/10.1017/S0954579412000028
Songprakun, W., & McCann, T. V. (2012). Effectiveness of a self-help manual on the promotion of resilience in individuals with depression in Thailand: A randomised controlled trial. *BMC Psychiatry, 12*, Article 12. https://doi.org/10.1186/1471-244X-12-12

Resources

Literature

Brownlee, K., Rawana, J., Franks, J., Harper, J., Bajwa, J., O'Brien, E., & Clarkson, A. (2013). A systematic review of strengths and resilience outcome literature relevant to children and adolescents. *Child and Adolescent Social Work Journal, 30*(5), 435–459.
Hass, M., & Graydon, K. (2009). Sources of resiliency among successful foster youth. *Child and Youth Services Review, 31*(4), 457–463. https://doi.org/10.1016/j.childyouth.2008.10.001
Hulme, J. (2017). *The school of wellbeing: 12 extraordinary projects promoting children and young people's mental health and happiness*. Jessica Kinsley.
Larson, S. (2010). Strength-based discipline that taps into the resilience of youth. *Reclaiming Children and Youth, 18*(4), 22.
Leppert, K., & Strauss, B. (2011). The role of resilience for coping in different age groups. *Zeitschrift für Gerontologie und Geriatrie, 44*(5), 313. https://doi.org/10.1007/s00391-011-0193-2
Maddi, S. R., Harvey, R. H., Khoshaba, D. M., Fazel, M., & Resurreccion, N. (2009). The personality construct of hardiness. IV: Expressed in positive cognitions and emotions concerning oneself and developmentally relevant activities. *Journal of Humanistic Psychology, 49*(3), 292–305.
Masten, A. S. (2001). Ordinary magic: Resilience processes in development. *American Psychologist, 56*(3), 227–238. https://doi.org/10.1037/0003-066X.56.3.227
McGrath, R. E. (2015). Character strengths in 75 nations: An update. *Journal of Positive Psychology, 10*(1), 41–52. https://doi.org/10.1080/17439760.2014.888580
Nickolite, A., & Doll, B. (2008). Resilience applied in school: Strengthening classroom environments for learning. *Canadian Journal of School Psychology, 23*(1), 338–348. https://doi.org/10.1177/0829573508316596
Prince-Embury, S., & Saklofske, D. H. (Eds.). (2014). *Resilience interventions for youth in diverse populations*. Springer. https://doi.org/10.1007/978-1-4939-0542-3
Reivich, K., & Shatté, A. (2002). *The resilience factor: 7 keys to finding your inner strength and overcoming life's hurdles*. Broadway Books.
Shoshani, A., & Slone, M. (2016). The resilience function of character strengths in the face of war and protracted conflict. *Frontiers in Psychology, 6*, Article 2006. https://doi.org/10.3389/fpsyg.2015.02006
Southwick, S. M., & Charney D. S. (2018). *Resilience: The science of mastering life's greatest challenges* (2nd ed.). Cambridge University Press. https://doi.org/10.1017/9781108349246
Ungar, M. (2008). Resilience across cultures. *British Journal of Social Work, 38*(2), 218–235. https://doi.org/10.1093/bjsw/bcl343
Ungar, M. (2019). *Change your world*. Sutherland House.
Ungar, M., Ghazinour, M., & Richter, J. (2013). What is resilience within the ecology of human development? *Journal of Child Psychology and Psychiatry, 54*(4), 348–366. https://doi.org/10.1111/jcpp.12025
Ungar, M., Russell, P., & Connolly, G. (2014). School-based interventions to enhance the resilience of participants. *Journal of Educational and Developmental Psychology, 4*(1), 66–83. https://doi.org/10.5539/jedp.v4n1p66

Story of Resilience

Bauer, J. J., McAdams, D. P., & Sakaeda, A. R. (2005). Interpreting the good life: Growth memories in the lives of mature, happy people. *Journal of Personality and Social Psychology, 88*(1), 203–217. https://doi.org/10.1037/0022-3514.88.1.203

Burns, G. (2001). *101 healing stories: Using metaphors in therapy.* Wiley.

King L. A, & Miner K. N. (2000). Writing about the perceived benefits of traumatic events: Implications for physical health. *Personality and Social Psychology Bulletin. 26*(2), 220–230. https://doi.org/10.1177/0146167200264008

McAdams, D. P. (2001). The psychology of life stories. *Review of General Psychology, 5*(2), 100–122. https://doi.org/10.1037/1089-2680.5.2.100

Nagabhushan, P. (2011). Narrative development in adolescence: Creating the storied self. *Journal of Youth and Adolescence, 40,* 756–758.

Websites

Teach Resiliency
https://phecanada.ca/programs/teach-resiliency/home
With support from Canada's Young Health Program (YHP) Physical and Health Education Canada (PHE Canada), this 2012 research project examined child and youth mental health in Canadian schools.

Center on the Developing Child, Harvard University
https://developingchild.harvard.edu/science/key-concepts/resilience/
The objectives of this center are to develop science-based innovations that achieve breakthrough outcomes for children facing adversity.

Academic Resilience Consortium
https://academicresilience.org/
The Academic Resilience Consortium (ARC) is an association of faculty, professionals, and students in higher education who are dedicated to understanding and promoting student resilience.

Multimedia

The Three Secrets of Resilient People
https://youtu.be/NWH8N-BvhAw
In this powerful and courageous talk, Lucy Hone shares the three strategies that got her through an unimaginable tragedy – and offers a profound insight into human suffering.

Resilience in Kids Created by First to Draw
https://youtu.be/HYsRGe0tfZc
This video teaches resilience skills to adults so they can pass them on to children and young people.

The Power of Resilience
https://youtu.be/isfw8JJ-eWM
This TEDx talk by Sam Goldstein focuses on how to foster strength, hope, and optimism in our children.

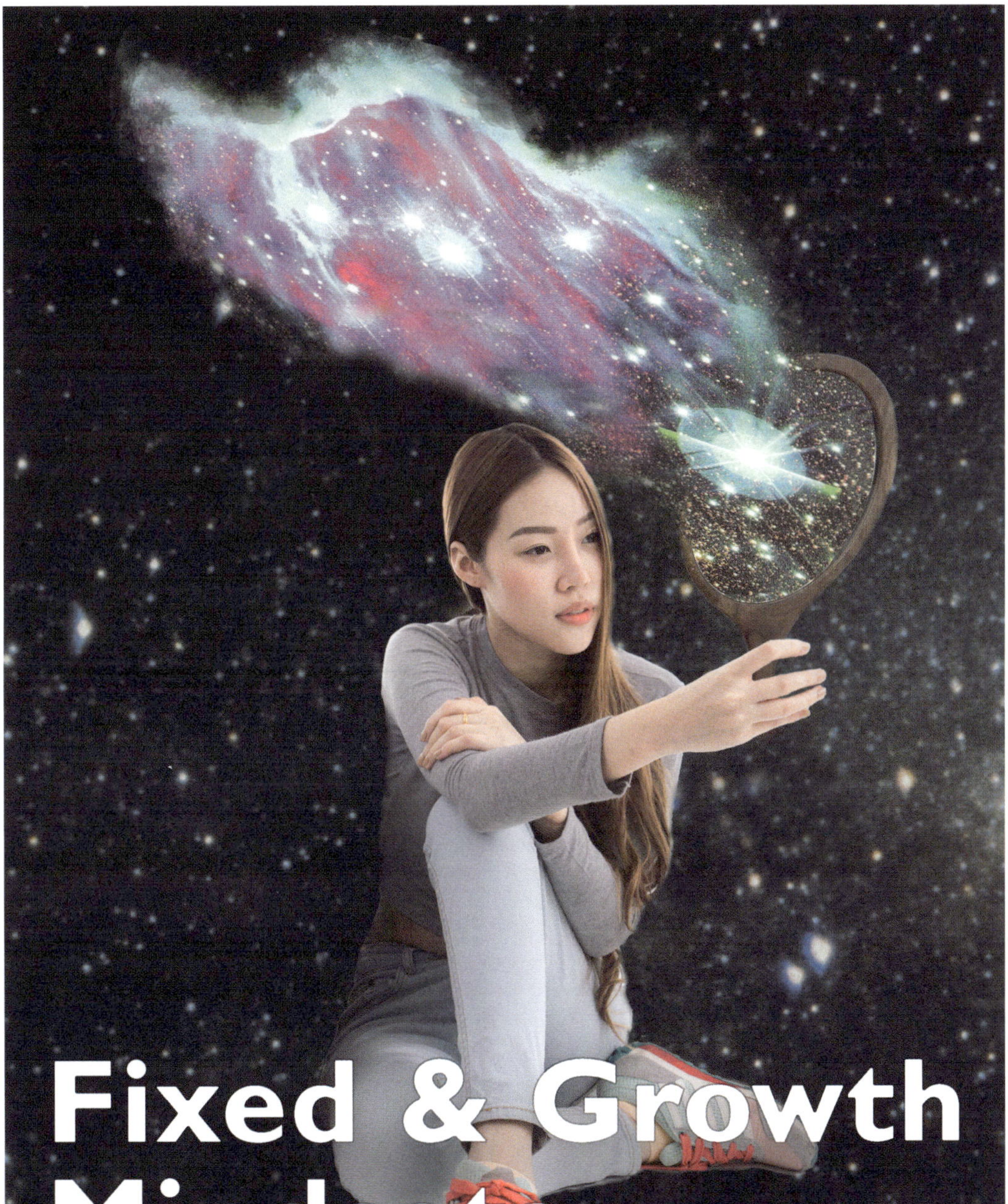
Fixed & Growth
Mindsets

Module 2: Fixed and Growth Mindsets

In Module 2, participants explore the differences between a fixed mindset and a growth mindset. They become attuned to how their mindset can impact how they confront challenges, perceive obstacles and effort, receive criticism, and ultimately achieve their full potential.

Module Topic	Minutes to Allot	
Learning Outcomes By reflecting on and responding to six scenarios regarding markers of fixed and growth mindsets, participants: • Distinguish between fixed and growth mindsets • Examine and assess their mindset patterns • Explore ways to nurture a growth mindset	5	5
Opening Activities Start the module with a relaxation or mindfulness practice Invite participants to share a few events from their gratitude journal that have occurred since the last session Invite questions about the previous module and practice(s)	10	15
Illustration of Core Concepts Review core concepts and show video illustrations Facilitate reflection and discussion: • *What are the key messages in the video(s) you just watched?* • *How might these concepts be relevant in your life?*	15	15
Practice: Identify Your Mindset Reactions Invite participants to share examples of situations in which they tend to rely on either a fixed or growth mindset Have participants complete *Worksheet: Common Situations and Reactions* Debrief learning from the practice using the questions: • *Which situations in everyday life did you find yourself approaching with a fixed mindset?* • *Which ones did you approach with a growth mindset?* • *What did you learn about yourself in relation to fixed and growth mindsets?*	20	30
Closing Activities Invite discussion of everyday applications Remind participants of relevant resources at the end of the module Guide participants in a 3-minute closing relaxation or mindfulness practice	10	10
Total	60 minutes	75 minutes

Core Concepts of Fixed and Growth Mindsets

Many of the themes here are also presented in the Core Concepts section of the Workbook (p. 43):

- A *mindset* is an attitude or belief that determines how individuals interpret a situation and how they respond (Dweck, 2006).
- A *fixed mindset* regards skills, abilities, and personal qualities as largely *unchangeable*, whereas a *growth mindset* regards skills, abilities, and personal qualities as *changeable*. The differences between a fixed and growth mindset are summarized in Figure 2, which is based on the

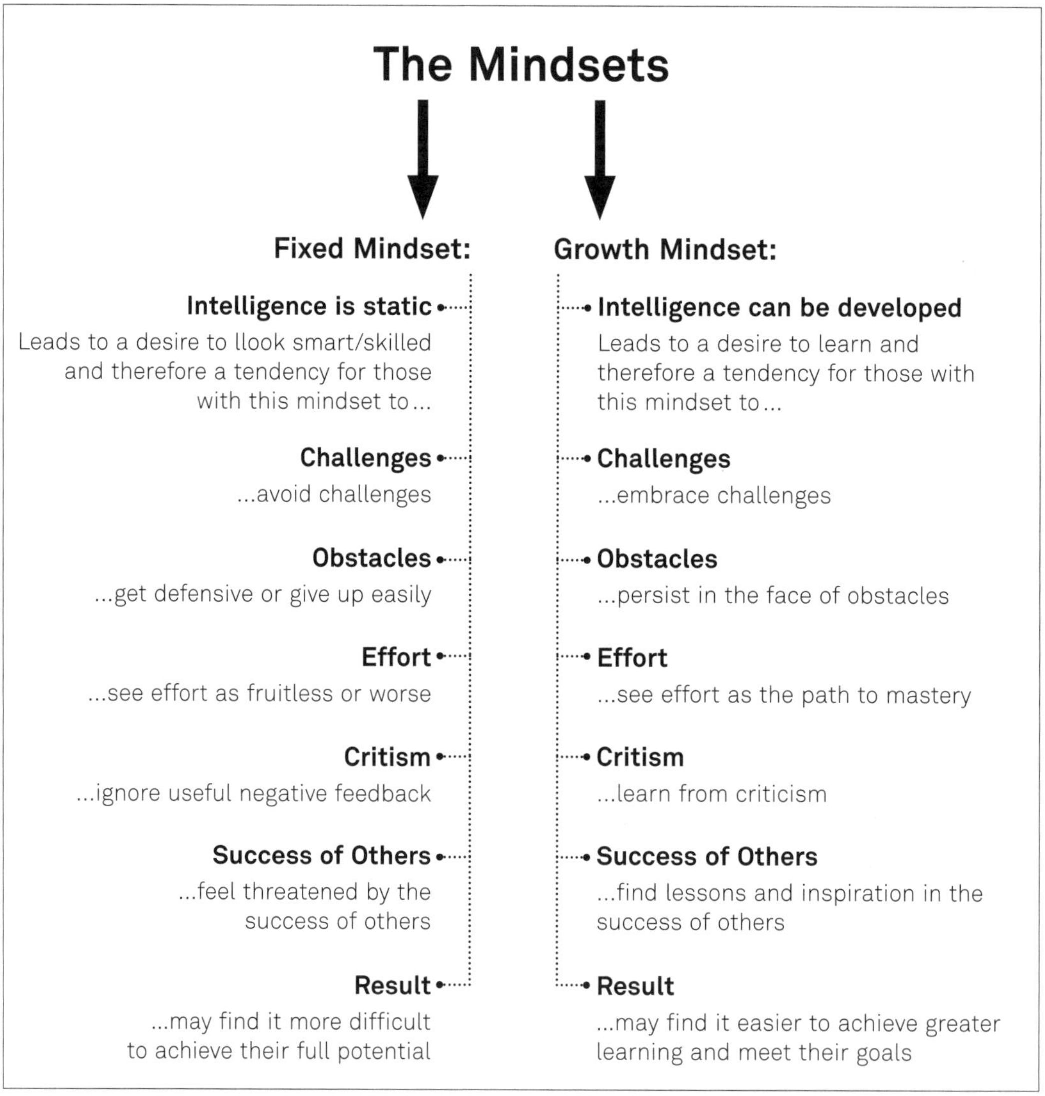

Figure 2. Differences between fixed and growth mindsets (Figure WB1 on p. 43 in the Workbook). Based on Figure 3.5 in Scarbrough (2023) by Ian Joslin licensed under CC BY 4.0, https://creativecommons.org/licenses/by/4.0/

pioneering work of Carol Dweck (2006). These mindsets, in turn, affect how we think about opportunities, efforts, and obstacles. A growth mindset tends to be associated with strengths such as persistence, prudence, humility, self-regulation, and curiosity.

- Individuals with a fixed mindset believe their basic abilities, intelligence, and talents are fixed characteristics or traits. They have a certain amount, and their goal is to look smart or competent all the time and never look stupid or unskilled. Individuals with a growth mindset understand that their talents and abilities can be developed through effort, good teaching, and persistence. They don't necessarily think everyone's the same or anyone can be Einstein, but they believe everyone can get smarter if they work at it (Dweck, 2012).
- Interventions based on a growth mindset have been applied in schools and other settings. Some studies have found significant benefits of interventions on students' achievement, behavior, and symptoms of depression and anxiety (e.g., Schleider & Weiss, 2018; Yeager et al., 2019; Yeager & Dweck, 2012). Although a recent meta-analysis found only small effects on achievement and no overall effect on mindsets (Macnamara & Burgoyne, 2022), another meta-analytic review suggests that growth mindset interventions positively impact academic achievement, mental health, and social abilities when they are delivered with high fidelity and target individuals who are likely to show the greatest benefits (e.g., groups experiencing substantial challenges) (Burnette et al., 2023).
- Mindset is also important in many other areas of life, including interpersonal relationships, resilience, and developing strengths and skills (Martin, 2015). People with a growth mindset, for example, are more likely to believe that refugees can assimilate into a host society and are more likely to support them (Madan et al., 2019). Research has found that the belief that social attributes can be developed is linked to lower levels of aggression in adolescents (Yeager & Dweck, 2012). Interventions that teach a growth mindset have been found to reduce students' behavior problems (Yeager & Dweck, 2012) and symptoms of depression (Miu & Yeager, 2015; Schleider & Weisz, 2018).
- Our mindsets can differ across situations. We may have more of a growth mindset in some situations but less in others. For example, a person may have a fixed mindset concerning mathematics skills and a growth mindset for learning a new language. Our mindset in new situations may differ from that in regularly occurring situations. We may have more of a growth mindset if the activity or challenge utilizes our existing strengths, talents, and abilities. However, if the task requires us to develop our skills and strengths further, we may initially be hesitant due to a fixed mindset.
- For participants, a growth mindset is critical because it helps them develop their personality and optimize their potential. Although committing to this growth mindset can be challenging, it eventually builds resilience. Participants with a growth mindset are more likely to cultivate their personality by acquiring specific skills. They tend to learn from the constructive criticism of their teachers and peers rather than ignore it or perceive it as an attack on them. They find inspiration in the success of others rather than feel threatened by their success (Gutshall, 2013; Hochanadel & Finamore, 2015; Richards & Huppert, 2011).

Illustrations of Fixed and Growth Mindsets

Play at least one of the three video illustrations of the core concept.

MINDSET
https://youtu.be/2nF90sAW-Yg
(Duration: 7:22 minutes)
The video shows an animated message that explains core beliefs about a fixed mindset.

Growth Mindset vs. Fixed Mindset
https://youtu.be/KUWn_TJTrnU
(Duration: 5:03 minutes)
This hand-drawn video explains the two mindsets in an easy-to-understand and educational manner.

Identify: Growth or Fixed Mindset?
(Duration: 4:53 minutes)
https://youtu.be/3vz6HU1LlOU
This video clip tests your understanding of growth and fixed mindsets by showing six popular media clips that display the main character using one or the other.

Reflection and Discussion

Ask the participants to complete the Reflection and Discussion section in their Workbook (p. 45) and to address the following question:

What are the key messages in the video(s) you just watched?

How might these concepts be relevant in your life?

Practice: Identify Your Mindset Reactions

The goal of this module's practice is to build participants' ability to distinguish between a fixed mindset and a growth mindset. The practice invites participants to explore their own tendencies to employ a fixed or growth mindset depending on the learning situation.

Worksheet: Common Situations and Reactions (below, also on p. 46 of Workbook) is a fill-in-the-blank worksheet that asks participants to reflect on how they might typically respond to three common learning situations. It also prompts them to think about their own definitions of success and failure. Together these six queries provide a foundation for the group to discuss aspects of fixed and growth mindsets.

Facilitate the practice by adapting the following steps to your audience and program:

- Refer participants to the Worksheet on p. 46 of their Workbook, which lists six brief scenarios/situations. Allow sufficient time for participants to read these and respond to these scenarios in writing.

- Read each scenario aloud, taking time to discuss participants' responses before moving to the next scenario. Discuss how our responses to various situations are influenced by our mindset. Also discuss how our mindset is influenced by our cultural context (e.g., familial, extended family, cultural, ethnic, or national community).
- Underscore the point that most of us fall on a continuum, with growth and fixed mindsets at the poles. Therefore, it is normal to find it hard to locate themselves on one side of the continuum. Also note that people can have different mindsets in different academic subjects or domains of life.
- Emphasize that our mindset can either help or hinder our resilience and well-being.

Worksheet: Common Situations and Reactions (WB, p. 46)

	Situations and reactions in everyday life	F/G
1	My instructor wrote a lot of comments on my assignment, highlighting areas that I need to improve. My reaction was: ____________ ____________	
2	When I struggle with a subject at school or a project at work, my first thought is: ____________ ____________	
3	When I think about trying something new, I feel ____________ and think ____________	
4	People who excel at something do so because: ____________ ____________	
5	When I see other people accomplishing something noteworthy, my first reaction is: ____________ ____________	
6	To me, failure means: ____________ ____________	

Practice Debrief

After participants have completed the worksheet (p. 46), invite them to complete the Practice Debrief in their Workbook (p. 47). To debrief this activity, discuss the following questions:

Which situations in everyday life did you find yourself approaching with a fixed mindset?
Which ones did you approach with a growth mindset?
What did you learn about yourself in relation to fixed and growth mindsets?

Learning and Cultural Fit

Adapt this practice to the learning and cultural needs of your participants' and their unique values and demographics. Keep the following in mind:

- Rarely does anyone have a fixed or growth mindset in all situations. Someone can have a fixed mindset in one domain (e.g., self-sufficient and not willing to accept help at home) but have a growth mindset in another domain (e.g., co-operative learner at work). These mindset differences can sometimes also be attributed to cultural norms.
- Mindset can also vary by the type of situation. We may find that we have more of a growth mindset in some situations, but less in others. These differences could be due to our family, culture, or socioeconomic factors. Furthermore, our mindset in new situations might differ from that in regularly occurring situations. During the initial stages of a task, we may be hesitant due to a fixed mindset. As the task evolves, we may show more of a growth mindset.
- Recognize the limits of focusing on effort alone when promoting a growth mindset. For example, when encouraging a growth mindset for a participant with a specific learning disability (SLD), increasing effort alone may not lead to anticipated success without additional support or learning new strategies.
- Equating growth mindset with effort, for the most part, would be erroneous. Effort indeed is critical, but effort alone may not be enough for success. One needs innovative strategies and different solutions which are contextually relevant. Also, one needs to know when and how to apply one specific strategy and when to switch to a different one, according to situational demands. Asking for advice or help can also signify a growth mindset in that we are open to different perspectives and approaches.
- A growth mindset can to be fostered by structuring tasks in manageable steps that help participants to start, continue, and complete them. It helps to provide clear instructions for how the participant should think about their own progress throughout the completion of the task.
- Encouraging a persistent and focused effort will motivate participants to continue learning. Avoid using general or overused statements such as "do your best" or "keep working." Instead, have participants set learning and task goals that help them realize they may not be at their best "*yet*." Table 4 shows some "yet" examples.

Table 4. Examples of "not yet" language to get to a growth mindset (adapted from Dweck, 2012)

Fixed mindset	Growth mindset
My assignments/projects are so disorganized	*I have not yet started to organize my assignments and projects.*
I am not good at origami.	*I have not yet taken time to learn origami.*
Math makes me really anxious.	*I have yet to learn strategies to cope with my math anxiety.*
I am extremely reluctant to submit my assignment or project until it is perfect.	*I have yet to learn how to distinguish between perfect and good-enough work.*
I eat junk food when I am stressed.	*I have not yet learned ways of coping with stress.*
I will never be able to forgive my ex-boyfriend.	*I have not yet forgiven my ex-boyfriend.*

Closing Activities

The goal of closing the module is to help participants integrate their understanding of fixed and growth mindsets and to take their new learning into everyday life.

Discuss with participants the Everyday Applications section, also found on p. 48 in their Workbook. Invite participants to be mindful in their day-to-day lives by noticing actions and habits which show their mindset habits or those of others. Encourage them to use relevant resources found at the end of this module, some of which are included in their workbooks starting on p. 49.

Choose a 3-minute mindfulness activity from Regular Practice 1: Mindfulness and Relaxation to close the module.

Everyday Applications

- When facing new situations, remind yourself: "I'm just new at this." Recall that learning new skills can be challenging. It feels comfortable to do what we already know how to do. Going outside our comfort zone can help us to grow and develop new skills.
- Peers, family members, teachers, and the media can make us think we have to be the best, the smartest, the most talented, the most popular. You can nurture a growth mindset in everyday life by refocusing; rather than aiming to be the best, we can discover that many everyday life endeavors can be more satisfying if we consider only our own personal improvement. This makes our efforts fulfilling, focused, and, most importantly, flexible in responding to challenges.
- Many challenges require that we learn or modify our habits of mind. There is no shortcut to practice. Break down everyday challenges (especially ones you are less confident about) into discrete steps that need to be practiced. This will help you to understand and improve each aspect of the task. Continue doing this and you will develop patience for practice. For instance, if you are unable to master one specific step, you can tell yourself, "While I have mastered the previous one, I need to practice this specific component." This will help you to quiet the inner critic ("I am not good at this and can never be" or "this is too hard"). You can foster a healthier approach by saying to yourself, "I need more practice on this specific aspect of the task, and then I will improve."
- You can nurture your growth mindset in pursuing everyday challenges by having multiple paths, multiple approaches, and multiple resources. For example, if one strategy for approaching a difficult task is not working, then try a different strategy. Be willing to ask knowledgeable others for help in coming up with new strategies. The more strategies you learn, the more strategies you will have available to you in approaching other challenges.
- Notice when and where you use more fixed-mindset statements. Try using "yet" statements when trying to motivate yourself or others. For example, "I have not mastered this specific theorem yet" reminds us that effort causes positive change and can influence what kind of person we will be in the future.
- It is critical when working with others in a team, or in any collaborative endeavor, that we provide positive feedback to the group regarding effort and process, as much as we do for the outcomes. This helps to promote a growth mindset in others.

References

Burnette, J. L., Billingsley, J., Banks, G. C., Knouse, L. E., Hoyt, C. L., Pollack, J. M., & Simon, S. (2023). A systematic review and meta-analysis of growth mindset interventions: For whom, how, and why might such interventions work? *Psychological Bulletin, 149*(3-4), 174–205. https://doi.org/10.1037/bul0000368

Dweck, C. S. (2006). *Mindset: The new psychology of success*. Random House.

Dweck, C. S. (2012). *Mindset: How you can fulfil your potential.* Constable & Robinson.

Gutshall, C. A. (2013). Teachers' mindsets for participants with and without disabilities. *Psychology in the Schools, 50*(10), 1073–1083. https://doi.org/10.1002/pits.21725

Hochanadel, A., & Finamore, D. (2015). Fixed and growth mindset in education and how grit helps participants persist in the face of adversity. *Journal of International Education Research, 11*(1), 47.

Macnamara, B. N., & Burgoyne, A. P. (2022). Do growth mindset interventions impact students' academic achievement? A systematic review and meta-analysis with recommendations for best practices. *Psychological Bulletin*. Advance online publication. https://doi.org/10.1037/bul0000352

Madan, S., Basu, S., Rattan, A., & Savani, K. (2019). Support for resettling refugees: The role of fixed versus growth mind-sets. *Psychological Science, 30*(2), 238–249. https://doi.org/10.1177/0956797618813561

Martin, A. J. (2015). Growth approaches to academic development: Research into academic trajectories and growth assessment, goals, and mindsets. *British Journal of Educational Psychology, 85*(2), 133–137. https://doi.org/10.1111/bjep.12071

Miu, A. S., & Yeager, D. S. (2015). Preventing symptoms of depression by teaching adolescents that people can change: Effects of a brief incremental theory of personality intervention at 9-month follow-up. *Clinical Psychological Science, 3*(5), 726–743. https://doi.org/10.1177/2167702614548317

Richards, M., & Huppert, F. A. (2011). Do positive children become positive adults? Evidence from a longitudinal birth cohort study. *Journal of Positive Psychology, 6*(1), 75–87. https://doi.org/10.1080/17439760.2011.536655

Scarbrough, S. (2023). *Psychology of human relations*. Open Oregon Educational Resources. https://openoregon.pressbooks.pub/psychologyofhumanrelations/

Schleider, J., & Weisz, J. (2018). A single-session growth mindset intervention for adolescent anxiety and depression: 9-month outcomes of a randomized trial. *Journal of Child Psychology and Psychiatry, and Allied Disciplines, 59*(2), 160–170. https://doi.org/10.1111/jcpp.12811

Yeager, D. S., & Dweck, C. S. (2012). Mindsets that promote resilience: When students believe that personal characteristics can be developed. *Educational Psychologist, 47*(4), 302–314. https://doi.org/10.1080/00461520.2012.722805

Yeager, D. S., Hanselman, P., Walton, G. M., Murray, J. S., Crosnoe, R., Muller, C., Tipton, E., Schneider, B., Hulleman, C. S., Hinojosa, C. P., Paunesku, D., Romero, C., Flint, K., Roberts, A., Trott, J., Iachan, R., Buontempo, J., Man Yang, S., Carvalho, C. M, ... Dweck, C. S. (2019). A national experiment reveals where a growth mindset improves achievement. *Nature, 573*(7774), 364–369. https://doi.org/10.1038/s41586-019-1466-y

Resources

Literature

Chan, D. W. (2012). Life satisfaction, happiness, and the growth mindset of healthy and unhealthy perfectionists among Hong Kong Chinese gifted participants. *Roeper Review, 34*(4), 224–233. https://doi.org/10.1080/02783193.2012.715333

Dweck, C. (2014). Teachers' mindsets: "Every student has something to teach me": Feeling overwhelmed? Where did your natural teaching talent go? Try pairing a growth mindset with reasonable goals, patience, and reflection instead. It's time to get gritty and be a better teacher. *Educational Horizons, 93*(2), 10–15. https://doi.org/10.1177/0013175X14561420

Dweck, C. S. (2012). *Mindset: How you can fulfil your potential.* Constable & Robinson.

Gutshall, C. A. (2013). Teachers' mindsets for participants with and without disabilities. *Psychology in the Schools, 50*(10), 1073–1083. https://doi.org/10.1002/pits.21725

Hildrew, C. (2018). *Becoming a growth mindset school: The power of mindset to transform teaching, leadership and learning.* Routledge. https://doi.org/10.4324/9781315179506

Hochanadel, A., & Finamore, D. (2015). Fixed and growth mindset in education and how grit helps participants persist in the face of adversity. *Journal of International Education Research, 11*(1), 47.

Jennifer, A. S., Shumow, L., & Kackar-Cam, H. (2015). Exploring teacher effects for mindset intervention outcomes in seventh-grade science classes. *Middle Grades Research Journal, 10*(2), 17.

Martin, A. J. (2015). Growth approaches to academic development: Research into academic trajectories and growth assessment, goals, and mindsets. *British Journal of Educational Psychology, 85*(2), 133–137. https://doi.org/10.1111/bjep.12071

Nebolsine, E. (2020). *The grit workbook for kids: CBT skills to help kids cultivate a growth mindset and build resilience.* New Harbinger.

Nottingham, J., & Larsson, B. (2018). *Challenging mindset: Why a growth mindset makes a difference in learning – and what to do when it doesn't.* Crown.

Richards, M., & Huppert, F. A. (2011). Do positive children become positive adults? Evidence from a longitudinal birth cohort study. *Journal of Positive Psychology, 6*(1), 75–87. https://doi.org/10.1080/17439760.2011.536655

Sheehan, K., & Ryan, J. (2017). *Growing a growth mindset: Unlocking character strengths through children's literature.* Rowman & Littlefield.

Websites

Growth Mindset vs. Fixed Mindset
https://youtu.be/KUWn_TJTrnU
This animation distinguishes between two mindsets with helpful examples from daily life.

The Power of Believing That You Can Improve
https://www.ted.com/talks/carol_dweck_the_power_of_believing_that_you_can_improve
In this TEDxNorrkoping series talk, Carol Dweck, the researcher who introduced the concept of mindset, argues that learning about our mindset can help to increase our brain's capacity to learn and solve problems.

Mindset Kit
https://www.mindsetkit.org/
This free online resource offers lessons and practices that teach adaptive thinking skills.

Multimedia

Growth Mindset Introduction: What It Is, How It WORKS, and Why It Matters
https://youtu.be/75GFzikmRY0
A growth mindset creates the foundation for greater learning, and research shows that it can improve our ability to grow and develop, in all areas of life.

The Most Powerful Mindset for Success
https://youtu.be/qjBdcyueom8
The video explains how a growth mindset is associated with success.

Seven Reasons Why Smart Hardworking People Don't Become Successful
https://www.youtube.com/watch?v=cqINcpbcZqs
The video explains seven reasons one might not be finding success despite being smart and hardworking.

Change Your Mindset, Change the Game
https://youtu.be/0tqq66zwa7g
Alia Crum presents solid scientific evidence to show the influence of mindset on the body, and how changing one's mindset can produce significantly different results.

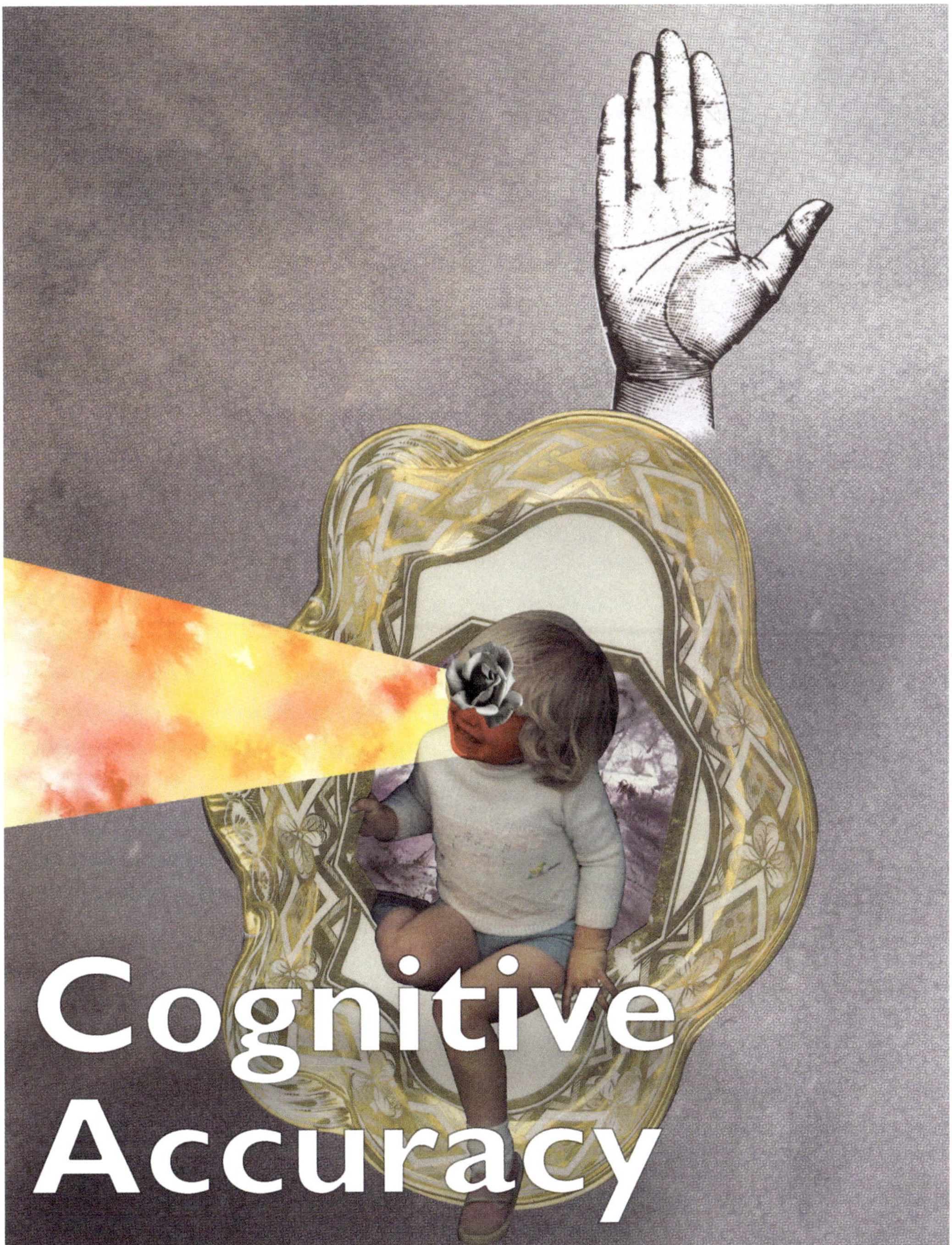
Cognitive
Accuracy

Module 3: Cognitive Accuracy

In Module 3, participants examine more closely thought patterns that can distort their perception of experiences. By learning about common thinking shortcuts that can lead to faulty conclusions, participants can check their thinking and develop more accurate and helpful cognitive responses.

Module Topic	Minutes to Allot	
Learning Outcomes By writing about a recent challenge, and noticing emotions, actions and thoughts associated with it, participants: • Recognize thinking tendencies that can lead to inaccurate interpretations and affect their reactions • Develop more accurate and helpful perceptions about their thoughts, emotions, and reactions	5	5
Opening Activities Start the module with a relaxation or mindfulness practice Invite participants to share a few events from their gratitude journal that have occurred since the last session Invite questions about the previous module and practice(s)	10	15
Illustration of Core Concepts Review core concepts and show video illustrations Facilitate reflection and discussion: • *What are the key messages in the video(s) you just watched?* • *How might these concepts be relevant in your life?*	15	15
Practice: 1) Unpack Experiences to Understand Challenges Invite participants to brainstorm challenges they have yet to overcome Have participants complete *Worksheet: Unpack Experiences to Understand Challenges*, detailing their challenge, and their associated thoughts or beliefs and reactions **Practice: 2) Explore Your Thinking Shortcuts** Review the seven thinking shortcuts with participants and invite them to share examples of each shortcut Invite participants to assess each challenge identified in Practice 1 in relation to thinking shortcuts Debrief learning from practice with question: • *Which shortcuts do you use most frequently?* • *What might be the consequences of relying on these shortcuts?*	20	30
Closing Activities Invite discussion of everyday applications Remind participants of relevant resources at the end of the module Guide participants in a 3-minute closing relaxation or mindfulness practice	10	10
Total	60 minutes	75 minutes

Core Concepts of Cognitive Accuracy

Many of the themes here are also presented in the Core Concepts section of the Workbook (p. 51):

- Cognitive Accuracy (Module 3) and Cognitive Flexibility (Module 4) are based on the premise that the human mind is not a passive container of information. In fact, it is inundated with information that comes from a number of sources, including external environmental stimuli and internal bodily sensations. To manage this information, the human mind tries to process this information in its own way. Thus, our thinking preferences and patterns develop.
- Emotions are as important to our perceptual apparatus as thinking is. Humans respond to events that happen around them. For example, the sound of a police siren, a gunshot, or a thunderstorm elicit emotions in us. Our emotional reactions are largely influenced by our thinking that takes place in the heat of the moment. If we interpret the sound of the police siren as alarming, as many people do, a range of emotions associated with fear may arise. If we work for the police, we may not interpret the siren as alarming and experience fear, but rather vigilance or readiness to act. Likewise, in the interpersonal realm, two individuals can react differently to the same situation. For example, a partner leaving the relationship: One may feel depressed and lonely if the relationship was valued, another may feel relieved if the relationship was toxic and stressful.
- Thoughts and feelings influence each other. Our feelings can also color our interpretations. Cognitive behavioral therapy (CBT), in essence, deals with the cluster of thoughts, feelings, and behaviors. The causal order may not be as important as recognizing that they influence each other. Often these thoughts, feelings, and behaviors are habitual responses or shortcuts, which may be inaccurate and out of proportion to the situation. Relying on these shortcuts can make it difficult for us to respond thoughtfully in ways that reflect our goals.
- The average healthy adult experiences about 6,000 thoughts in a day (Tseng & Poppenk, 2020). If we attended to all thoughts, we would be overwhelmed. So, we rely on habits of filtering these thoughts. For example, we focus on what appears most salient to us and conclude that this is particularly meaningful. This automatic filtering can lead us to biases, such as focusing on certain aspects of information while ignoring other parts. Some of these biases may be shaped by sociocultural circumstances, i.e., socioeconomic status, family, school, and community. This may lead to making thinking errors which are called cognitive distortions or in SBR's framework, thinking shortcuts.
- We may assume that challenges, setbacks, failures, and adversities determine our reactions (feelings or actions; Figure 3).
- However, scientific research shows it is our thinking that determines our reactions (Ellis, 1962). When we unpack an experience, we find the following three parts – challenge, thought, and reaction (Figure 4):
  - **Challenge:** A setback, failure, or difficulty. Table 5 lists examples (Table WB1 in the Workbook).
  - **Thought:** Thinking habits or beliefs about causes of the setback, failure, or difficulty. These are sometimes related to thinking patterns/habits or to deeper beliefs that may or may not be accurate or helpful (Helmond et al., 2015). Thoughts generate reactions. Table 6 lists some thoughts that can be associated with these challenges.
  - **Reaction:** Our feelings and actions that result from our thoughts or beliefs about a particular challenge. Table 5 illustrates emotions or reactions that can result from these thoughts.

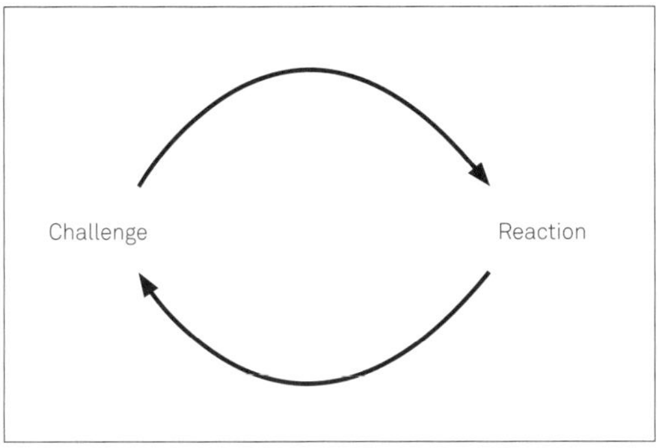

Figure 3. Challenge and reaction cycle (Figure WB2 in the Workbook).

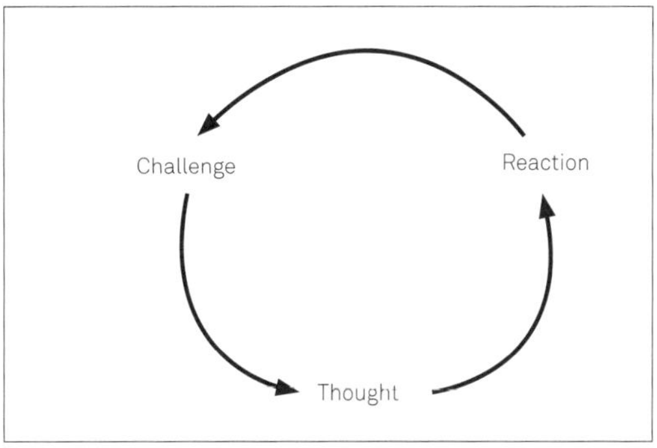

Figure 4. Cognitive-behavioral model: Challenge, thought, and reaction cycle (Figure WB3 in the Workbook).

Table 5. Unpacking experiences (Table WB1 in the Workbook)

Challenge	Thought or belief	Reaction
A friend spreads misinformation online about you.	I have been treated unfairly.	Anger
You are not selected for this year's award or promotion, which you believe you deserve.	I am not good enough; I do not think that I will ever be selected.	Sadness
During exams or project presentations, despite preparing well, you become nervous and are unable to recall material.	I am going to fail the exam. Due to my poor presentation, I am not going to do well on this project.	Fear, anxiety
Your friend tells you that they are hurt by something you said.	I cannot be a loyal friend.	Guilt, shame

- Our reactions in turn impact how we perceive challenges. When we stop to identify thoughts, especially when they are inaccurate or unhelpful, we can prevent reactions that can worsen a situation.
- Unpacking our challenges can help us identify thinking shortcuts – automatic assumptions we tend to make, often without much evidence to support them! We use shortcuts automatically to get through life. Shortcuts allow us to avoid having to think long and deeply about our experiences and decisions. So shortcuts are helpful in some situations, but sometimes they can get us into trouble, especially when they lead us to make interpretations that are not accurate or helpful.
- Thinking shortcuts affect a wide range of interpretations, including thoughts about what is happening in the present moment, what has happened in the past to cause an event, what will happen in the future, or what a particular experience means about us, others, or the world.
- When we are dealing with challenges, our attention becomes narrow, and we tend to focus on protecting ourselves. In this defensive mode, we focus more on aspects of the situation which threaten us. It is normal and often necessary to use thinking shortcuts. However, we need self-awareness to know where their usage may not be helpful.

Illustrations of Cognitive Accuracy

After watching one or more of the following videos, facilitate a group discussion to make sure that everyone understands automatic thoughts and related cognitive traps. This understanding is important for the next activity.

The ABCs of CBT: Thoughts, Feelings and Behavior
https://youtu.be/Stw9P38ePVI?si=cCUEU7L9ND63WcZt
(Duration: 6:44 minutes)
This clip explains the ABCs of cognitive behavioral therapy (CBT) – that is, the relationship between thoughts, feelings, and behavior.

Automatic Thoughts
http://www.youtube.com/watch?v=m2zRA5zCA6M
(Duration: 4:53 minutes)
This video explains the concept of automatic thoughts – negative thinking patterns that can creep into our mind and be harmful for our health. It then goes through an exercise to replace these thoughts with healthier options.

Identifying Automatic Thoughts
https://youtu.be/6uklmsylb54
(Duration: 3:29 minutes)
In this video, a cognitive behavioral therapist describes the process of identifying emotions and related automatic thoughts.

Rethinking Thinking
(Duration: 5:21 minutes)
https://www.ted.com/talks/trevor_maber_rethinking_thinking
This TED-Ed video explains how we develop beliefs about the world through the "ladder of inference."

Thoughts, Feelings and Behaviors
https://youtu.be/PcFmrVZ0e-I?si=a2_THD4Z518GzQ9Q
(Duration: 3:16 minutes)
This video clip distinguishes between thoughts, feelings, and behaviors. It describes how these three elements influence each other and impact our mental health.

Paul Potts sings Nessun Dorma
https://www.youtube.com/watch?v=1k08yxu57NA
(Duration: 4:10 minutes)
In a clip from *Britain's Got Talent*, a socially shy salesman, Paul Potts, receives feedback that indicates several thinking shortcuts by the judges.

Dr. David Burns on How Our Thoughts Can Shape Our Lives
https://youtu.be/3AeLhieSyJw
(Duration: 4:14 minutes)
David Burns, author of *The Feeling Good Handbook*, discusses how our thoughts can shape our lives.

Reflection and Discussion

Invite participants to complete the Reflection and Discussion section of their Workbook (p. 54) regarding the video(s) they have watched. Discuss the questions:

What are the key messages in the video(s) you just watched?

How might these concepts be relevant in your life?

Practice 1: Unpack Experiences to Understand Challenges

Vividly recalling accompanying thoughts, beliefs, and emotions from negative events is not easy. Often our recall is influenced by situational factors such as our mood before or at the time of recall, or the events that transpired after the challenge. Therefore, in everyday life, it can sometimes be helpful to pause the flow of events and deliberate in order to unpack our negative experiences. It appears simple but can be challenging for participants. It takes time and practice to master the skills of cognitive accuracy.

Module 3: Cognitive Accuracy is designed to help participants understand their negative experiences by parsing them into challenges, reactions (emotional and behavioral), and underlying thoughts or thinking patterns that might be driving their reactions. Participants learn that by identifying their thoughts associated with negative experiences, they will be able to make better sense of them. In the coming modules, they will learn to deploy other resources to mitigate the impact of negative reactions.

This practice helps participants to disentangle beliefs, thoughts, and reactions systematically. Using the cognitive behavioral framework (Figure 4), participants apply cognitive behavioral skills to understand their challenges, reactions, thoughts, and beliefs about negative experiences.

Facilitate this practice by adapting the following steps to your audience and program:

- Start the practice by having participants take a couple of deep breaths, with their eyes either closed or fixed on an object close to the floor.
- Refer participants to their worksheet, Practice 1: Unpack Experiences to Understand Challenges (Workbook, p. 55). Ask them to brainstorm challenges they are trying to overcome. These could be recent situations in daily life that are stressful or that they would like to handle better. Encourage them to search for challenges that cause strong negative emotions, such as anger, anxiety, sadness, or guilt, or a mix of these emotions. See sample situations in Table 5 (Table WB1 in Workbook) and Table 6.
- Challenge: Encourage participants to be specific and factual in writing about these challenges. They should report only the facts of the situation, i.e., what would be observable to another person. For example, "I didn't complete an important assignment on time" or "a friend has told me a few times that I should lose weight." or "I lose my temper quickly when explaining something to my younger sibling." Invite them to recall, as vividly as possible, the accompanying thoughts they had in their head when the challenge took place.

- Thought/belief: Ask participants to recall and write about the thoughts they experienced at the time of the challenge. As discussed in the Core Concepts, a typical person, on average, experiences at least 6,000 thoughts in a day.
- Reaction: Ask participants to write about their feelings and behaviors.
- When facilitating this practice, ensure that participants are able to connect their feelings with thoughts that make sense to them and help them understand why they become angry. Notice when participants are able to recall thoughts that accompanied the negative emotions they experienced. For example, consider a participant who is angry that someone is spreading slanderous news about them on social media. Ask the person to think back to the moment they first learned about the gossip. What were their thoughts at that moment? Are they typically associated with anger, e.g., my rights have been violated; I have been treated unfairly (see Table 6).

Table 6. Sample challenges for Practice 1

Challenges	Thoughts and beliefs	Reactions
Someone says and does something offensive. You are accused or implicated for doing something that you have not done. Someone steals or deprives you of something without your consent or permission.	*I have been treated unfairly. My rights have been violated.*	Angry, annoyed, frustrated, outraged, offended, exasperated
You lose a loved one, or a cherished relationship breaks down. You lose an important object or position for which you have worked hard.	*I wonder if I will ever be able to regain this relationship or position.* *I am not good enough. I am not competitive enough.*	Sad, grieving, blue, melancholic, dismayed
Despite preparing for the important presentation, you find in the moment that you forget a couple of key points. As an event you organized is unfolding, you notice some hiccups that will likely mean it doesn't go as well as you hoped. You find yourself preoccupied about the outcome of an event or situation about which you now can't do much.	*I am not a good presenter. I cannot handle the pressure of presentation, no matter how well I prepare.* *I cannot successfully organize an event.* *I always expect the worst possible outcome.*	Afraid, anxious, panicked, alarmed, doubtful, ambivalent
You say something that brings your loved one to tears. A friend tells you that they are hurt by a comment you made about them.	*Despite my good intentions, I end up hurting my loved ones. I am unable to live up to my own standards.*	Guilty, ashamed, regretful, self-blaming

Worksheet: Unpack Experiences to Understand Challenges

Challenge	Thought/belief	Reaction

Practice 2: Explore Your Thinking Shortcuts

Practice 2 builds on Practice 1, helping participants to understand patterns of errors in their thinking by exploring seven habitual thinking shortcuts that we rely on given the fast pace of life. These shortcuts can lead us to draw conclusions that do not always reflect the facts of the situation.

Understanding our thinking shortcuts is especially important when we react strongly to a challenge (or experience the same challenge repeatedly). This practice provides insight to seven common shortcuts that people use in everyday life. It also invites participants to consider their unique tendencies or signature patterns.

Facilitate this practice by adapting the following steps to your audience and program:

- Have participants read the seven thinking shortcuts listed in the box below (Workbook pp. 56–57), allowing them time to reflect and write their reactions in the space beneath each thinking shortcut. Encourage participants to also think about the consequences of relying on thinking shortcuts.
- Ask participants to pair up and discuss their reflections for about five minutes.
- Alternatively, facilitators can discuss each of the seven thinking shortcuts with the entire group. Ask the group which thinking shortcuts are most common and which ones cause most distress.
- Invite participants to reflect on how they can develop accurate thinking (cognitive accuracy) after completing Practice 1 and Practice 2.

Examples of Common Thinking Shortcuts for Practice 2

1. Jumping to Conclusions
Coming to a firm conclusion even though you have no information to support it.
Example: I will fail this class because I did poorly on the test.

2. Tunnel Vision
Selecting only one piece of information and dwelling on it exclusively, ignoring other important information.
Example: My school experience is terrible because I don't like math class.

3. Magnifying and Minimizing
Magnifying is perceiving a positive or a negative to be bigger than it is. Minimizing is perceiving a positive or a negative to be smaller than it is. Both are distortions of reality.
Examples: Magnifying: I look ugly because of my nose.
Minimizing: I only won this spelling trophy because I got lucky.

4. Personalizing
Holding yourself personally responsible for negative outcomes, even blaming yourself, even though several factors are responsible.
Example: She did not come to my birthday because she doesn't like me.

5. Externalizing
Holding others responsible for your problems and overlooking your role in the situation.
Example: I failed my math test because the instructor made the questions overly confusing.

6. Overgeneralizing
Drawing conclusions about all cases or situations based on one case or situation.
Example: My classmate from Holland is mean, so all Dutch people must be mean.

7. Mind Reading
Concluding what another person is thinking (usually negative) without consulting the person.
Example: I assume my friend is upset with me because of her facial expressions.

Practice Debrief

Invite participants to complete the reflection on Explore Your Thinking Shortcuts (WB, p. 58). To debrief cognitive accuracy, discuss the following questions:

> *Which shortcuts do you use most frequently? Think about this in different contexts, e.g., school, work, family, friends, leisure. What might be the consequences of relying on these shortcuts?*

Learning and Cultural Fit

Adapt this practice to the learning and cultural needs of your audience, its unique values and demographics. Possible adaptations include:

- Although the skills discussed in this module are helpful in understanding many problems, it is important to remember that not all emotions can be fully understood or controlled by rational thought alone. It is important that before trying to change an emotion, the instructor understands that they should avoid making participants feel that their emotional reactions are "right" or "wrong." Make sure that the goal of this exercise is to help participants to understand the relationship between their thoughts, emotions, and actions when they face challenges (Ready & Wright, 2011).
- Some participants may struggle to link their thoughts, emotions, and actions, and understand how they interact with each other in response to challenges, setbacks, and failures. To make it more concrete, encourage participants to practice that linking skill with the help of Table 6.
- Consistent with Table 5, Table 6 lists sample challenges in the four most commonly experienced negative emotions (anger, sadness, anxiety, and guilt). Also listed are common reactions and sample underlying thoughts and beliefs. It should be noted that negative emotions are not completely independent of each other. That is, the negative event may produce anger and sadness at the same time or sadness initially, followed by anger or guilt. The sample challenges, reactions, and thoughts and beliefs are also influenced by familial or larger cultural contexts.
- During Practice 1 and 2, some participants may struggle to accurately recall what they thought as the challenge unfolded. To support their accurate recall, probe participants about their emotional reaction: How strong was it? What did they do in response? Sometimes the reaction is inaction – that is, we do not do anything. Help them to use their emotional and behavioral reactions to explore their thoughts. Help them make the connections. For example, after being made fun of (challenge), Emma became quiet (reaction), and said to herself, "I am an unlikeable person" (thought).
- Participants from diverse backgrounds, e.g., culture, ethnicity, gender, may have learned different ways of understanding their own emotions, thoughts, and behaviors. Some may prioritize rational thought; others may emphasize emotional and somatic experiences. Furthermore, participants may have learned a specific way to interpret and respond to challenges. Invite participants to consider their family's models of and responses to emotional expression, their family's approach to problem-solving, and the power dynamics in decisions that suppress emotions.
- Be aware that many behaviors and emotional reactions are shaped by years of cultural/familial practices and habits and are not easy to change. However, this exercise can provide the first step of awareness.

Closing Activities

The goal of closing this module is to help participants integrate their understanding of cognitive accuracy and to take their new learning into everyday life.

Discuss with participants the Everyday Applications section, also found on p. 58 in their Workbook. Invite participants to be mindful in their day-to-day lives by noticing actions and habits which show their thinking shortcut habits or those of others. Encourage them to use relevant resources found at the end of this module and included in their workbooks starting on p. 59.

Choose a 3-minute mindfulness activity from Regular Practice 1: Mindfulness and Relaxation to close the module.

Everyday Applications

- Thinking is something we do every minute of every day. Our thinking can cause us problems and help us resolve them. Observe your thinking shortcuts. When you unpack your challenges, you may discover that you handle some situations well, while others test you. You may also discover specific patterns in how you handle certain challenges.
- Notice which thinking shortcuts you tend to rely on for clues about your own common thinking traps. Exploring one's thinking shortcuts offers individuals an opportunity to become aware of the specific patterns they use to understand and solve their problems. For example, a person who often uses the thinking shortcut of personalization is likely to be quite a sensitive person, while one using jumping to conclusions predominantly could be an anxious person. The thinking shortcut you use more often can offer you valuable insights into yourself and your specific approaches to solving problems. We all rely on these thinking shortcuts to make sense of complex experiences in a short period of time. Although these shortcuts help us, they can also trick us into thinking they are correct because they "popped into our heads" first. It can be helpful to remember that these are just our first thoughts about the situation, and ask ourselves, "How else can I look at this?"
- Notice how situations change your choice of thinking shortcut. Awareness of the shortcuts you use most often can also offer you a better understanding of specific situations and challenges that you want to resolve. You may jump to conclusions with your romantic partner, while you take the time to explore situations when you have conflicts with your friends. At the same time, you may be using tunnel vision with a peer with whom you have had conflicts, while being more open-minded with another peer who shares some common interests.
- There are many everyday ways to make your thinking more accurate:
  - Take your time and admit to not knowing the answer.
  - Avoid holding beliefs that are too rigid.
  - Get comfortable with unknowns.
  - Be curious. Ask questions.
  - Talk to trusted people.
  - Interact with people from diverse backgrounds.
  - Be your own devil's advocate. Question yourself.
  - Try to be open-minded. Think about other ways of interpreting the situation.
  - Look for evidence for and against your beliefs.
  - Treat yourself like a friend. What would you tell a friend in the same situation?

References

Ellis, A. (1962). *Reason and emotion in psychotherapy.* Lyle Stuart.

Helmond, P., Overbeek, G., Brugman, D., & Gibbs, J. (2015). A meta-analysis on cognitive distortions and externalizing problem behavior: Associations, moderators, and treatment effectiveness. *Criminal Justice and Behavior, 42*(3), 245–262. https://doi.org/10.1177/0093854814552842

Ready, D. D., & Wright, D. L. (2011). Accuracy and inaccuracy in teachers' perceptions of young children's cognitive abilities: The role of child background and classroom context. *American Educational Research Journal, 48*(2), 335–360. https://doi.org/10.3102/0002831210374874

Tseng, J., & Poppenk, J. (2020). Brain meta-state transitions demarcate thoughts across task contexts exposing the mental noise of trait neuroticism. *Nature Communications, 11*(1), 1–12. https://doi.org/10.1038/s41467-020-17255-9

Resources

Literature

Burns, D. D. (1993). *The feeling good handbook.* Plume.

Clark, D. A., & Beck, A. T. (2012). *The anxiety and worry workbook: The cognitive behavioral solution.* Guilford Press.

Ellis, A. (1962). *Reason and emotion in psychotherapy.* Lyle Stuart.

Gibbs, J. C., Overbeek, G., Helmond, P., & Brugman, D. (2014). A meta-analysis on cognitive distortions and externalizing problem behavior: Associations, moderators, and treatment effectiveness. *Criminal Justice and Behavior, 42*(3), 245–262.

Helmond, P., Overbeek, G., Brugman, D., & Gibbs, J. (2015). A meta-analysis on cognitive distortions and externalizing problem behavior: Associations, moderators, and treatment effectiveness. *Criminal Justice and Behavior, 42*(3), 245–262. https://doi.org/10.1177/0093854814552842

Iwamasa, G. Y., & Hays, P. A. (2019). *Culturally responsive cognitive behavior therapy: Practice and supervision.* American Psychological Association. https://doi.org/10.1037/0000119-000

Mindful, B. (2019). *Manage your emotions: How to be aware of yourself, control your anger and thoughts, grow resilience thinking and empathy skills to improve communication for a happy and successful life* (Eva H., Narr.) [Audiobook]. https://tinyurl.com/y8sp927e

Ready, D. D., & Wright, D. L. (2011). Accuracy and inaccuracy in teachers' perceptions of young children's cognitive abilities: The role of child background and classroom context. *American Educational Research Journal, 48*(2), 335–360. https://doi.org/10.3102/0002831210374874

Websites

Beck Institute
https://beckinstitute.org
Beck Institute was founded by Aaron Beck, one of the most influential psychologists of the 20th century. The institute advances CBT, which has been shown in more than 1,000 randomized trials to be effective for many different psychiatric disorders, psychological problems, and medical conditions with psychological components.

Association for Behavioral and Cognitive Therapies
http://www.abct.org
The Association for Behavioral and Cognitive Therapies is a multidisciplinary organization which aims to advance the scientific understanding, assessment, prevention, and treatment of human problems through behavioral, cognitive, and biological evidence-based principles.

Positive CBT
https://positivepsychology.com/category/positive-cbt/
This website offers resources which attempt to integrate positive psychology within the cognitive behavioral therapy model.

Beyond Blue
https://www.beyondblue.org.au/home
This Australian website provides information and support to understand cognitive behavioral therapy and to recognize signs and symptoms of various mental health conditions. Please note, some content of the website is restricted to an Australian audience.

Multimedia

SenseAbility
https://www.youtube.com/user/SenseAbilityOfficial/featured
This Australian strengths-based program teaches high-school students resilience by enhancing six senses: self-worth, control, belonging, purpose, future, and humor. The website hosts a number of brief videos illustrating concepts of resilience, well-being, positive communication, and self-talk.

APA PsycTherapy
https://www.apa.org/pubs/databases/psyctherapy/
APA PsycTherapy offers the opportunity to observe over 500 unscripted therapy sessions led by prominent therapists. Please note, this is a subscription-only service.

What Is Cognitive Behavioral Therapy?
https://youtu.be/q6aAQgXauQw
This video explains what cognitive behavioral therapy is and how it works.

Strength-Based Resilience & Positive Psychology
https://youtu.be/NsGfgRkz0AQ
A clinical psychologist, therapist, and researcher, Tayyab Rashid (one of the authors of the present work) focuses on strength-based resilience, and how it helps people improve their life by focusing on their strengths.

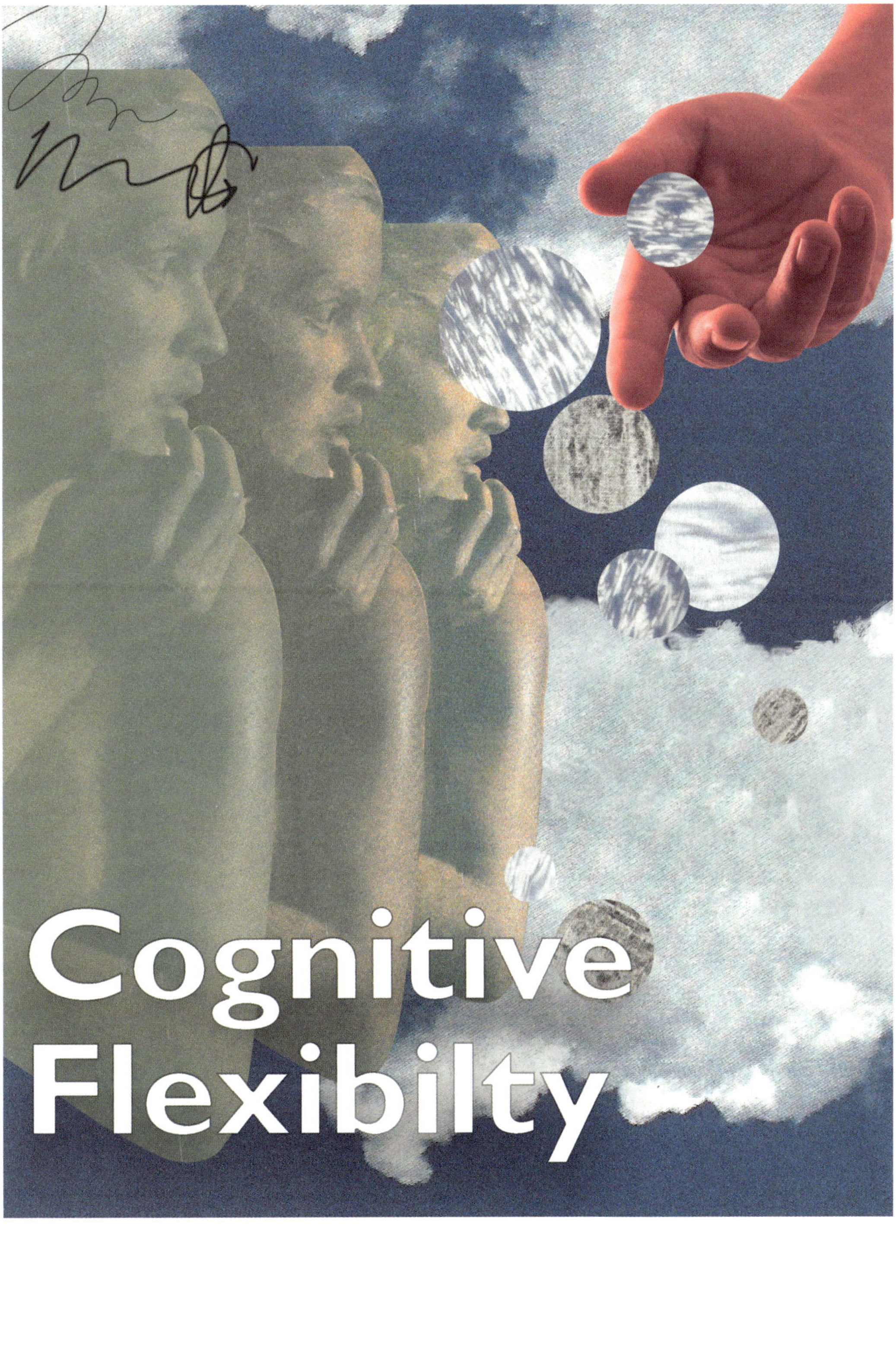
Cognitive
Flexibilty

Module 4: Cognitive Flexibility

This module introduces awareness of our habitual ways of explaining events to ourselves, whether positive or negative. The module draws from theories related to hopelessness, depression, and optimism, using the concept of explanatory style to help participants experience greater flexibility in interpreting and responding flexibly to daily situations and setbacks.

Module Topic	Minutes to Allot	
Learning Outcomes By learning about their explanatory style – that is, the way they explain the causes of an event to themselves – participants: • Explore their habitual patterns of explaining the causes of challenges • Assess the extent to which causes are personal, permanent and pervasive • Cultivate a flexible thinking style in response to challenging events	5	5
Opening Activities Start the module with a relaxation or mindfulness practice Invite participants to share a few events from their gratitude journal that have occurred since the last session Invite questions about the previous module and practice(s)	10	15
Illustration of Core Concepts Review core concepts and show video illustrations Facilitate reflection and discussion: • *What are the key messages in the video(s) you just watched?* • *How might these concepts be relevant in your life?*	15	15
Practice: Tune in to Your Explanatory Style Review sample challenges illustrating explanatory style Have participants complete Worksheet: Explanatory Style Practice Activity to assess their explanatory style through three experiences Debrief learning from practice(s) using questions: • *What did you learn about your explanatory style?* • *What is the evidence for your explanatory style?* • *On which dimension could you make changes?*	20	30
Closing Activities Invite discussion of everyday applications Remind participants of relevant resources at the end of the module Guide participants in a 3-minute closing relaxation or mindfulness practice	10	10
Total	60 minutes	75 minutes

Core Concepts of Cognitive Flexibility

Many of the themes here are also presented in the Core Concepts section of the Workbook (p. 61):

- *Cognitive flexibility* is the skill of examining an event or its causes or implications from multiple perspectives; in other words, considering multiple causes rather than just one. Considering alternatives helps us respond more flexibly to life challenges.
- The way we explain the causes of an event, positive or negative, is known as *explanatory style*. It is the way we tend to explain causes of an event to ourselves (Abramson et al., 1989; Seligman, 1975, 1991).
- Research by Abramson, Seligman, and their colleagues (Abramson et al., 1978; Alloy et al., 1984) has identified three dimensions of explanatory style (Figure 5; see Figure WB4 in the Workbook):
  - **Personal (me vs. not me):** Individuals hold themselves responsible for a setback, or they attribute setbacks to external or situational factors.
  - **Permanent (always vs. not always):** Individuals believe that setbacks are caused by permanent and unchangeable factors, rather than causes that are temporary and changeable.
  - **Pervasive (everything vs. not everything):** Individuals believe that setbacks are caused by factors that impact all aspects of their life, or they see the cause as affecting only one or two areas of life.
- Of the three dimensions, permanent and pervasive associations in relation to negative events are especially important to examine more closely. If we think the consequences of a negative event are permanent and pervasive, we can lose hope, feel helpless, and give up on our goals. Beliefs about both causes and consequences of negative events are important and can affect our well-being. According to the reformulated learned helplessness and hopelessness theories of depression (Abramson et al., 1978; Abramson et al., 1989), beliefs that causes are permanent and pervasive can lead to depression. This is similar to Aaron Beck's theory of depression (Beck, 1976), in which negative beliefs about self, world, and the future maintain one's depressive feelings.

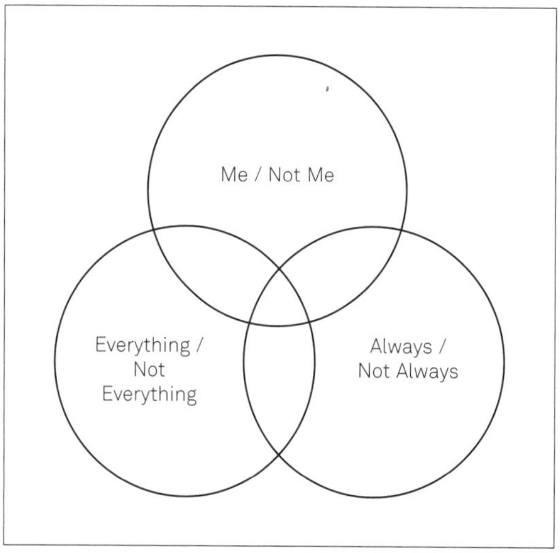

Figure 5.
Three dimensions of explanatory style (Figure WB4 in the Workbook). Adapted from Seligman (1991)

- The way you explain the causes of events and experiences impacts you. However, this impact differs from person to person and from situation to situation. Research has shown that pessimistic or hopeless thinking styles (particularly the tendency to attribute negative events to permanent and pervasive causes) are associated with increased feelings of hopelessness, depression, and anxiety, and also increased risk for these difficulties over time. Depressive symptoms can be prevented through interventions that teach skills for identifying and countering a pessimistic or hopeless explanatory style (Houston, 2016).
- Another related factor in explanatory style is one's perceived level of control in a situation. Imagine if someone keeps experiencing failures and challenges that they cannot control. For example, this can happen to young people in countries in conflict or at war. Individuals in such environments may adopt an explanatory style that blames the environment for all of their problems, including the problems over which they did have some control. Furthermore, irrespective of sociocultural milieu, the ways that parents' habitually explain negative events that their children experience may impact the way children explain events to themselves (Garber & Flynn, 2001).
- Fortunately, our explanatory style can be identified and changed. As much as sociocultural milieu impacts attributional style, so does awareness and practice. Careful observations and cognitive practices can change attributional style.

Illustrations of Cognitive Flexibility

Play at least one of the three videos below to illustrate the core concepts of cognitive flexibility and encourage discussion.

Explanatory Style
https://youtu.be/OCuiziwASEM?si=MUqFZNWWeWpHCyA
(Duration: 10:36 minutes)
This video describes the Three Ps of explanatory style, i.e., the degree to which we explain an outcome as permanent, personal, and pervasive. People can identify their explanatory style to help combat negative and pessimistic thinking.

Dangerous Minds 1995 Choice
https://www.youtube.com/watch?v=QNkTZUS80eo
(Duration: 4:16 minutes)
A teacher gives a moving speech to her high-school class that invites participants to actively choose their actions rather than succumb to circumstances.

How Can I Be More Creative? Exercise Cognitive Flexibility With a Mini Creative Thinking Workshop
(Duration: 3:33 minutes)
https://youtu.be/c3v0dK0NMsA
This short video shows how you can start exercising cognitive flexibility.

Reflection and Discussion

Invite participants to complete the Reflection and Discussion section of their Workbook (p. 63) regarding the video(s) they have watched. Discuss the questions:

What are the key messages in the video(s) you just watched?

How might these concepts be relevant in your life?

Practice: Tune in to Your Explanatory Style

Cognitive accuracy helps us to see the connections between our thoughts and reactions following negative events. It is a first step in understanding whether we are interpreting situations accurately and whether our thoughts and reactions make sense given the facts of the situation. By learning to recognize our habitual ways of explaining problems in our lives (explanatory style), we can learn to identify a wide range of possible and likely causes for negative events. This can be especially helpful for individuals with a more pessimistic explanatory style (a tendency to believe negative events have permanent and pervasive causes).

Practice: Tune in to Your Explanatory Style builds on skills of cognitive accuracy. It provides participants an opportunity to think about three specific challenges that had a negative outcome, then reflect on them in a more accurate and flexible manner.

Facilitate this practice by adapting the following steps to your audience and program:

- Refer participants to worksheets (Workbook pp. 65–67) and have them write down three recent challenges. These challenges could be similar to the ones that participants wrote about for Module 3, Practice 1: Unpack Experiences to Understand Challenges.
- Ask participants to recall as accurately as possible their thoughts in the moment. That is: "What did you think in the heat of the moment, as the cause of the challenge, problem, or setback?" Emphasize that their aim is to identify the thought they had in the moment about the cause of the challenge. Then, have them consider to what extent the cause was personal (me/not me), permanent (always/not always), and pervasive (everything/not everything).
- Some participants may have difficulty articulating their thoughts about the cause in relation to these three dimensions. Some situations are unclear, and we may not have all necessary information to identify a clear cause. Provide additional examples that can help participants narrow down challenges to those they can attribute somewhat clear causes.

Examples of Explanatory Style Practice Activity

Challenge Example 1

I met with my guidance counselor and because I failed a required course, I am not going to be able to graduate from high school this year.

Thoughts:

I thought it was all my fault. I believed that I would never go to college and would likely end up living on the streets.

Mostly **me**	①..... 3..... 5..... 7	Mostly **other people or circumstances**
Will **always** be present	1..... ③..... 5..... 7	Will **not always** be present
Influences **everything** in my life	1..... 3..... ⑤..... 7	Influences **just this one** situation

Reflection:

Looking back, a lot was going on in my life that was distracting me from my studies. My situation has improved. I know I can do better, so that I will graduate next year and I can choose whether I want to go on to college.

Challenge Example 2

I was unable to complete a project at work and I will not get the promotion I deserve.

Thoughts:

I am always unlucky. My team on this project was not cooperative

Mostly due to **me**	1..... 3..... ⑤..... 7	Mostly due to **other people or circumstances**
Will **always** be present	1..... ③..... 5..... 7	Will **not always** be present
Influences **everything** in my life	①..... 3..... 5..... 7	Influences **just this one** situation

Reflection:

Putting things in perspective, two of my team members have recently started their jobs. They are not familiar with the team dynamics. I will have other opportunities in the coming months to prove my abilities.

Worksheet: Explanatory Style – Challenge 1 (from the Workbook, p. 65)

Your challenge:

____

____

What did you think at that moment about the cause of the challenge?

____

____

Explanatory Style Dimensions

Mostly **me**	1..... 3..... 5..... 7	Mostly **other people or circumstances**
Will **always** be present	1..... 3..... 5..... 7	Will **not always** be present
Influences **everything** in my life	1..... 3..... 5..... 7	Influences **just this one** situation

Reflection:
What did you learn about your explanatory style? What is the evidence for your explanatory style?
On which dimension could you make changes?

____

____

____

____

____

____

____

____

____

Practice Debrief

Invite participants to complete the Reflection section for each of their three challenges on pp. 65–67 in their Workbook. To debrief the cognitive flexibility activity, discuss the following questions:

What did you learn about your explanatory style?
What is the evidence for your explanatory style?
On which dimension could you make changes?

Learning and Cultural Fit

Adapt this practice to the learning and cultural needs of your audience, its unique values and demographics. Possible adaptations include:

- Be mindful that the notion of flexibility may not be readily applicable to some participants who may be facing challenging circumstances that are beyond their immediate control, such as the death of a loved one, dysfunctional family dynamics, or socioeconomic challenges (Mezulis et al., 2004).
- Although cognitive flexibility is desirable in general, it may have serious limitations when addressing particular circumstances, for example, a debilitating disability, an abusive family, significant trauma and grief, or poverty.
- Sometimes our first thoughts are not accurate or helpful. Skills of cognitive flexibility and accuracy can help us come to more realistic conclusions about our experiences. Other times, our first thoughts may be accurate, and the situation may be as bad (or has potential to be as bad) as we are fearing. In those situations, it can be important to think about whether there is anything we can do to solve the problem and also about how we can take care of ourselves and of others.

Closing Activities

The goal of closing this module is to help participants integrate their understanding of cognitive flexibility and to take their new learning into everyday life.

Discuss with participants the Everyday Applications section, also found on p. 68 in their Workbook. Invite participants to be mindful in their day-to-day lives by noticing actions and habits which show their explanatory style or those of others. Encourage them to use relevant resources found at the end of this module and included in their workbooks, starting on p. 68.

Choose a 3-minute mindfulness activity from Regular Practice 1: Mindfulness and Relaxation to close the module.

Everyday Applications

- Cognitive flexibility can help you to fine-tune your understanding of yourself. This skill helps you to reflect on everyday problems and your beliefs about them, and to learn ways to recover from a setback.
- Unpacking our challenges into thoughts about their causes can help us to understand that it is not just the severity of the setback, failure, or difficulty that determines our resilience. It is also the way that we explain it to ourself. Whenever you next face a setback, failure, or difficulty, use the practice mentioned in the module to become aware of your habitual way of explaining the causes of events to yourself.
- The flexibility framework of Me vs. Not Me, Always vs. Not Always, and Everything vs. Not Everything can help you to view a challenge in a specific, contextualized, and nonthreatening way. This can help you deal with problems. Work to uncover your pattern: Are you typically a Me person or a Not Me person? Always or Not Always? Everything or Not Everything? Reflect on your typical explanatory style to be more balanced in resolving your challenges. Ask yourself, "What is the evidence for this belief? Are there other ways of looking at this situation?"
- Whenever you find yourself stuck in solving a problem, approach the problem in a flexible manner to view the situation in an open-minded, understanding, and clear way.

References

Abramson, L., Metalsky, G. I., & Alloy, L. B. (1989). Hopelessness depression: A theory-based subtype of depression. *Psychological Review, 96*(2), 358–372. https://doi.org/10.1037/0033-295X.96.2.358

Abramson, L. Y., Seligman, M. E., & Teasdale, J. D. (1978). Learned helplessness in humans: Critique and reformulation. *Journal of Abnormal Psychology, 87*(1), 49–74. https://doi.org/10.1037/0021-843X.87.1.49

Alloy, L. B., Peterson, C., Abramson, L. Y., & Seligman, M. E. P. (1984). Attributional style and the generality of learned helplessness. *Journal of Personality and Social Psychology, 46*, 681–687. https://doi.org/10.1037/0022-3514.46.3.681

Beck, A. T. (1976). *Cognitive therapy and the emotional disorders.* International University Press.

Garber, J., & Flynn, C. (2001). Predictors of depressive cognitions in young adolescents. *Cognitive Therapy and Research, 25*, 353–376. https://doi.org/10.1023/A:1005530402239

Houston, D. M. (2016). Revisiting the relationship between attributional style and academic performance. *Journal of Applied Social Psychology, 46*(3), 192–200. https://doi.org/10.1111/jasp.12356

Mezulis, A. H., Abramson, L. Y., Hyde, J. S., & Hankin, B. L. (2004). Is there a universal positivity bias in attributions? A meta-analytic review of individual, developmental, and cultural differences in the self-serving attributional bias. *Psychological Bulletin, 130*(5), 711–747. https://doi.org/10.1037/0033-2909.130.5.711

Seligman, M. E. P. (1975). *Helplessness: On depression, development, and death.* Freeman.

Seligman, M. E. P. (1991). *Learned optimism: How to change your mind and your life.* Vintage Books.

Resources

Literature

Abramson, L., Metalsky, G. I., & Alloy, L. B. (1989). Hopelessness depression: A theory-based subtype of depression. *Psychological Review, 96*(2), 358–372. https://doi.org/10.1037/0033-295X.96.2.358

Bein, A. M. (2008). *The Zen of helping: Spiritual principles for mindful and open-hearted practice.* John Wiley.

Dobelli, R. (2013). *The art of thinking clearly.* HarperCollins.

Ellis, A. (1988). *A rational emotive behavior therapy.* Allyn & Bacon.

Hayes, S. C., & Deakins, M. (2019). *A liberated mind: How to pivot toward what matters* [Audiobook]. Penguin.

Hirt, E. R., Devers, E. E., & McCrea, S. M. (2008). I want to be creative: Exploring the role of hedonic contingency theory in the positive mood-cognitive flexibility link. *Journal of Personality and Social Psychology, 94*(2), 214–230. https://doi.org/10.1037/0022-3514.94.2.94.2.214

Huizinga, M., Smidts, D. P., & Ridderinkhof, K. R. (2014). Change of mind: Cognitive flexibility in the classroom. *Perspectives on Language and Literacy, 40*(2), 31–35.

Leary, R. (2020). *Neuroplasticity: Overthinking & rewire your brain: How to declutter and unfu*k your anxious mind, build mental toughness, stop worrying and become a better version of yourself.*

Liu, Y., & Wang, Z. (2014). Positive affect and cognitive control: Approach-motivation intensity influences the balance between cognitive flexibility and stability. *Psychological Science, 25*(5), 1116–1123. https://doi.org/10.1177/0956797614525213

Neenan, M., & Dryden, W. (2004). *Cognitive therapy 100 key points and techniques* (1st ed.). Brunner-Routledge.

Peterson, C. (1991). The meaning and measurement of explanatory style. *Psychological Inquiry, 2*(1), 1–10. https://doi.org/10.1207/s15327965pli0201_1

Reivich, K., & Shatte, A. (2002). *The resilience factor: 7 essential skills for overcoming life's inevitable obstacles.* Broadway Books.

Seligman, M. E. P. (1975). *Helplessness: On depression, development, and death.* Freeman.

Seligman, M. E. P. (1991). *Learned optimism: How to change your mind and your life.* Vintage Books.

Seligman, M. E. P. (1998). Optimism: The difference it makes. *Science and Spirit, 9,* 6–19.

Yeager, J. M., Fisher, S. W., & David, D. N. (2011). *Building character, resilience and relationships in youth.* Kravis.

Wilding, C., & Milne, A. (2008). *Teach yourself cognitive behavioural therapy.* Teach Yourself Books.

Websites

Developing Psychological Flexibility
https://www.psychologytools.com/resource/developing-psychological-flexibility/
This website offers techniques for developing psychological flexibility according to the acceptance commitment therapy model. A downloadable handout is available in eight languages.

Importance of Psychological Flexibility in Happy Relationships
https://www.inc.com/jessica-stillman/happiness-relationships-psychological-flexibility.html
Learn insight from a review of 174 studies that link low psychological flexibility to weak family ties, less satisfying relationships, and less effective parenting. Psychological flexibility is the key to thriving relationships.

Flexible Thinking: How to Encourage Kids to Go With the Flow
https://www.pbs.org/parents/thrive/flexible-thinking-how-to-encourage-kids-to-go-with-the-flow
This webpage from American Public Broadcasting Service (PBS Kids) discusses strategies to help children learn flexible thinking skills.

Multimedia

Learned Optimism Positive Psychology
https://youtu.be/6tN9wMbdqZU
Reviewing Martin Seligman's book *Learned Optimism*, this video explains the difference between optimistic and pessimistic explanations.

Psychological Flexibility: How Love Turns Pain Into Purpose
https://youtu.be/o79_gmO5ppg
Psychologist Steven Hayes explains in this TEDx University of Nevada how one can develop psychological flexibility.

5 Tips to Improve Your Critical Thinking
https://www.ted.com/talks/samantha_agoos_5_tips_to_improve_your_critical_thinking
From a sea of decisions, it is impossible to make a perfect choice. Samantha Agoos describes in this TED-Ed a 5-step process that may help us in making better decisions.

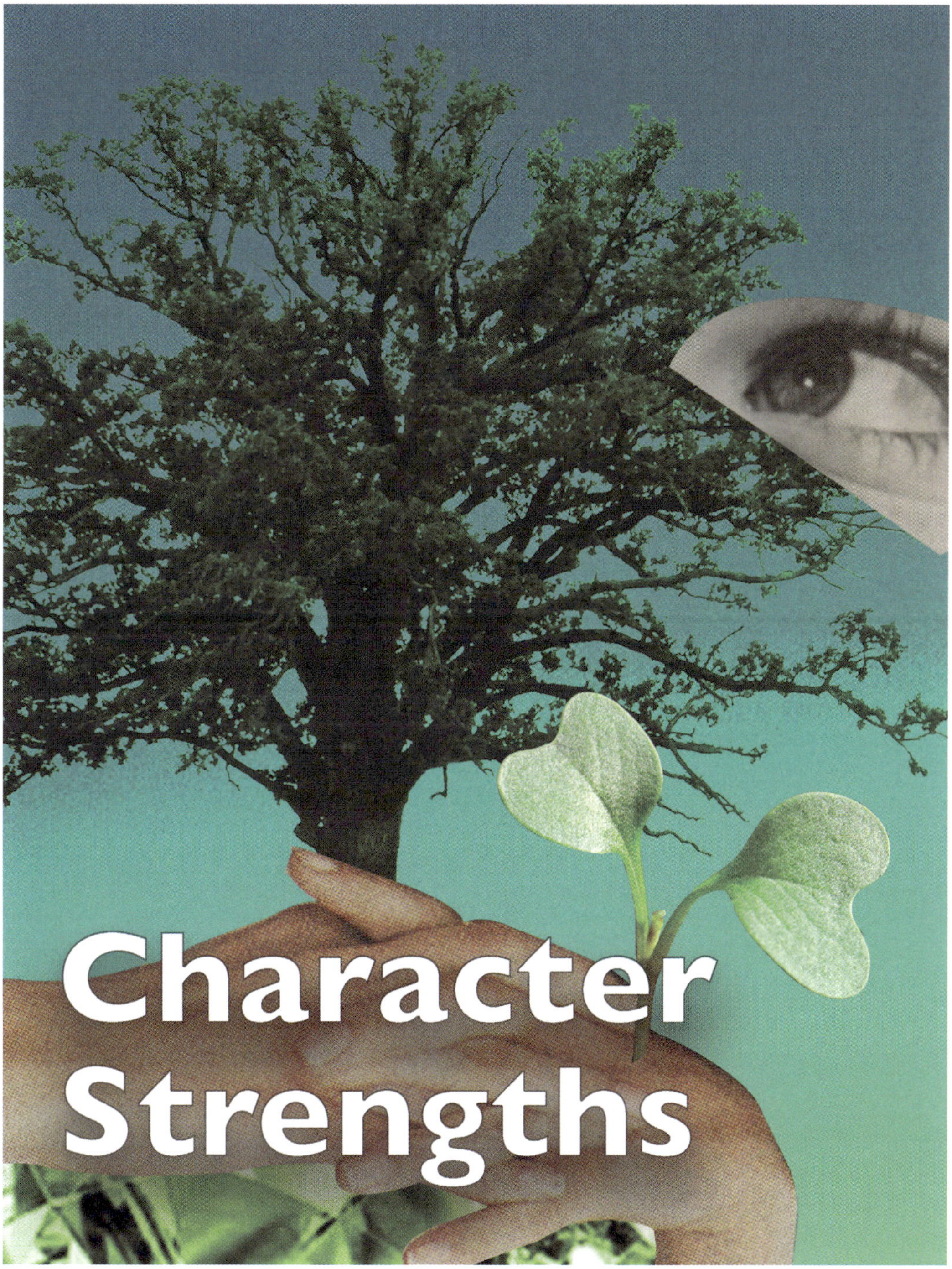
Character
Strengths

Module 5: Character Strengths

The first of three modules focusing on character strengths, this module introduces the framework of 24 strengths or positive traits that contribute to our well-being and the well-being of those around us. It orients participants to the definitions of and research into character strengths and their distinctive potential to be inherent resources for well-being and resilience.

Module Topic	Minutes to Allot	
Learning Outcomes By identifying their character strengths from multiple perspectives, including emotional, cognitive, and relational, participants: • Value character strengths as intrinsic attributes that can be used, refined, and developed to boost resilience • Understand that character strengths are as real and impactful in our lives as weaknesses • Hone skills to acknowledge one's own strengths as well as spot strengths in others	5	5
Opening Activities Start the module with a relaxation or mindfulness practice Invite participants to share a few events from their gratitude journal that have occurred since the last session Invite questions about the previous module and practice(s)	10	15
Illustration of Core Concepts Review core concepts and show video illustrations Facilitate reflection and discussion: • *What are the key messages in the video(s) you just watched?* • *How might these concepts be relevant in your life?*	15	15
Practice: Spot Your Character Strengths Have participants identify their top character strengths through two activities: pictures of each strength and word descriptions Debrief learning from practice(s) using questions: • *How well do these strengths describe your personality?* • *What did you learn from identifying your strengths?* • *What might explain differences in the strengths you selected from each activity?* Assign homework tasks	20	30
Closing Activities Invite discussion of everyday applications Remind participants of relevant resources at the end of the module Guide participants in a 3-minute closing relaxation or mindfulness practice	10	10
Total	60 minutes	75 minutes

Core Concepts of Character Strengths

Many of the themes here are also presented in the Core Concepts section of the Workbook (p. 71).

- *Character strengths* are positive traits that manifest through our feelings, thoughts, and actions (Box 1, p. 25). Character strengths enable us to act in ways that contribute to our well-being and the well-being of those around us (Peterson & Seligman, 2004).
- Christopher Peterson and Martin Seligman spearheaded the endeavor of compiling and publishing a comprehensive classification of strengths, titled, *Classification of Strengths and Virtues* (CSV; Peterson & Seligman, 2004). CSV is the strengths framework most widely used by positive psychology practitioners. More than 1,000 studies on the CSV Classification have been published, and surveys based on this model have been administered in more than 40 languages to more than 30 million people (www.viacharacter.org; VIA Institute, 2023).
- Whereas examining weaknesses, deficits, dysfunctions, and disorders helps us gauge our psychological stress and symptoms, exploring character strengths help us understand and discover many different ways of doing good (Grant & Sonnentag, 2010; Linley et al., 2010).
- Peterson and Seligman (2004), two pioneers of positive psychology, define character strengths through the following criteria:
  - Character strengths are widely recognized and valued across cultures.
  - Character strengths are good for you and others; they increase your life satisfaction and happiness.
  - When someone displays character strengths, such as courage, honesty, gratitude, kindness, self-regulation, or playfulness, others usually admire these traits and do not become jealous. In other words, character strengths do not diminish others.
  - Specific character strengths have real-life role models, such as Malala Yousafzai (bravery), Greta Thunberg (leadership), Nelson Mandela (forgiveness), Stephen Hawking (love of learning), and Terry Fox (persistence). Real-life role models help to inspire young people to emulate their strengths. Everyday interactions, especially in classroom settings which spot, genuinely acknowledge, and support strengths of each other are critical in boosting resilience and well-being among students (Norrish, 2015; Quinlan et al., 2014; White & Waters, 2015).
  - While character strengths are positive, it is possible that overuse or underuse of specific strengths can cause problems and strain relationships (Niemiec, 2019; Peterson, 2006). Too much kindness for example can lead to leniency. Too little prudence can expose us to risky situations. Balanced use of strengths are important – we will discuss this topic in Module 7: Problem Solving and Strengths.
  - Character strengths are concrete enough to be measured reliably, and they vary between individuals. For example, some individuals are high on curiosity, while others are low on curiosity; some are more interested in creativity, while others are passionate about showing kindness to others (Niemiec, 2019; Rust et al., 2009).
  - Character strengths are not fixed. They can be built and developed through repeated actions and transmission of societal values (Proyer et al., 2015; Rashid & Seligman, 2018).

- In cultivating resilience, character strengths offer three distinct advantages, including
  - Knowing and using your strengths helps you to reinterpret and reframe challenges from a strength perspective rather than from a weakness perspective.
  - Character strengths are resources to help us to understand and build resilience better. Knowing and relying on strengths provide additional options to manage or overcome challenges, adversities, and setbacks. Working on character strengths can motivate us to be proactive whereas working on deficits can deplete our energy.
- Some participants may feel that this list of 24 strengths does not capture their own strengths, particularly those that are more culturally relative (e.g., tolerance, familial duty, balance, amiability). Acknowledge that there likely is a much wider variety of strengths valued in different families, communities, and cultures.

Illustrations of Character Strengths

Play at least one of the three videos below to illustrate the core concepts of character strengths and encourage discussion.

The Science of Character
https://youtu.be/U3nT2KDAGOc
(Duration: 8:04 minutes)
This educational video explores the neuroscience and social science that prove we can shape who we are and who we want to be in the world.

Know Your Character Strengths
https://youtu.be/JLUOlLRbazA
(Duration: 2:59 minutes)
This video describes the importance of knowing, using, and developing your strengths.

An Adaptable Mind
https://youtu.be/937iCwJd3fI
(Duration: 11:02 minutes)
This short documentary examines the skills and strengths we need in the 21st century.

Reflection and Discussion

Invite participants to complete the Reflection and Discussion section of their Workbook (p. 72) regarding the video(s) they have watched. Discuss the questions:

What are the key messages in the video(s) you just watched?

How might these concepts be relevant in your life?

Practice: Spot Your Character Strengths

The purpose of this practice is to help participants identify their top (or signature) character strengths. This is a multistep process.

As discussed in Chapter 1, our inherent negativity bias prevents us from focusing on positives – our own and others. One of the central premises of SBR is that we can draw on our strengths to address challenges. The practice in this module lays the foundation for participants to understand the CSV character strengths model, which consists of 24 strengths. By inviting them to notice their top character strengths, they can begin the habit of using them as problem-solving resources.

There are three steps to this practice which guide participants in spotting their top strengths: (1) spotting strengths through visual images of each character strength; (2) spotting strengths through word descriptions; and (3) creating a consolidated list showing results of the first two steps. Of all the positive psychology practices and interventions, this remains one of the most used exercises (Carr, 2022). Facilitators will benefit from reviewing the steps and by practicing at least once, on themselves, before they facilitate it.

Step 1. Character Strengths Pictures Worksheet (Workbook p. 73)

- After discussing the core concepts of character strengths, facilitators should ensure they have access to the video clip available with the online material of the Workbook. The video clip can be downloaded free of charge once you register on the website (for instructions see p. 171 in the Workbook).
- Cue the video clip at the start. Ask participants to have Worksheet: Character Strengths Pictures ready.
- Facilitators can also download this worksheet and print a copy for each participant. After cuing the video and worksheet, facilitators can use the following script:

The video will play a sequence of pictures that illustrate strengths, in the order listed on your worksheet. Each picture will appear for a few seconds only. Without focusing on whether the picture best represents the strength or not, tune in to your emotions as sharply as you can. Consider whether the strength pictured is one you believe to be central to who you are. If so, circle the name of the strength promptly or put an "✓" in the column next to it. Try to limit your selection to five or six strengths that best describe you.

Worksheet: Character Strengths Pictures

1	Creativity	
2	Curiosity	
3	Open-mindedness	
4	Love of learning	
5	Perspective	
6	Bravery	
7	Persistence	
8	Integrity	
9	Vitality	
10	Love	
11	Kindness	
12	Social intelligence	
13	Citizenship	
14	Fairness	
15	Leadership	
16	Forgiveness	
17	Humility	
18	Prudence	
19	Self-regulation	
20	Appreciation of beauty & excellence	
21	Gratitude	
22	Hope	
23	Humor	
24	Spirituality	

Step 2. Character Strengths Descriptions Worksheet (Workbook p. 74)

- Next, ask participants to follow the directions on the Character Strengths Descriptions Worksheet. Participants will read descriptions of 24 strengths (without their titles) and select five or six that most often characterize them.

Worksheet: Character Strengths Descriptions

	Character strengths	✓
1	I am good at thinking of new and better ways of doing things.	
2	I love to explore things and ask questions; I am open to different experiences and activities.	
3	I am flexible and open-minded; I think through and examine all sides before deciding.	
4	I love to learn many new ideas, concepts, and facts in school or on my own.	
5	Friends consult with me on important matters as they consider me to be wise beyond my age.	
6	I do not give up in the face of hardship or challenge, even when I am afraid.	
7	I finish most things; even if I get distracted, I am able to refocus and complete tasks.	
8	I consider myself to be a genuine and honest person, known to be trustworthy and to act consistently with my values.	
9	I am energetic, cheerful, and full of life.	
10	Showing and receiving genuine love and affection come naturally to me.	
11	I love to do acts of kindness for others, often without being asked.	
12	I manage myself well in social situations and am known to have good interpersonal skills.	
13	I am an active community or team member and contribute to the success of my group.	
14	I stand up for others when they are treated unfairly, bullied, or ridiculed.	
15	Others often choose me as a leader, as I am known to lead well.	
16	I do not hold grudges; I easily forgive those who offend me.	
17	I don't like to be the center of attention and prefer others to shine.	
18	I am careful and cautious; I can anticipate risks and consequences of my actions and respond accordingly.	
19	I manage my feelings and behaviors even in challenging situations; I generally follow rules and routines.	
20	I am moved deeply by beauty in nature and in art (e.g., painting, music, theater, etc.), and/or by excellence in many fields of life.	
21	I express thankfulness for good things through words and actions.	
22	I hope and believe that more good things will happen than bad ones.	
23	I am playful and funny and use humor to connect with others.	
24	I believe in a higher power and participate in religious or spiritual practices (e.g., prayer, meditation, etc.) willingly.	

Step 3. Character Strengths Pictures and Descriptions Worksheet (Workbook p. 75)

- After completing the two worksheets above, ask participants to summarize their responses using the Character Strengths Pictures and Descriptions Worksheet.
- In the Character Strengths Pictures column, participants place a checkmark "✓" next to the 5 or 6 strengths that they selected after watching the video clip.
- In the next column, participants place a checkmark "✓" next to the 5 or 6 strengths that they selected from the Character Strengths Description Worksheet, in which the row numbers correspond with the name of the strength.

Worksheet: Character Strengths Pictures Compared With Descriptions

	Character strength	Worksheet: Character Strengths Pictures	Worksheet: Character Strengths Descriptions
1	Creativity & originality		
2	Curiosity & interest in the world		
3	Open-mindedness, judgement, & critical thinking		
4	Love of learning		
5	Perspective & wisdom		
6	Bravery & valor		
7	Persistence, diligence, & industry		
8	Integrity, authenticity, & honesty		
9	Vitality, zest, enthusiasm, & energy		
10	Love: capacity to love & be loved		
11	Kindness & generosity		
12	Social intelligence		
13	Citizenship, teamwork, & loyalty		
14	Fairness, equity, & justice		
15	Leadership		
16	Forgiveness & mercy		
17	Humility & modesty		
18	Prudence, caution, & discretion		
19	Self-regulation & self-control		
20	Appreciation of beauty & excellence		
21	Gratitude		
22	Hope & optimism		
23	Humor & playfulness		
24	Spirituality & religiousness		

Practice Debrief

Have the participants reflect on and discuss the following questions in their Workbook (p. 76):

How well do these strengths, as revealed in the Worksheet: Character Strengths Pictures Compared With Descriptions, describe your personality?

What did you learn from identifying your strengths from the perspectives of pictures and descriptions?

Were there differences in the strengths you selected in the Pictures activity versus those in the Descriptions activity? Reflect on these differences.

Are there any strengths, not listed above, that are important to your core personality?

Homework

Assign Signature Strengths Homework. Ask participants to complete the following activities before the next meeting:
- Complete the Signature Strengths Questionnaire-72 (SSQ-72), print the feedback, and bring it to the next session. Find SSQ-72 at: http:// www.strengthsbasedresilience.com/assessment
- Ask them to identify three people who know them well (including a friend or peer, family member, and/or teacher or colleague) and have them complete the relevant Friend/Peer, Family Member, or Teacher/Colleague worksheet on pp. 82–84 (Workbook). (Note: Facilitators can view these worksheets in the next module on pp. 178–180).

Anticipate problems that participants might encounter with this homework. If you are teaching the course and know the student, you can complete the Teacher worksheet. If participants cannot get people to complete the worksheet for them in writing, they can ask them to identify their strengths verbally. Alternatively, participants can imagine what their friends, family members, and teachers/colleagues might perceive to be their top strengths.

Learning and Cultural Fit

Adapt this practice to the learning and cultural needs of your audience, its unique values and demographics. Possible adaptations include:
- Perhaps due to cultural norms, some participants may not value their character strengths, especially if their strengths are relatively more self-focused (e.g., love of learning, curiosity, or creativity) rather than other-focused (e.g., social intelligence, kindness, love). These participants may benefit from identifying rituals and traditions that celebrate strengths in relating with others. For example, families, regardless of their religion or ethnicity, utilize the individual strengths of family members. One person may cook using their strength of creativity, another may clean and decorate using their strength of appreciation of beauty, a third may meet and greet family members, using their strength of social intelligence.

- Some participants may view strengths as fixed qualities and wonder why they should explore or build strengths, as they are already intact resources. Remind them that we can always become stronger. Just like strength or weight training, we develop strengths and become stronger through practice. It will help to link this to having a growth mindset. Nonetheless, we need to be mindful about the pace and specific expectations of being stronger.
- Action is important. Strengths show up in our behavior. For example, often when describing someone being kind, we also mention ways in which someone acts in kindness or their actions show kindness.
- For participants who are having trouble identifying their strengths (perhaps because of modesty), it can help to invite them to think about what their parents or siblings or close friends would say about them. For example: "What would your best friends say if I asked them about your top strengths?"

Closing Activities

The goal of closing this module is to help participants integrate their understanding of character strengths through interactive practices and to take their new learning into everyday life.

Discuss with participants the Everyday Applications section, also found on p. 77 in their Workbook. Invite participants to be mindful in their day-to-day lives by noticing actions and habits which show their character strengths or those of others. Encourage them to use relevant resources found at the end of this module and included in their workbooks starting on p. 78.

Choose a 3-minute mindfulness activity from Regular Practice 1: Mindfulness and Relaxation to close the module.

Everyday Applications

- We are geared to look for negatives, as we discussed in Regular Practice 2: Gratitude Journal. As a result, we end up spending a lot of time trying to remediate or improve our weaknesses or shortcomings, such as not being smart enough, athletic enough, popular enough, good-looking enough, creative enough, or productive enough. Using what you have just learned about your strengths, think of ways in which you can improve yourself by working on activities you are good at that exercise your strengths.
- Think of an activity that you find interesting or meaningful that you can do and that allows you to build on your strengths. Find time every week to do this activity. Activities that use your strengths contribute to your well-being and help you build your abilities.
- To deepen your understanding of character strengths in everyday life, think in terms of analogies, such as:
  The term "curiosity" reminds me of ____________________.
  Bravery is like ____________________.
  Another word for kindness is ____________________.
- Start with yourself. Think of everyday situations which show character strengths you identified about yourself in this module. For example, when you clean your room, kitchen or garage, help loved ones with a task they cannot do on their own, or pay bills on time, ask yourself which strength you are using. Spot these actions, and think of how these behaviors and habits may be genuine and authentic manifestations of your strengths. Let them boost your confidence, especially when everyday stressors drain you. Likewise, recognize and appreciate the strengths of your loved ones that you see, in their everyday actions and experiences. This can help you to see your loved ones more realistically and in a positive manner.
- Most character strengths have an interpersonal dimension. Notice which strengths in your day-to-day life support your ability to cultivate and maintain relationships with others.

References

Carr, A. (2022). *Positive psychology: The science of wellbeing and human strengths* (3rd ed.). Routledge. https://doi.org/10.4324/9781003082866

Grant, A. M., & Sonnentag, S. (2010). Doing good buffers against feeling bad: Prosocial impact compensates for negative task and self-evaluations. *Organizational Behavior and Human Decision Processes, 111*(1), 13–22. https://doi.org/10.1016/j.obhdp.2009.07.003

Linley, P. A., Nielsen, K. M., Gillett, R., & Biswas-Diener, R. (2010). Using signature strengths in pursuit of goals: Effects on goal progress, need satisfaction, and well-being, and implications for coaching psychologists. *International Coaching Psychology Review, 5*(1), 6–15. https://doi.org/10.53841/bpsicpr.2010.5.1.6

Niemiec, R. M. (2019). Finding the golden mean: The overuse, underuse, and optimal use of character strengths. *Counselling Psychology Quarterly, 32*(3–4), 453–471. https://doi.org/10.1080/09515070.2019.1617674

Norrish, J. (2015). *Positive education: The Geelong Grammar School journey*. Oxford University Press. https://doi.org/10.1093/acprof:oso/9780198702580.001.0001

Peterson, C. (2006). *Primer in positive psychology*. Oxford University Press.

Peterson, C., & Seligman, M. E. P. (2004). *Character strengths and virtues: A handbook and classification*. Oxford University Press / American Psychological Association.

Proyer, R. T., Gander, F., Wellenzohn, S., & Ruch, W. (2015). Strengths-based positive psychology interventions: A randomized placebo-controlled online trial on long-term effects for a signature strengths- vs. a lesser strengths-intervention. *Frontiers in Psychology, 6*, Article 456. https://doi.org/10.3389/fpsyg.2015.00456

Quinlan, D. M., Swain, N., Cameron, C., & Vella-Brodrick, D. A. (2014). How other people matter in a classroom-based strengths intervention: Exploring interpersonal strategies and classroom outcomes. *Journal of Positive Psychology, 10*(1), 77–89. https://doi.org/10.1080/17439760.2014.920407

Rashid, T., & Seligman, M. E. P. (2018). *Positive psychotherapy: Clinician manual.* Oxford University Press. https://doi.org/10.1093/med-psych/9780195325386.001.0001

Rust, T., Diessner, R., & Reade, L. (2009). Strengths only or strengths and relative weaknesses? A preliminary study. *Journal of Psychology, 143*(5), 465–476. https://doi.org/10.3200/JRL.143.5.465-476

VIA Institute (2023). *What the research says about character strengths.* https://www.viacharacter.org/research/findings

White, M. A., & Waters, L. E. (2015). A case study of "The Good School": Examples of the use of Peterson's strengths-based approach with students. *The Journal of Positive Psychology, 10*(1), 69–76. https://doi.org/10.1080/17439760.2014.920408

Resources

Literature

Brown, W. K. (2006). The value of role models in inspiring resilience. *Reclaiming Children & Youth, 14*(4), 199–202.

Burke, J., & McGuckin, C. (2022). Bullying and character development: An examination of character strengths associated with bullying and cyberbullying in postprimary schools in Ireland. *Journal of Character Education, 18*(1), 51–68.

Ferragut, M., Blanca, M. J., & Ortiz-Tallo, M. (2014). Psychological virtues during adolescence: A longitudinal study of gender differences. *European Journal of Development Psychology, 11*(5), 521–531. https://doi.org/10.1080/17405629.2013.876403

Linkins, M., Niemiec, R. M., Gillham, J., & Mayerson, D. (2014). Through the lens of strength: A framework for educating the heart. *Journal of Positive Psychology, 10*(1), 64–68. https://doi.org/10.1080/17439760.2014.888581

Linley, A. (2008). *Average to A+: Realising strengths in yourself and others.* CAPP Press.

Linley, A., & Bateman, T., (2018). *The strengths profile book: Finding what you can do + love to do and why it matters.* CAPP Press.

Madden, W., Green, S., & Grant, A.M. (2011). A pilot study evaluating strengths-based coaching for primary school participants: Enhancing engagement and hope. *International Coaching Psychology Review, 6*(1), 71–83. https://doi.org/10.53841/bpsicpr.2011.6.1.71

McGovern, T. V., & Miller, S. L. (2008). Integrating teacher behaviors with character strengths and virtues for faculty development. *Teaching of Psychology, 35*(4), 278–285. https://doi.org/10.1080/00986280802374609

Naddaf, S. A., & Lavy, S. (2022). Character strengths' change during COVID-19. *Journal of Happiness Studies, 24*, 185–210. https://doi.org/10.1007/s10902-022-00575-6

O'Byrne, R., Thompson, R., Friedmann, J. S., & Lumley, M. N. (2022). Parent engagement with an online, school-based, character strengths promotion program. *International Journal of Applied Positive Psychology, 7*, 355–377. https://doi.org/10.1007/s41042-022-00072-4

Oppenheimer, M. F., Fialkov, C., Ecker, B., & Portnoy, S. (2014). Teaching to strengths: Character education for urban middle school participants. *Journal of Character Education, 10*(2), 91–105.

Park, N., & Peterson, C. (2006). Moral competence and character strengths among adolescents: The development and validation of the Values in Action Inventory of Strengths for Youth. *Journal of Adolescence, 29*(6), 891–905. https://doi.org/10.1016/j.adolescence.2006.04.011

Park, N., & Peterson, C. (2009). Strengths of character in schools. In R. Gilman, E. S. Huebner, & M. J. Furlong (Eds.), *Handbook of positive psychology in schools* (pp. 65–76). Routledge.

Polly, S., & Britton, K. (2015). *Character strengths matter: How to live a full life.* Positive Psychology News.

Proctor, C., Tsukayama, E., Wood, A. M., Maltby, J., Fox Eades, J., & Linley, P. A. (2011). Strengths gym: The impact of a character strengths-based intervention on the life satisfaction and well-being of adolescents. *Journal of Positive Psychology, 6*(5), 377–388. https://doi.org/10.1080/17439760.2011.594079

Proyer, R. T., Sidler, N., Weber, M., & Ruch, W. (2012). A multi-method approach to studying the relationship between character strengths and vocational interests in adolescents. *International Journal for Educational and Vocational Guidance, 12*(2), 141–157. https://doi.org/10.1007/s10775-012-9223-x

Rousso, J. (2016). *The little book of character strengths.* VIA Institute.

Seider, S., Novick, S., & Gomez, J. (2013). The effects of privileging moral or performance character development in urban adolescents. *Journal of Early Adolescence, 33*(6), 786–820. https://doi.org/10.1177/0272431612468318

Shoshani, A., & Ilanit Aviv, I. (2012). The pillars of strength for first-grade adjustment: Parental and children's character strengths and the transition to elementary school. *Journal of Positive Psychology, 7*(4), 315–326. https://doi.org/10.1080/17439760.2012.691981

Steen, T. A., Kachorek, L. V., & Peterson, C. (2003). Character strengths among youth. *Journal of Youth & Adolescence, 32,* 5–16. https://doi.org/10.1023/A:1021024205483

Tough, P. (2012). *How children succeed: Grit, curiosity, and the hidden power of character.* Houghton Mifflin Harcourt.

Wagner, L., & Ruch, W. (2015). Good character at school: Positive classroom behavior mediates the link between character strengths and school achievement. *Frontiers in Psychology, 6,* Article 610. https://doi.org/10.3389/fpsyg.2015.00610

Weber, M., & Ruch, W. (2012). The role of a good character in 12-year-old school children: Do character strengths matter in the classroom? *Child Indicators Research, 5,* 317–334. https://doi.org/10.1007/s12187-011-9128-0

Weziak-Bialowolska, D., Lee, M. T., Bialowolski, P., Chen, Y., VanderWeele, T. J., & McNeely, E. (2022). Prospective associations between strengths of moral character and health: Longitudinal evidence from survey and insurance claims data. *Social Psychiatry and Psychiatric Epidemiology, 58,* 163–176. https://doi.org/10.1007/s00127-022-02344-5

Character Strengths: Definitions and Conceptualization

Peterson, C., & Seligman, M. E. P. (2004). *Character strengths and virtues: A handbook and classification.* Oxford University Press; American Psychological Association.

Park, N., & Peterson, C. (2006). Moral competence and character strengths among adolescents: The development and validation of the Values in Action Inventory of Strengths for Youth. *Journal of Adolescence, 29*(6), 891–905. https://doi.org/10.1016/j.adolescence.2006.04.011

Steen, T. A., Kachorek, L. V., & Peterson, C. (2003). Character strengths among youth. *Journal of Youth & Adolescence, 32,* 5–16. https://doi.org/10.1023/A:1021024205483

Distinguishing Character Strengths From Talents, Abilities, and Values

Peterson, C. (2006). *A primer in positive psychology.* Oxford University Press.

Character Strengths in Educational Settings

Norrish, J. (2015). *Positive education: The Geelong Grammar School journey.* Oxford University Press. https://doi.org/10.1093/acprof:oso/9780198702580.001.0001

Quinlan, D. M., Swain, N., Cameron, C., & Vella-Brodrick, D. A. (2014). How other people matter in a classroom-based strengths intervention: Exploring interpersonal strategies and classroom outcomes. *Journal of Positive Psychology, 10*(1), 77–89. https://doi.org/10.1080/17439760.2014.920407

White, M. A., & Waters, L. E. (2015). A case study of "The Good School": Examples of the use of Peterson's strengths-based approach with students. *The Journal of Positive Psychology, 10*(1), 69–76. https://doi.org/10.1080/17439760.2014.920408

Websites

Bring Your Strengths to Life & Live More Fully

https://www.viacharacter.org/

This website of the VIA Institute on Character (previously the Values in Action Institute) offers invaluable resources on both the science and practice of character, with a free measure of character strengths.

How Do CliftonStrengths and the VIA Survey Compare?

https://www.gallup.com/cliftonstrengths/en/249878/compare-via-survey-cliftonstrengths.aspx

The Gallup Strengths Finder measures 34 themes related to personal development in the workplace.

Be Your Best SELF With STRENGTHS

https://www.strengthsprofile.com/en-gb

The Realise2 strengths assessment measures 60 different strengths.

Greater Good Magazine: Science-Based Insights for a Meaningful Life

https://greatergood.berkeley.edu/

The Greater Good Science Center studies the psychology, sociology, and neuroscience of well-being and teaches skills that foster a thriving, resilient, and compassionate society.

Character Labs

https://characterlab.org/about/

Co-founded by Angela Duckworth, Rosa Lee, and Egbert Chang, this nonprofit organization supports educators and researchers by providing knowledge that fosters the emotional, social, intellectual, and physical well-being of young people.

Multimedia

The Gift and Power of Emotional Courage

https://www.ted.com/talks/susan_david_the_gift_and_power_of_emotional_courage

Psychologist Susan David shares how we deal with our emotions.

Grit: The Power and Passion of Perseverance

https://www.ted.com/talks/angela_lee_duckworth_grit_the_power_of_passion_and_perseverance

Angela Lee Duckworth argues that grit is a better predictor of success than IQ.

Ignite Your Character Strengths with Ryan Niemiec and Robert McGrath

https://youtu.be/Q2AfyO-2yhM

Two distinguished scholars of character strengths, Ryan Niemiec and Robert McGrath, discuss how the power of character strengths can ignite one's positive personality.

What Are Your Character Strengths? A Brief Video to Assess Character Strengths

https://www.facebook.com/NZIWR/videos/235350247696599/

The New Zealand Institute of Wellbeing and Resilience provides a brief video to assess character strengths.

Structured Debriefing of the VIA Character Strengths Profile

https://youtu.be/2ZZ74Gy6UWI

This brief video walks viewers through how to interpret and set goals related to their VIA Character Strengths Profile.

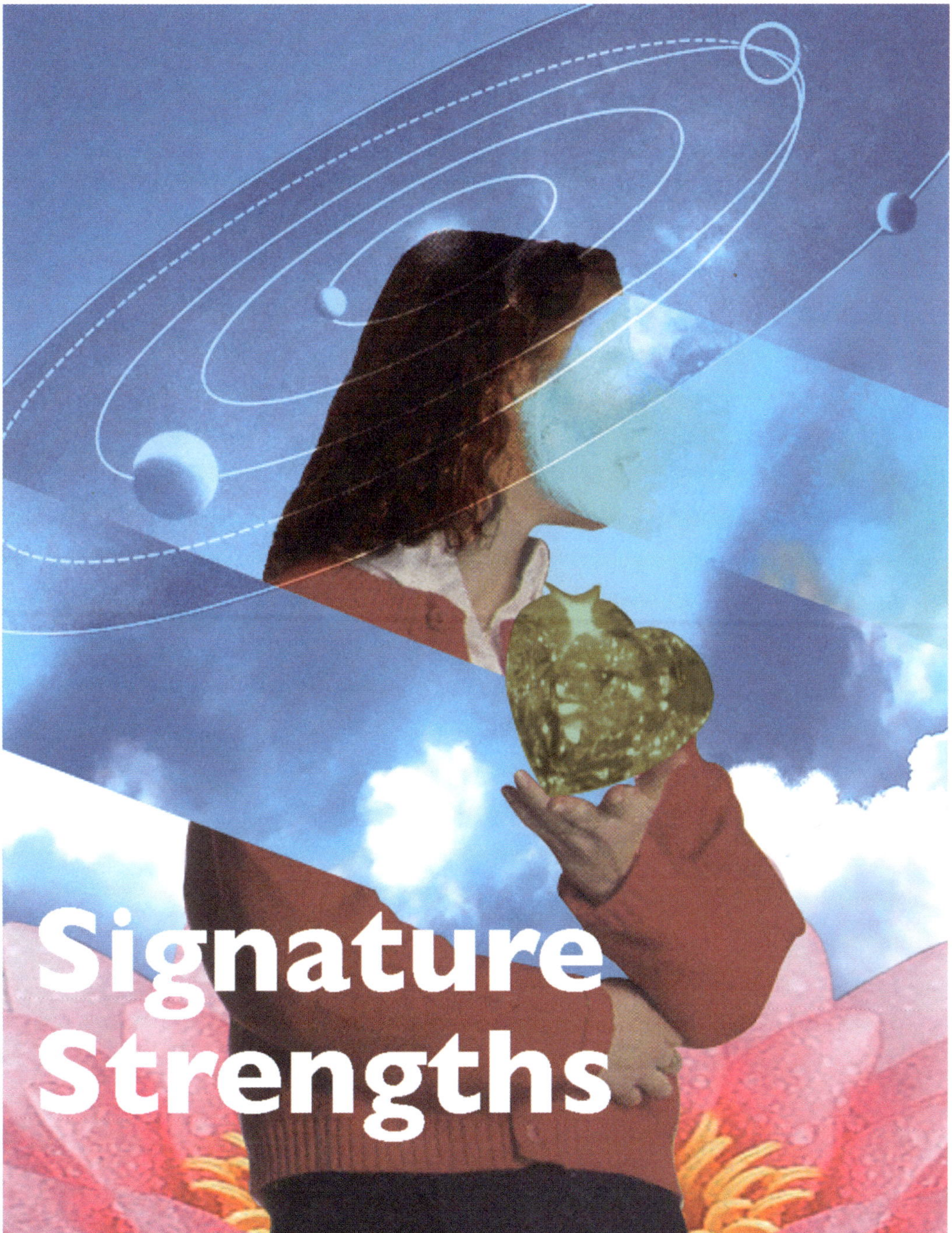
Signature
Strengths

Module 6: Signature Strengths

The second of three modules on character strengths teaches participants about the concept of signature strengths or top strengths that are central to who one is. The module explores the value of gaining perspective from others to increase awareness of top strengths. It also introduces the importance of practical wisdom, adapting expressions of strengths to situational demands by considering relevance, conflict, and specificity.

Module Topic	Minutes to Allot	
Learning Outcomes By inviting people who know them well to assess their strengths, as well as examining their use, underuse, overuse, and the desirability of strengths, participants: • Own their cluster of top strengths as sources of energy and learning • Identify opportunities to set personal goals for improvement • Apply strengths adaptively to the unique demands of various situations	5	5
Opening Activities Start the module with a relaxation or mindfulness practice Invite participants to share a few events from their gratitude journal that have occurred since the last session Invite questions about the previous module and practice(s)	10	15
Illustration of Core Concepts Review core concepts and show video illustrations Facilitate reflection and discussion: • *What are the key messages in the video(s) you just watched?* • *How might these concepts be relevant in your life?*	15	15
Practice: Compile Your Signature Strengths Profile Walk participants through the Signature Strengths Profile Once compiled, have participants assess their use, overuse, underuse, and the desirability of each strength and discuss practical wisdom strategies Debrief learning from practice(s) using questions: • *How well do your signature strengths reflect your personality?* • *Are there significant differences between your perspective and those of your peer, family member and teacher or colleague?* • *Did multiple people identify the same specific strength?* • *If different people identified different strengths, what accounts for this?* • *Do you display your signature strengths more often with specific people or in specific situations?*	20	30
Closing Activities Invite discussion of everyday applications Remind participants of relevant resources at the end of the module Guide participants in a 3-minute closing relaxation or mindfulness practice	10	10
Total	60 minutes	75 minutes

Core Concepts of Signature Strengths

The themes here are also presented in the Core Concepts section of the Workbook (p. 79):

- Everyone has strengths but to varying degrees: high, medium, and low. Our highest strengths are called *signature strengths*. Some of your friends are more curious than others. Some may love learning or may be very socially intelligent. Some friends are always very kind and others are very playful and cheerful.
- According to Christopher Peterson (2006) and Martin Seligman (2011), signature strengths are the character strengths that come naturally to you. For example:
  - If kindness is one of your signature strengths, doing acts of kindness, even without being asked, gives you deep satisfaction.
  - If playfulness is a signature strength a person has and celebrates, they can experience greater happiness if they play games, joke around, or otherwise have fun with others in life.
- According to Peterson (2006) and Seligman (2011), signature strengths are also your core character strengths, and when you use them:
  - You feel a sense of ownership and authenticity (e.g., "This is the real me").
  - You are excited when you are displaying this strength. For example, if prudence is one of your signature strengths, you feel at ease and comfortable while being prudent. If you are brave, you don't shrink from challenges.
  - You learn rapidly when you use your signature strengths.
  - You look for new ways to use your signature strengths.
  - You find that it is almost impossible to stop using your signature strengths.
  - You do not feel exhausted when you use your signature strengths. Tasks do not seem a burden to you, and you do not tire quickly. You feel happier.
- Research shows that strengths-based interventions increase positive affect, happiness, and life satisfaction, and decrease depressive symptoms (Schutte & Malouff, 2019). Strengths can help you achieve your goals. You can use your strengths toward goals that people expect you to achieve, such as getting good grades, getting along with others, being a leader, etc. However, you are more likely to use your strengths to achieve goals that are personally important and meaningful to you. These goals could be creative, athletic, academic, or anything that is meaningful to you. Several studies (Schutte & Malouff, 2019) have shown that people who use their strengths frequently:
  - Are happier and more satisfied with life
  - Are more resilient and handle stress better
  - Are more assertive and confident
  - Are more engaged and productive at work
  - Have a greater sense of self-worth and self-respect
  - Are more energetic
  - Are more likely to accomplish their goals
- Character strengths are expressed in degree, not in categories (McGrath et al., 2010; Niemiec & Pearce, 2021). That is, we have degrees of gratitude, prudence, and curiosity. It is highly unlikely that we are completely devoid of these strengths. Strengths should not be considered independent concepts. For example, strengths of gratitude and hope often appear as the top strengths of some individuals. Likewise, persistence often accompanies

self-regulation and hope, and optimism. Moreover, the character strengths and virtues framework is just one of many models of strengths. Finally, strengths are both being and doing. That is, strengths are part of being and also what we do (Niemiec & McGrath, 2019).

Illustrations of Signature Strengths

Play at least one of the three videos below to illustrate the core concepts of signature strengths and encourage discussion.

Resilience Through Your Signature Strengths
https://youtu.be/xcLmzuEsXcI
(Duration: 6:17 minutes)
Maria Sirois, a clinical psychologist, discusses the importance of amplifying your resilience, by identifying and using your core strengths; that is, your signature strengths. She recommends that we lean on our strengths and thus discover who we are – a revelation which offers us a greater sense of control.

How to Identify and Use Your Signature Character Strengths
https://youtu.be/Icar7lb2KIA
(Duration: 3:32 minutes)
Clinical psychologist and author Chris Mackey discusses the benefits of identifying and utilizing your top character strengths. He underscores the importance of knowing your strengths and using them in concert with others.

Signature Strengths
https://youtu.be/2Kc32NxxrVQ
(Duration: 5:35 minutes)
With the help of a car trunk packing analogy, David Pollay helps us to understand the importance of knowing what you are really good at (i.e., what your signature strengths are) and how to look for and spot signature strengths in others.

Reflection and Discussion

Invite participants to complete the Reflection and Discussion section of their Workbook (p. 80) regarding the video(s) they have watched. Discuss the questions:

What are the key messages in the video(s) you just watched?

How might these concepts be relevant in your life?

Practice: Compile your Signature Strengths Profile

Building on the previous practice where participants identified their character strengths through pictures and descriptions, this practice deepens participants' understanding of their character strengths through a process of gathering feedback from significant others, including loved ones, about their top five or six signature strengths.

Participants can experience several benefits as a result of compiling their Signature Strengths Profile. Labeling positive attributes of oneself in an authentic manner, as participants did in Module 5, can be helpful to mitigate self-criticism and self-deprecation. However, when other people acknowledge and spot our strengths, they improve their relationship with us. When they genuinely acknowledge our strengths, abilities, and talents, our self-concept improves, our self-confidence gets a boost, and we feel empowered. Strengths-spotting by loved ones can lift our mood when we feel down or demotivated.

The Signature Strengths Profile compiles participants' own perception of their top 5 strengths with opinions of others who know them well. By looking at their strengths from multiple perspectives, participants can get a more rounded view of their signature strengths, i.e., those strengths that are a core part of them.

Refer participants to the Practice: Compile your Signature Strengths Profile on p. 81 in the Workbook. There are nine steps in compiling the Signature Strengths Profile, the first six involve checking off in the respective column the different perspectives on the participants top five strengths: self-reported from pictures (1) and word descriptions (2), a friend (3), a family member (4), a teacher or colleague (5), and the results from the online SSQ-72 (6). After tallying the most commonly observed strengths (7), with each check having a unitary value of "1", participants reflect on their under and overuse of strengths (8) as well as which strengths they need to develop further (9).

Table 7 walks practitioners through the 9 steps of facilitating this practice. Following these instructions, we discuss in more detail how to approach Column 8, under and overuse of strengths.

Table 7. Instructions for practice: Compile Your Signature Strengths

Columns	Instructions to participants
Column 1: Pictures Column 2: Descriptions	In the first two columns of the Signature Strengths Profile on p. 85, check "✓" your top 5 strengths from the Worksheets you completed in Module 5: Character strengths pictures compared with descriptions (p. 75).
Columns 3–5: Friend or Peer Family Member Teacher or Colleague	Identify three people who know you well in the above categories. Ask them to complete one of the three worksheets on the next three pages. Record their perceptions of your top 5–6 strengths by checking "✓" selected strengths in the respective columns. Note that if you can't get people to complete the worksheet for you, you can ask them to talk with you about their perceptions of your strengths. Alternatively, can you imagine what they might perceive to be your top strengths?
Column 6: SSQ-72	Complete the Signature Strengths Questionnaire-72 (SSQ-72) at https://www.strengthsbasedresilience.com/assessment. Check "✓" your top five or six strengths.
Column 7: Totals	For each checkmark "✓" assign a unitary value of "1" across each strength and tally each row. Your top five scores are considered Signature strengths.
Column 8: U/O	Review all 24 strengths. Mark a U or an O in this column next to any strength you underuse (U) or overuse (O). Aim to limit your selection to five. See discussion below.
Column 9: Desired	Identify five strengths that you want to develop. Think about other strengths on the list that you value and would like to strengthen. These could be strengths that would help you: • Be the kind of person you would like to be • Reach your goals • Have even better relationships with others If you are uncertain about your underuse or overuse of strengths (Column 8), or the strengths you want to develop (Column 9), return to this activity after Module 7: Problem-Solving and Strengths.

Underuse and Overuse of Strengths (Column 8)

The goal of compiling the Worksheet: Signature Strengths Profile is not only to equip participants with knowledge of what their strengths are – assessed from multiple perspectives – but also to develop the skill of "know how" to use them. Aristotle calls this "know how" skill the master virtue – Wisdom. According to Barry Schwartz and Kenneth Sharpe in their book *Practical Wisdom – The Right Way to Do the Right Thing* (Schwartz & Sharpe, 2010), without the wisdom of knowing how to use one's strengths, our strengths can be like unruly children: they want to do well, but their actions can result in doing more harm than good. For example, without knowing how to use courage, one can easily drift into recklessness. Persisting with a task that has fundamental flaws may lead someone to waste resources.

After participants have tallied their signature strengths in Column 7, their reflection in Column 8 enables them to assess how well they are using strengths. Are they overusing their signature strengths? Are they underutilizing some strengths for which they did not receive high scores? Can they cultivate their strengths by developing their know-how or practical wisdom?

Balanced Use of Strengths

This program teaches participants to use their signature strengths and values in a balanced way, based on the notion of practical wisdom proposed by Schwartz and Sharpe (2010) that considers the three factors of relevance, conflict, and specificity. The workbook provides brief descriptions and examples of relevance, conflict, and specificity (Workbook page 87). You can facilitate a discussion on the application of practical wisdom to deploy strengths using the scenario and questions below. Start your discussion by describing the following scenario:

> A good friend of yours asks for your opinion about an important presentation they are about to do in a couple of days. You are well versed on this topic, and you believe aspects of the presentation need significant improvement. How can you use an understanding of these three factors of practical wisdom to guide your response and use your strengths adaptively? Let's assume your signature strengths include honesty, social intelligence, appreciation of beauty and excellence, prudence, and love of learning.

Relevance

Which of your signature strengths are more relevant to this situation? Honesty? Social intelligence? Appreciation of beauty and excellence? Prudence? Love of learning?

Depending on the person and your relationship with them, as well as your goal in supporting them, any of them might be relevant. Let's say you decide both honesty and social intelligence are the most relevant.

Conflict

What do you do when two strengths come into conflict? How can being mindful of the context of the situation guide you toward an adaptive use of strengths?

For context, you know your friend is sensitive. This can create a conflict for you. Should you provide candid feedback using your honesty or could it be perceived as criticism? Or should you use your social intelligence and provide more positive feedback. Your concern is that while it may not improve the presentation, it will keep the relationship intact.

Both strengths are applicable. Honest feedback can help the person address deficits in the presentation. However, at the same time, not everyone is able to receive honest feedback. Therefore, being too honest risks damaging the relationship. Social intelligence on the other hand can preserve the relationship, but an overuse of it may lead one to being overly cautious, even inauthentic by providing socially desired praise.

Specificity

How will you translate the selected strength(s) into action? Which specific actions will demonstrate appropriate use of strengths like honesty and social intelligence?

In this case, you might choose to lead with social intelligence by asking your friend what kind of feedback will be helpful to them and how much time they have to make changes, i.e., high level or detailed, positive or constructive, exploratory or directive. You might begin your honest feedback by pointing out what works well, and gauge how much feedback you provide based on their earlier answers.

Developing practical wisdom requires being attuned to the situation at hand and calibrating strengths accordingly.

Worksheet: Signature Strengths Profile

Strengths		WS: Character strength pictures	WS: Character strength descriptions	WS: Friend or peer	WS: Family member	WS: Teacher or colleague	SSQ-72	Totals	U/O	Desired
Wisdom & Knowledge: Cognitive strengths that entail the acquisition and use of knowledge										
1	Creativity & originality									
2	Curiosity & interest in the world									
3	Open-mindedness, judgement, & critical thinking									
4	Love of learning									
5	Perspective & wisdom									
Courage: Emotional strengths that involve accomplishing goals in the face of internal or external opposition										
6	Bravery & valor									
7	Persistence, diligence, & industry									
8	Integrity, authenticity, & honesty									
9	Vitality, zest, enthusiasm, & energy									
Humanity: Interpersonal strengths that involve tending to and befriending others										
10	Love: capacity to love & be loved									
11	Kindness & generosity									
12	Social intelligence									
Justice: Civic strengths that support healthy community life										
13	Citizenship, teamwork, & loyalty									
14	Fairness, equity, & justice									
15	Leadership									
Temperance: Strengths that protect against excess										
16	Forgiveness & mercy									
17	Humility & modesty									
18	Prudence, caution, & discretion									
19	Self-regulation & self-control									
Transcendence: Strengths that forge connections to the larger universe and provide meaning										
20	Appreciation of beauty									
21	Gratitude									
22	Hope & optimism									
23	Humor & playfulness									
24	Spirituality & religiousness									

SSQ-72 = Signature Strengths Questionnaire–72; U/O = underused versus overused strengths; WS = Worksheet.

Worksheet: Friend or Peer

Place a check "✓" in the Signature Strengths column for the **five to six** attributes that you think most often characterize your friend or peer.

		Signature strengths
1	Are good at thinking of new and better ways of doing things.	
2	Love to explore things and ask questions; are open to different experiences and activities.	
3	Are flexible and open-minded; think through and examine all sides before deciding.	
4	Love to learn many new ideas, concepts, and facts in school or on their own.	
5	Are considered to be wise beyond their age - friends consult them regarding important matters.	
6	Do not give up in the face of hardship or challenge, even when afraid.	
7	Finish most things, even when distracted; are able to refocus and complete tasks.	
8	Are genuine and honest, known to be trustworthy; act consistently with their values.	
9	Are energetic, cheerful, and full of life.	
10	Showing and receiving genuine love and affection comes naturally to them.	
11	Love to do kind acts for others, often without being asked.	
12	Manage themself well in social situations and are known to have good interpersonal skills.	
13	Are an active community or team member; contribute to the success of their group.	
14	Stand up for others when they are treated unfairly, bullied, or ridiculed.	
15	Are often chosen by others as a leader; known to lead well.	
16	Do not hold grudges; forgive easily those who offend them.	
17	Don't like to be the center of attention and prefer others to shine.	
18	Are careful and cautious, can anticipate risks and problems of their actions and respond accordingly.	
19	Manage feelings and behaviors well in challenging situations; generally follow rules and routines.	
20	Are moved deeply by beauty in nature and in art (e.g., painting, music, theater, etc.), and/or by excellence in many fields of life.	
21	Express thankfulness for good things through words and actions.	
22	Hope and believe that more good things will happen than bad ones.	
23	Are playful, funny, and use humor to connect with others.	
24	Believe in a higher power and participate in religious or spiritual practices (e.g., prayer, meditation, etc.) willingly.	

Worksheet: Family Member

Place a check "✓" in the Signature Strengths column for the **five to six** attributes that you think most often characterize your family member.

		Signature strengths
1	Are good at thinking of new and better ways of doing things.	
2	Love to explore things and ask questions; are open to different experiences and activities.	
3	Are flexible and open-minded; think through and examine all sides before deciding.	
4	Love to learn many new ideas, concepts, and facts in school or on their own.	
5	Are considered to be wise beyond their age - friends consult them regarding important matters.	
6	Do not give up in the face of hardship or challenge, even when afraid.	
7	Finish most things, even when distracted; are able to refocus and complete tasks.	
8	Are genuine and honest, known to be trustworthy; act consistently with their values.	
9	Are energetic, cheerful, and full of life.	
10	Showing and receiving genuine love and affection comes naturally to them.	
11	Love to do kind acts for others, often without being asked.	
12	Manage themself well in social situations and are known to have good interpersonal skills.	
13	Are an active community or team member; contribute to the success of their group.	
14	Stand up for others when they are treated unfairly, bullied, or ridiculed.	
15	Are often chosen by others as a leader; known to lead well.	
16	Do not hold grudges; forgive easily those who offend them.	
17	Don't like to be the center of attention and prefer others to shine.	
18	Are careful and cautious, can anticipate risks and problems of their actions and respond accordingly.	
19	Manage feelings and behaviors well in challenging situations; generally follow rules and routines.	
20	Are moved deeply by beauty in nature and in art (e.g., painting, music, theater, etc.), and/or by excellence in many fields of life.	
21	Express thankfulness for good things through words and actions.	
22	Hope and believe that more good things will happen than bad ones.	
23	Are playful, funny, and use humor to connect with others.	
24	Believe in a higher power and participate in religious or spiritual practices (e.g., prayer, meditation, etc.) willingly.	

Worksheet: Teacher or Colleague

Place a check "✓" in the Signature Strengths column for the five attributes that you think most often characterize your participant or colleague.

		Signature strengths
1	Are good at thinking of new and better ways of doing things.	
2	Love to explore things and ask questions; are open to different experiences and activities.	
3	Are flexible and open-minded; think through and examine all sides before deciding.	
4	Love to learn many new ideas, concepts, and facts in school or on their own.	
5	Are considered to be wise beyond their age – friends consult them regarding important matters.	
6	Do not give up in the face of hardship or challenge, even when afraid.	
7	Finish most things, even when distracted; are able to refocus and complete tasks.	
8	Are genuine and honest, known to be trustworthy; act consistently with their values.	
9	Are energetic, cheerful, and full of life.	
10	Showing and receiving genuine love and affection comes naturally to them.	
11	Love to do kind acts for others, often without being asked.	
12	Manage themself well in social situations and are known to have good interpersonal skills.	
13	Are an active community or team member; contribute to the success of their group.	
14	Stand up for others when they are treated unfairly, bullied, or ridiculed.	
15	Are often chosen by others as a leader; known to lead well.	
16	Do not hold grudges; forgive easily those who offend them.	
17	Don't like to be the center of attention and prefer others to shine.	
18	Are careful and cautious, can anticipate risks and problems of their actions and respond accordingly.	
19	Manage feelings and behaviors well in challenging situations; generally follow rules and routines.	
20	Are moved deeply by beauty in nature and in art (e.g., painting, music, theater, etc.), and/or by excellence in many fields of life.	
21	Express thankfulness for good things through words and actions.	
22	Hope and believe that more good things will happen than bad ones.	
23	Are playful, funny, and use humor to connect with others.	
24	Believe in a higher power and participate in religious or spiritual practices (e.g., prayer, meditation, etc.) willingly.	

Practice Debrief

Invite participants to complete the Practice Debrief section in their Workbook on p. 88. To debrief signature strengths, discuss the following questions:

How well do the signature strengths you identified through this activity reflect your personality?

Are there significant differences between your perspective and those of your peer, family member, and teacher or colleague? Did multiple people identify the same specific strengths? If different people identified different strengths, what might account for this?

Do you display your signature strengths more often with specific people or in specific situations?

Learning and Cultural Fit

Adapt this practice to the learning and cultural needs of your audience, its unique values and demographics. Possible adaptations include:

- Some participants do not acknowledge their strengths for fear of coming across as arrogant. This program encourages them to acknowledge and express their strengths in a prosocial and respectful manner. Not acknowledging our signature strengths may limit our awareness, not only of our own assets and resources but also those of others.
- If participants are unsure which signature strength to use in what context, help them to understand that they can rely on their emotions to first hear and feel what the situation demands. Encourage them to make their emotions an ally of their reasoning.
- Know that signature strengths may not be useful in all situations. Encourage participants not to be afraid of experimenting with alternative strengths, skills, and strategies.
- Encourage participants to consult with people they consider to be wise about what is the right thing to do in a given situation. Consulting and seeking counsel from friends and older persons is a critical part of almost all non-Western cultural traditions. This often results in shared decision making, resulting in shared responsivity, in case the expression of the strength was not relevant.

Closing Activities

The goal of closing this module is to help participants integrate their cognitive understanding of signature strengths and to take their new learning into everyday life.

Discuss with participants the Everyday Applications section, also found on p. 90 in their Workbook. Invite participants to be mindful in their day-to-day lives by noticing actions and habits which show their signature strength or those of others. Encourage them to use relevant resources found at the end of this module and included in their workbooks starting on p. 90.

Choose a 3-minute mindfulness activity from Regular Practice 1: Mindfulness and Relaxation to close the module.

Everyday Applications

- Notice in your everyday activities when you are using your signature strengths. Pay attention to how using them makes you feel excited, energized, or more authentic. Celebrate their use.
- Begin to reflect on your behavior in strengths terms. When facing an everyday challenge, ask yourself two questions: (1) Are you unintentionally creating problems for yourself by overusing or underusing particular strengths? (2) How could you solve your problems using strengths? When thinking in strengths terms, do not belittle the problems: The problems are real, and they need a solution. Thinking in strengths terms should not be equated with looking at the world through "rose-colored glasses." Instead, view strengths as valuable resources to improve the quality of your actions and interactions.
- Work on spotting strengths in the actions of other people. Instead of describing the behavior of others in terms of weaknesses, try to describe them in terms of their strengths. Ask yourself whether their application of strengths is a balanced use, overuse, or underuse.
- Assess if signature strengths are being used to do the right thing. Consult with wise minds about what is the right thing to do, within the circumstances. If one signature strength poses conflicts, consider another one that may resolve it. If you are still unsure which signature strength to use in what context, rely on emotions to first hear and feel what the situation demands. Before you act, make emotion a partner of reason. For example, we often face situations where we "think" the right thing to do is to tell the truth, but we "feel" this would cause harm to someone else. By noticing and valuing this "feeling" caution, we may use strengths of kindness and social intelligence to tailor our approach.
- Know that not all situations can be addressed through your signature strengths. Experiment with alternative strengths, skills, abilities, and talents.
- Bring a mindful approach to your daily challenges. Notice how your signature strengths become resources to challenge troubling thoughts and feelings as well as to overcome difficult experiences. Through this deepened awareness, you can enhance your signature strengths and develop new strengths through practice.

References

McGrath, R., Rashid, T., Park, N., & Peterson, C. (2010). Is optimal functioning a distinct state? *The Humanistic Psychologist, 38*, 159-169. https://doi.org/10.1080/08873261003635781

Niemiec, R. M., and McGrath, R. E. (2019). *The power of character strengths: Appreciate and ignite your positive personality*. VIA Institute on Character.

Niemiec, R. M., & Pearce, R. (2021). The practice of character strengths: Unifying definitions, principles, and exploration of what's soaring, emerging, and ripe with potential in science and in practice. *Frontiers in Psychology, 11*, Article 590220. https://doi.org/10.3389/fpsyg.2020.590220

Peterson, C. (2006). *A primer in positive psychology*. Oxford University Press.

Schutte, N. S., & Malouff, J. M. (2019). The impact of signature character strengths interventions: A meta-analysis. *Journal of Happiness Studies, 20*(4), 1179–1196. https://doi.org/10.1007/s10902-018-9990-2

Schwartz, B., & Sharpe, K. (2010). *Practical wisdom: The right way to do the right thing*. Penguin.

Seligman, M. E. P. (2011). *Flourish: A visionary new understanding of happiness and well-being*. Free Press.

Resources

Literature

Buschor, C., Proyer, R. T., & Ruch, W. (2013). Self- and peer-rated character strengths: How do they relate to satisfaction with life and orientations to happiness? *Journal of Positive Psychology, 8*(2), 116–127. https://doi.org/10.1080/17439760.2012.758305

Doman, F. (2020). *Authentic resilience: Bringing your strengths to life.* Authentic Strengths Advantage.

Forest, J., Mageau, G. V. A., Crevier-Braud, L., Bergeron, L., Dubreuil, P., & Lavigne, G. V. L. (2012). Harmonious passion as an explanation of the relation between signature strengths' use and well-being at work: Test of an intervention program. *Human Relations, 65*(9), 1233–1252. https://doi.org/10.1177/0018726711433134

Lavy, S., Littman-Ovadia, H., & Bareli, Y. (2014). Strengths deployment as a mood-repair mechanism: Evidence from a diary study with a relationship exercise group. *Journal of Positive Psychology, 9*(6), 547–558. https://doi.org/10.1080/17439760.2014.936963

Linley, P. A., Nielsen, K. M., Gillett, R., & Biswas-Diener, R. (2010). Using signature strengths in pursuit of goals: Effects on goal progress, need satisfaction, and well-being, and implications for coaching psychologists. *International Coaching Psychology Review, 5*(1), 6–15. https://doi.org/10.53841/bpsicpr.2010.5.1.6

Niemiec, R. M. (2018). *Character strengths interventions: A field guide for practitioners.* Hogrefe.

Niemiec, R. M., & McGrath, R. E. (2019). *The power of character strengths: Appreciate and ignite your positive personality.* VIA Institute on Character.

Proyer, R. T., Gander, F., Wellenzohn, S., & Ruch, W. (2015). Strengths-based positive psychology interventions: A randomized placebo-controlled online trial on long-term effects for a signature strengths- vs. a lesser strengths intervention. *Frontiers in Psychology, 6,* Article 456. https://doi.org/10.3389/fpsyg.2015.00456

Roberts, F., & Wright. (2018). *Character toolkit for teachers: 100+ classroom and whole school character education activities for 5- to 11-year-olds.* Jessica Kingsley Publishers.

Rust, T., Diessner, R., & Reade, L. (2009). Strengths only or strengths and relative weaknesses? A preliminary study. *Journal of Psychology, 143*(5), 465–476. https://doi.org/10.3200/JRL.143.5.465-476

Toner, E., Haslam, N., Robinson, J., & Williams, P. (2012). Character strengths and well-being in adolescence: Structure and correlates of the Values in Action Inventory of Strengths for Children. *Personality and Individual Differences, 52*(5), 637–642. https://doi.org/10.1016/j.paid.2011.12.014

Wood, A. M., Linley, P. A., Matlby, J., Kashdan, T. B., & Hurling, R. (2011). Using personal and psychological strengths leads to increases in well-being over time: A longitudinal study and the development of the strengths use questionnaire. *Personality and Individual Differences, 50*(1), 15–19. https://doi.org/10.1016/j.paid.2010.08.004

Yeager, J., Fisher, S., & Shearon, D., (2008). *Smart strengths: Building character, resilience and relationship in youth.* VIA Institute.

Young, K. C., Kashdan, T. B., & Macatee, R. (2014). Strength balance and implicit strength measurement: New considerations for research on strengths of character. *Journal of Positive Psychology, 10*(1), 17–24. https://doi.org/10.1080/17439760.2014.920406

Websites

VIA Institute on Character Section on Signature Strengths
https://www.viacharacter.org/research/findings/signature-strengths
Explore signature strengths-related research on the website of the VIA Institute on Character (was the Values in Action Institute).

Positive Psychology's Emphasis on Strengths
https://healthypsych.com/learning-center-identify-strengths/
Explore why signature strengths are important in positive psychology.

Discovering Your Signature Strengths
https://www.goodtherapy.org/blog/discovering-your-signature-strengths-0624135
Marla B. Cohen writes, "Discover your own signature strengths and align your life with their expression. Become aware of your weaknesses, too, if only to learn forgiveness and a better understanding of where you may be challenged."

Multimedia

What Are You Good at?
https://youtu.be/Q6W5IrZH7tc
Tayyab Rashid discusses the importance of character strengths in psychology and their use in psychotherapy.

Happify: How to Tap into Your Character Strengths to Change Your Life
https://www.happify.com/hd/character-strengths-infographic/
Happify is a popular app for well-being and resilience. This infographic includes background on character strengths and practical tips on how to increase your well-being.

The Surprising Science of Happiness
https://www.ted.com/talks/dan_gilbert_the_surprising_science_of_happiness
Dan Gilbert provides a humorous summary of his research on happiness. His findings show that getting what we want does not necessarily lead to happiness. Rather, as humans, we can manufacture happiness from experiences we neither planned for nor chose.

Happiness and Its Surprises
https://www.ted.com/talks/nancy_etcoff_happiness_and_its_surprises
Cognitive researcher Nancy Etcoff discusses brain structures and chemicals related to emotions and experiences of happiness. She explains how happiness is not merely the absence of unhappiness, but rather a result of our positive beliefs, thoughts, and actions.

The Happy Planet Index
https://www.ted.com/talks/nic_marks_the_happy_planet_index#t-58100
Statistician Nic Marks proposes that a nation's success ought to be measured by the happiness and well-being of its people, not by its productivity.

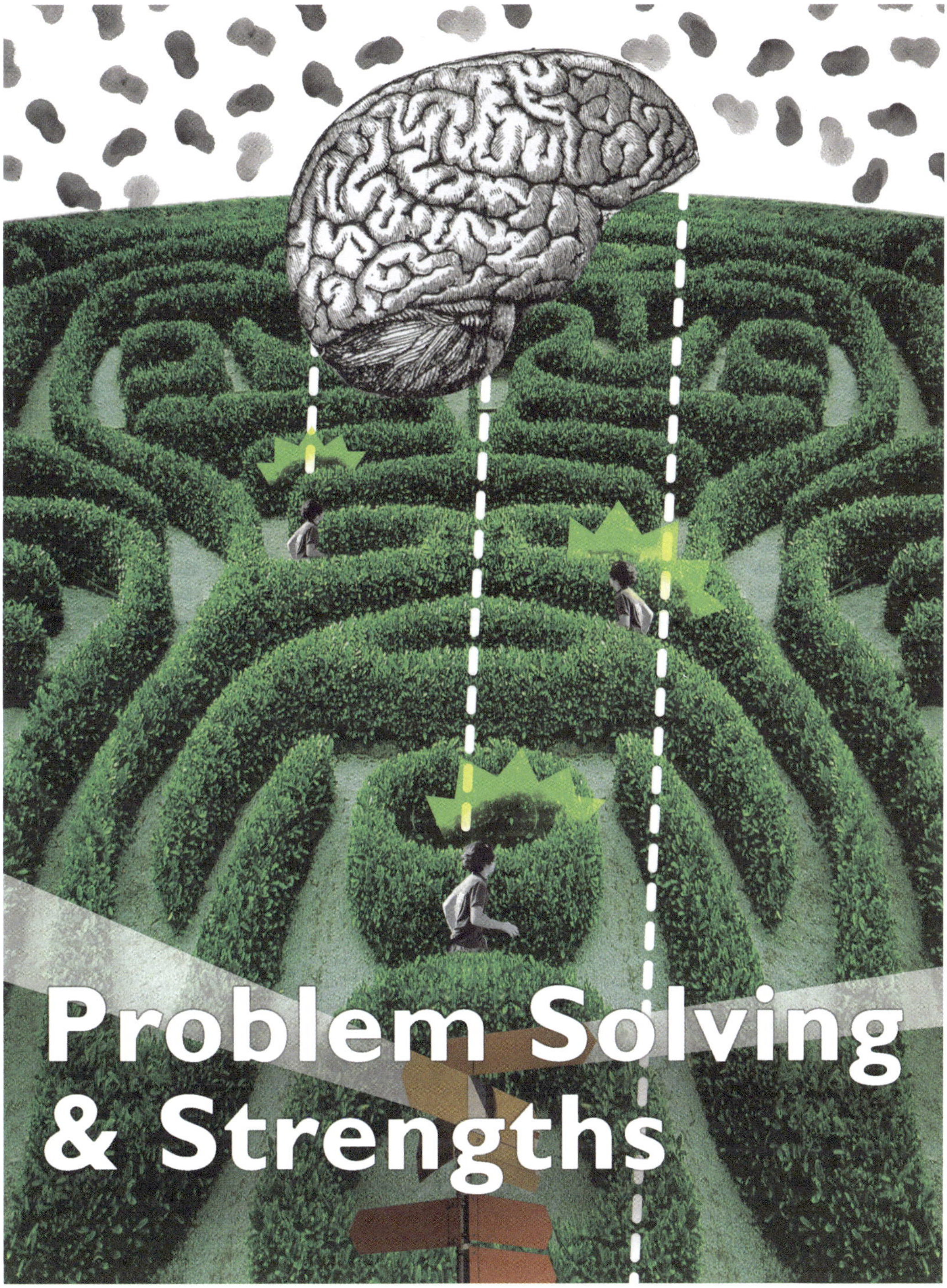
Problem Solving
& Strengths

Module 7: Problem Solving and Strengths

Building on practical wisdom concepts of relevance, conflict, and specificity introduced in Module 6, this module invites participants to practice using their strengths in a real-life problem-solving situation they are currently facing. Through multiple illustrations, it shows how they can recruit strengths to address common challenges that call for a resilient approach.

Module Topic	Minutes to Allot	
Learning Outcomes Considering relevance, conflict and specificity in relation to resolving a personal challenge, participants: • Calibrate their strengths according to the situational relevance and fit • Recruit strengths optimally to solve everyday problems and setbacks • Learn to use strengths in a balanced and adaptive way	5	5
Opening Activities Start the module with a relaxation or mindfulness practice Invite participants to share a few events from their gratitude journal that have occurred since the last session Invite questions about the previous module and practice(s)	10	15
Illustration of Core Concepts Review core concepts and show video illustrations Facilitate reflection and discussion: • *What are the key messages in the video(s) you just watched?* • *How might these concepts be relevant in your life?*	15	15
Practice: Use Strengths to Overcome Challenges Have participants think of a real-life problem or challenge they are currently facing Discuss the sample challenge with them, then have them complete *Worksheet: Your Challenge* to assess a personal problem Debrief learning from practice(s) using questions: • What strengths did you use (including overuse and underuse)? • How could you apply signature strengths to solve this challenge in a balanced way? • What specific actions will you take and what concrete outcomes will result?	20	30
Closing Activities Invite discussion of everyday applications Remind participants of relevant resources at the end of the module Guide participants in a 3-minute closing relaxation or mindfulness practice	10	10
Total	60 minutes	75 minutes

Core Concepts of Problem Solving and Strengths

Many of the themes here are also presented in the Core Concepts section of the Workbook (p. 93):

- When we understand and utilize our signature strengths, we gain insight to solve common everyday problems.
- The use of signature strengths enhances happiness and reduces psychological symptoms and distress. Studies are showing that the use of character strengths not only enhances well-being but also mitigates symptoms of obsessive-compulsive disorder (Littman-Ovadia & Freidlin, 2019), social anxiety (Freidlin & Littman-Ovadia, 2020; Kashdan et al., 2006), and depressive symptoms (Sin & Lyubomirsky, 2009; Uliaszek, Rashid, & Zarowsky, 2022).
- All 24 strengths can be used to solve problems in our daily lives. Using a strengths-based approach is generally associated with positive outcomes. Refinement of our strengths is an ongoing learning process which requires practice – of both our signature strengths as well as those strengths we want to develop.
- Adaptive use of strengths requires careful consideration of which strengths should be used and when. Neither underusing nor overusing these strengths provides a balance. Sometimes behaviors we consider negative in ourselves and others might instead be either over- or underuse of our signature strengths. Awareness of our and others' signature strengths can help us to reframe everyday stressors and negatives as either over- or underuse of signature strengths.
- Research shows that under- or overuse of any signature or non-signature strength is associated with negative emotions, whereas optimal use is associated with positive emotions (Kamushadze & Martskvishvili, 2021). Ryan Niemiec, who has done seminal work on character strengths, recommends the aware-explore-apply model for the optimal use of strengths (Niemiec, 2018). This model is described in the Everyday Applications section of this module (p. 98).
- The use of strengths for problem solving requires consideration of contextual and situational factors, where one strength might be more appropriate than another, especially when there is a conflict between two strengths. For example, teachers frequently find themselves in a conflict between using kindness toward one student versus fairness toward all students. Being aware of your diverse strengths and their occasional conflicts can help you to resolve challenges and move toward becoming an even better version of yourself.
- When using strengths to solve problems, the following four considerations can be helpful:
  - First, we need to perceive signature strengths as our deep psychological assets. Because signature strengths, when perceived as valued and recognized by others, predict well-being (Blanchard et al., 2020).
  - Second, we need to acknowledge that our or others' specific behaviors could also be an over- or underuse of their signature strengths. For example, forthright feedback or a direct remark could signify the overuse of courage or the underuse of someone's signature strengths of social intelligence or prudence. Repeated forgiving without behavioral change could be an overuse of signature strengths of forgiveness or love, or not confronting a close friend for serious ethical breaches could be an underuse of the signature strengths of integrity and bravery.

- Third, the under- and overuse of strengths depends on situational dynamics which determine the degree of strengths usage. For example, the degree of curiosity, creativity, or self-regulation one has and will use depends on situational context. Perhaps despite the desire to use one's creativity, one is unable to use it, as creativity generally or in specific situations is not supported by others.
- Fourth, one should also keep in mind that strengths are not singular and independent constructs. In most circumstances, people use several strengths together (for example, using strengths of love, social intelligence, kindness, courage, authenticity, and forgiveness when talking with a loved one about something they did that hurt you). Therefore, it is important to understand the signature strengths profile and the contextual features (Niemiec & Pearce, 2021).

Consider the following examples of the application of strengths to problem solving by participants in past workshops:

Strength: Playfulness

While working on a school project, Jack and his schoolmates start to disagree on details and get stuck. Jack uses his humor to reduce the tension, causing the group to laugh and focus on their mutual goals.

Strength: Capacity to Love and Be Loved

Jane was struggling with how to recognize her parents' anniversary in an authentic manner. She decided to digitally record her parents' earliest memories as a way of showing her love for them and their relationship.

Strength: Social Intelligence

Maliha noticed that her friend undervalued an important accomplishment. She used her social intelligence to pay closer attention to her friend's accomplishment and congratulate her on the specifics of the achievement. As a result, she improved and enhanced their bond.

Strength: Creativity

Mari was feeling bored and low in energy. She started taking classes ikebana (the Japanese art of flower arrangement) to tap into her creativity, then felt renewed and energized.

Strength: Love of Learning

Gerry reached out to a friend who was struggling with a concept related to a mathematics assignment. Together, they researched the topic, were able to understand the concepts, and enjoyed solving the problems in the assignment.

Illustrations of Problem Solving and Strengths

Play at least one of the three videos below to illustrate the core concepts of problem solving and strengths and encourage discussion.

Barry Schwartz on Practical Wisdom
https://youtu.be/kk973t2nhx0
(Duration: 4:54 minutes)
Practical wisdom is about using strengths adaptively. We are not born with wisdom; it is acquired.

Reel Wisdom – Lessons from 40 Films in 7 Minutes
https://youtu.be/G2wluTdf5FQ
(Duration: 7:00 minutes)
This video is a collage of lessons in wisdom from 40 popular films.

How Does Creativity Help Solve Problems?
https://youtu.be/zizkcQ1lXoA
(Duration: 2:40 minutes)
This video shares reflections on creativity and problem solving from distinguished individuals working in media, design, and the arts.

Reflection and Discussion

Invite participants to complete the Reflection and Discussion section of their Workbook (p. 95) regarding the video(s) they have watched. Discuss the questions:

What are the key messages in the video(s) you just watched?

How might these concepts be relevant in your life?

Practice: Use Strengths to Overcome Challenges

When we experience a stressor or challenge, our negativity bias often steers us to be defensive, aggressive, or avoidant. We believe this can be, in part, due to the power of the negativity bias and a lack of awareness about our strengths. Sometimes we intuitively know our strengths but lack specific strategies for action.

This activity follows Module 6: Signature Strengths, which is aimed at deepening participants' awareness of their signature strengths from multiple perspectives, as well as orienting them to practical wisdom, i.e., the adaptive use of strengths. The activity in this module encourages participants to put their signature strengths into action, in an adaptive manner, when dealing with everyday life challenges.

- Facilitators can start this practice with a brief centering exercise. Invite participants to close their eyes or fix their gaze near the floor. Ask them to take three deep breaths.

- Have them read the sample challenge below, which is also on p. 96 of the Workbook, then refer to the Worksheet: Your Challenge p. 97.
- Ask them to write about a recent real-life challenge or problem in "The Challenge." To help them brainstorm, encourage them to think of challenges which recur despite their repeated attempts to resolve them. Participants can also think of persistent problems which they have been trying to resolve without success. Also refer participants to Table WB2: 15 Common Challenges in their Workbook on pp. 99–101, included here as Table 8.
- Under "Strengths used (including overused and underused)," invite them to write about what might be a wise and balanced use of strengths for them as discussed in Module 6 (relevance, conflict, specificity).
- Have them outline specific actions and outcomes in the next two blank fields. Some participants may hesitate to undertake this activity as their Signature Strengths Profiles may not be complete due to missing input from others (e.g., family or friends). Encourage participants to use whatever data they have on their Signature Strengths Profile so far. They can always update which signature strengths can be used to overcome challenges, as additional data comes in.

The challenge:
I am not afraid to speak my mind. My colleagues describe me as rude. I think I am honest.

Strengths used (including overused and underused):
Using courage to speak my mind. I may be underusing social intelligence and overusing honesty.

Balanced use of strengths:
Use my honesty to ask for honest feedback from colleagues. Ask those who are high in social intelligence what strategies they would apply in similar circumstances or in relation to feedback. Use my courage to test out new ways to speak my mind that incorporate social intelligence strategies that I use with less confidence or frequency.

Specific actions:
I will reflect on my conduct, seek counsel, and modify my behavior. I will check in with my colleagues for feedback.

Concrete outcomes:
I will have a more equitable and respectful relationship with my colleagues.

Worksheet: Your Challenge

The challenge:

____

____

____

Strengths used (including overused and underused):

____

____

____

Balanced use of signature strengths:

____

____

____

Specific actions:

____

____

____

Concrete outcomes:

____

____

____

Practice Debrief

Note that the Workbook does not have a Practice Debrief section, however, you can discuss the following questions to debrief this practice.

- *After doing this exercise, do you have specific strategies for using your strengths to resolve the problem you identified?*
- *What did you learn about optimal use of strengths?*

Learning and Cultural Fit

Adapt this practice to the learning and cultural needs of your audience, its unique values and demographics. Possible adaptations include:

- Some participants may not be able to relate their strengths to problem solving. They may be more familiar with using remedial strategies to solve their problems. Therefore, it is important to discuss strengths as active means of problem solving with the help of concrete illustrations. For example, some participants may assume that hyperactivity can only be managed by learning techniques that make one less hyperactive - that is, reducing a perceived weakness. They may not entertain the notion that hyperactivity can also be managed by explicitly cultivating a state of relaxation or by harnessing hyperactivity in pursuits which benefit from its use, such as sports. Furthermore, if they can see hyperactivity as an overuse of zest, vitality, and enthusiasm, they may only need to tweak this strength to resolve an issue of perceived hyperactivity.
- In teaching participants to use strengths in problem solving, it is important to help them reflect on and discuss the impact of their strengths on others. For example, to ward off negativity, if a participant expresses gratitude for good things in a classroom setting, it is important that their description of good things does not make others feel deprived or less fortunate. Likewise, if a participant describes using curiosity and love of learning to master a difficult topic, this may discourage others, especially those who may not be able to master that topic due to a specific learning challenge.
- It is important to consider culturally informed ways of solving problems and using strengths. For example, the expression of a strength - let's say, zest - varies from culture to culture. Zest can be expressed in emotive ways in one culture and in a relatively quieter way in another culture. Likewise, prudence, humility, and self-regulation can have cultural nuances. Furthermore, some strengths may be more valued in one culture in comparison to other cultures.
- In teaching participants the use of specific strengths in solving a specific problem, it is important to ensure that participants are able to use or express their strengths with ease. Not all strengths come to all participants with the same degree of ease. Some participants may find it easier to use humor to deflate a stressful situation, while others may resolve the same situation better with social intelligence or with kindness. Some participants may be able to persevere individually with a challenge; others may overcome the same challenge by leveraging support from others, using their social intelligence, love, and teamwork. See Table 8 for 15 common challenges and the character strengths to address them (Workbook Table WB2).

Table 8. Fifteen common challenges and the character strengths to address them (see also Table WB2)

Challenge	Potential character strength(s)	Specific actions
1. Feeling isolated, lacking motivation to participate in social activities	Zest Self-regulation Appreciation of beauty	Start and maintain at least one outdoor activity weekly, such as hiking, biking, mountain biking, mountain climbing, brisk walking, or jogging. Invite a friend to accompany you.
2. Difficulty in finishing tasks, making careless mistakes, giving up easily	Persistence Love of learning	Identify factors that diminish your interest in daily activities. Brainstorm topics you'd like to learn more about and master. Set small and attainable goals, and share them with someone you trust so they can help you.
3. Experiencing sudden changes in emotions from being sullen to being angry	Self-regulation	Explore triggers of your emotional outbursts. Reflect on what you might be seeking to accomplish and what healthier reactions can achieve your desired outcome. For example, instead of lashing out or withdrawing, can you manage your emotions by engaging in soothing and calming behaviors or by engaging in healthier distracting actions? For example, you could practice a calming exercise guided by an app on your smartphone, or discussed earlier in this workbook, take calming breaths, or engage in a fun task to distract yourself.
4. Holding grudges, feeling deeply hurt, and finding it difficult to let go of or accept apologies from others	Forgiveness Social intelligence	Reflect on the emotional impact of holding onto grudges and their effect on your mental health. Also select at least one unresolved conflict and deliberately try to think from your "offender's" perspective. Recall times when you offended someone and were forgiven.
5. Not knowing how to respond to the friendly and light-hearted gestures of others, and feeling emotionally closed	Humor & playfulness Social intelligence	Observe others, especially your peers, engaging in light-hearted gestures and playful activities with a good-natured attitude. Also watch online video illustrations. Select a few interpersonal strategies you find fit best with your disposition and situation, and try them out with close friends with whom you feel most comfortable.

Table 8. continued

Challenge	Potential character strength(s)	Specific actions
6. Struggling to initiate meaningful social interactions; avoiding social situations and feeling isolated and listless	Social intelligence Bravery Curiosity	Start by attending social events where you feel safe and are not expected to engage in one-to-one interactions, such as attending an art class (e.g., photography, painting, graphic designing, cooking, knitting). Observe social interactions and look for ways people express their curiosity when interacting with others.
7. Thinking too much about failures and shortcomings, focusing more on potentially negative outcomes than positive ones	Hope & optimism Spirituality	Make a list of things that are currently working for you or at least working well enough. Reflect on their causes. Don't hesitate to credit yourself when and where it is due. You can also ask your trusted friends to identify things you have accomplished. Spend time in a spiritual practice to restore balance.
8. Spending a lot of time to be the best and feeling upset when others outperform you	Teamwork Perspective Humility	Put achievements and accomplishments in perspective. Develop awareness that material gains have diminishing returns – that is, if you are overly focused on being the best, you will most likely pay a heavy price in letting go of things that can make you happier and healthier. Read about and reflect on humility and identify at least one personal accomplishment, unknown to others, which you will deliberately not share, and will let speak for itself. Notice and appreciate strengths of others.
9. Having rigid and inflexible ways of thinking; struggling to adjust well to changes such as new settings, colleagues, and situations	Curiosity Open-mindedness	Systematically cultivate curiosity and open-mindedness by trying out new experiences. Play devil's advocate to build open-mindedness, deliberately examining all sides, reading and discussing contrary points of views to your own to better inform yourself.
10. Taking the good things in life and well-intentioned acts of others for granted; not appreciating good things in life to the extent they deserve to be appreciated	Gratitude Social intelligence Kindness	Write at least three things you are genuinely grateful for, but have not explicitly articulated. Reflect on whether there are things you take for granted. Notice and record (in writing or visually through photos on your smartphone) positive acts done by others throughout the day. Acknowledge the good deeds of others.

Table 8. continued

Challenge	Potential character strength(s)	Specific actions
11. Overestimating one's positive qualities and feeling the need to show accomplishments to others or on social media	Humility Authenticity	Recall and write about the experience of feeling authentic or genuine, without any external pretense; write statements acknowledging your imperfections and how you can still live with them.
12. Repeating mistakes, making decisions or acting out in ways that land one in trouble with others	Perspective Prudence Social intelligence	Recall a recent challenge and its unfavorable outcome. How did it impact you and others? What aspect of this challenge can you realistically change? Which specific strengths can help you resolve the situation? If needed, consult with those involved to make it a collaborative problem-solving approach.
13. Wanting to withdraw by isolating yourself or appearing uninterested	Capacity to love and be loved Social intelligence	Reflect on everyday gestures and actions of love and affection you experience from others. Think of the ways you could express them. Think of expressing your care and love for others in small ways, especially toward those who will appreciate them.
14. Experiencing difficulty in acknowledging and appreciating different points of view or cultural backgrounds	Fairness Curiosity Open-mindedness	Reflect that there are many ways of being and expressing oneself, and no one way is better than another. Find situations when you notice someone standing up for others when they are treated unfairly, bullied, or ridiculed. Think of ways you can support the person being bullied.
15. Getting stuck with daily routine; feeling bored and underchallenged	Creativity Persistence Leadership	Think of approaching routine tasks in a novel but creative manner, without fear of failure. Focus on the goal of trying, not necessarily the goal of being successful. Find ways to explore and express your creativity by starting or leading an activity outside of studies or work, something you always wanted to do but have not been able to do so far. If the first activity is not fulfilling, do not give up but keep trying until you find something fulfilling,

Note. Use of character strengths in dealing with these challenges is informed by the following works: Niemiec (2018); Schwartz & Sharpe (2010).

Closing Activities

The goal of closing this module is to help participants integrate their understanding of problem solving and strengths and to take their new learning into everyday life.

Discuss the everyday applications listed here and in the Workbook (p. 98). Invite participants to be mindful in their day-to-day lives by noticing their own and other's actions and habits which show the use of problem solving with strengths. Encourage them to use relevant resources found at the end of this module and included in their Workbook (p. 102).

Choose a 3-minute mindfulness activity from Regular Practice 1: Mindfulness and Relaxation to close the module.

Everyday Applications

- Everyday life challenges are often ambiguous and ongoing. We do not always have all the necessary information to decide which specific strengths to use, in what way, to overcome the challenges. Reflect on which strengths might lead to the optimal outcome. If in doubt, consult with a wise friend or family member. Table WB2 presents 15 specific problems and suggests strengths that can be applied and specific actions one can take to solve these problems.
- Not all daily life challenges can be resolved by your strengths alone. You can also draw on your talents, skills, abilities, and expertise. For instance, writing assignments can benefit from the strengths of persistence, curiosity, love of learning, and creativity. However, they also require writing and research skills as well as expertise in grammar and spelling. When faced with a challenge, assess the situation by first thinking about which specific strengths will support you and then identifying complementary talents, skills, and abilities.
- Monitor the use of your strengths especially noticing how your strengths help in overcoming a specific challenge, in both the short and long term. As an exercise, recall and reflect on three important decisions you made using your strengths in the past year. Would you still use the same strengths in the same ways or would you use different strengths in different ways to resolve the same or similar problems?
- List everyday stressors, hassles, and problems, which you have not been able to resolve despite your efforts. Reflect on how harnessing your strengths can help you to resolve them.
- Hardly any family does not experience conflict. Reflect on previous conflicts, sour interactions, and challenges. Think how you can use your strengths (and those of others) to negotiate similar issues if these reoccur.

References

Blanchard, T., Kerbeykian, T., & McGrath, R.E. (2020). Why are signature strengths and well-being related? Tests of multiple hypotheses. *Journal of Happiness Studies, 21*, 2095–2114. https://doi.org/10.1007/s10902-019-00170-2

Freidlin, P., & Littman-Ovadia, H. (2020). Prosocial behavior at work through the lens of character strengths. *Frontiers in Psychology, 10*, Article 3046. https://doi.org/10.3389/fpsyg.2019.03046

Kamushadze, T., & Martskvishvili, K. (2021). Character strength at its worst and best: Mediating effect of coping strategies. *Trends in Psychology, 29*(4), 655–669. https://doi.org/10.1007/s43076-021-00085-z

Kashdan, T. B., Julian, T., Merritt, K., & Uswatte, G. (2006). Social anxiety and posttraumatic stress in combat veterans: Relations to well-being and character strengths. *Behaviour Research and Therapy, 44*(4), 561–583. https://doi.org/10.1016/j.brat.2005.03.010

Littman-Ovadia, H., & Freidlin, P. (2019). Positive psychopathology and positive functioning: OCD, flourishing and satisfaction with life through the lens of character strength underuse, overuse and optimal use. *Applied Research in Quality of Life, 15,* 529–549. https://doi.org/10.1007/s11482-018-9701-5

Niemiec, R. M. (2018). *Character strengths interventions: A field guide for practitioners.* Hogrefe.

Niemiec, R. M., & Pearce, R. (2021). The practice of character strengths: Unifying definitions, principles, and exploration of what's soaring, emerging, and ripe with potential in science and in practice. *Frontiers in Psychology, 11,* Article 590220. https://doi.org/10.3389/fpsyg.2020.590220

Schwartz, B., & Sharpe, K. (2010). *Practical wisdom: The right way to do the right thing.* Penguin.

Sin, N., & Lyubomirsky, S. (2009). Enhancing well-being and alleviating depressive symptoms with positive psychology interventions: A practice-friendly meta-analysis. *Journal of Clinical Psychology, 65*(5), 467–487. https://doi.org/10.1002/jclp.20593

Uliaszek, A. A., Rashid, T., & Zarowsky, Z. (2022). The role of signature strengths in treatment outcome: Initial results from a large and diverse university sample. *Journal of Contemporary Psychotherapy, 52*(1), 15–21. https://doi.org/10.1007/s10879-021-09523-6

Resources

Literature

Bland, D. (2015). *Proverbs and the formation of character.* Cascade Books.

Brockman, J. (2012). *This will make you smarter: New scientific concepts to improve your thinking.* Harper Perennial.

Buschor, C., Proyer, R. T., & Ruch, W. (2013). Self- and peer-rated character strengths: How do they relate to satisfaction with life and orientations to happiness? *Journal of Positive Psychology, 8*(2), 116–127. https://doi.org/10.1080/17439760.2012.758305

Freidlin, P., Littman-Ovadia, H., & Niemiec, R. M. (2017). Positive psychopathology: Social anxiety via character strengths underuse and overuse. *Personality and Individual Differences, 108,* 50–54. https://doi.org/10.1016/j.paid.2016.12.003

Hammerness, P., & Margaret, M. (2011). *Organize your mind, organize your life train your brain to get more done in less time.* Harlequin.

Lavy, S., Littman-Ovadia, H., & Bareli, Y. (2014). Strengths deployment as a mood-repair mechanism: Evidence from a diary study with a relationship exercise group. *Journal of Positive Psychology, 9,* 1–12. https://doi.org/10.1080/17439760.2014.936963

Proyer, R. T., Sidler, N., Weber, M., & Ruch, W. (2012). A multi-method approach to studying the relationship between character strengths and vocational interests in adolescents. *International Journal for Educational and Vocational Guidance, 12,* 141–157. https://doi.org/10.1007/s10775-012-9223-x

Ricard, M., Andre, C., & Jollien, A. (2018). *In search of wisdom: A monk, a philosopher, and a psychiatrist on what matters most* (S. Chödzin Kohn, Trans.). Sounds True.

Schwartz, B., & Sharpe, K. E. (2010). *Practical wisdom: The right way to do the right thing.* Riverhead Books.

Sternberg, R. J. (Ed.). (1990). *Wisdom: Its nature, origins, and development.* Cambridge University Press. https://doi.org/10.1017/CBO9781139173704

Underuse and Overuse of Strengths, Psychological Flexibility, and Perspective

Biswas-Diener, R., Kashdan, T. B., & Minhas, G. (2011). A dynamic approach to psychological strength development and intervention. *Journal of Positive Psychology, 6*(2), 106–118. https://doi.org/10.1080/17439760.2010.545429

Glück, J., & Baltes, P. B. (2006). Using the concept of wisdom to enhance the expression of wisdom knowledge: Not the philosopher's dream but differential effects of developmental preparedness. *Psychology and Aging, 21*(4), 679–690.

Kamushadze, T., & Martskvishvili, K. (2021). Character strength at its worst and best: Mediating effect of coping strategies. *Trends in Psychology, 29*(4), 655–669. https://doi.org/10.1007/s43076-021-00085-z
Niemiec, R. M. (2019). Finding the golden mean: the overuse, underuse, and optimal use of character strengths. *Counselling Psychology Quarterly, 32*(3–4), 453–471. https://doi.org/10.1080/09515070.2019.1617674
Rust, T., Diessner, R., & Reade, L. (2009). Strengths only or strengths and relative weaknesses? A preliminary study. *Journal of Psychology, 143*(5), 465–476. https://doi.org/10.3200/JRL.143.5.465-476
Schwartz, B., & Sharpe, K. E. (2006). Practical wisdom: Aristotle meets positive psychology. *Journal of Happiness Studies, 7,* 377–395. https://doi.org/10.1007/s10902-005-3651-y

Character Strengths and Academic Achievement, Resilience, and Well-Being

Duckworth, A. L., & Seligman, M. E. P. (2005). Self-discipline outdoes IQ predicting academic performance in adolescents. *Psychological Science, 16*(12), 939–944. https://doi.org/10.1111/j.1467-9280.2005.01641.x
Karris Bachik, M. A., Carey, G., & Craighead, W. E. (2021). VIA character strengths among U.S. college students and their associations with happiness, well-being, resiliency, academic success and psychopathology. *Journal of Positive Psychology, 16*(4), 512–525. https://doi.org/10.1080/17439760.2020.1752785
Massingham, P. (2019). An Aristotelian interpretation of practical wisdom: The case of retirees. *Palgrave Communications, 5*(1), Article 123. https://doi.org/10.1057/s41599-019-0331-9
Nickolite, A., & Doll, B. (2008). Resilience applied in school: Strengthening classroom environments for learning. *Canadian Journal of School Psychology, 23*(1), 338–334. https://doi.org/10.1177/0829573508316596
Ouweneel, E., Le Blanc, P. M., & Schaufeli, W. B. (2011). Flourishing participants: A longitudinal study on positive emotions, personal resources, and study engagement. *Journal of Positive Psychology, 6*(2), 142–153. https://doi.org/10.1080/17439760.2011.558847
Peterson, C., & Seligman, M. E. P. (2004). *Character strengths and virtues: A handbook and classification.* Oxford University Press; American Psychological Association.
Tough, P. (2012). *How children succeed: Grit, curiosity and the hidden power of character.* Houghton Mifflin Harcourt.
Weber, M., & Harzer, C. (2022). Relations between character strengths, school satisfaction, enjoyment of learning, academic self-efficacy, and school achievement: An examination of various aspects of positive schooling. *Frontiers in Psychology, 13,* Article 826960. https://doi.org/10.3389/fpsyg.2022.826960

Websites

How Practical Wisdom Helps Us Cope with Radical Uncertainty
https://behavioralscientist.org/how-practical-wisdom-helps-us-cope-with-radical-uncertainty/
This paper by Schonbrun and Schwartz shows four ways we can lean on Aristotle's notion to guide us through uncertain terrain.

The Marginalian (previously Brain Pickings)
https://www.themarginalian.org/
Access free, interesting, and inspiring articles from across the arts, science, philosophy, creativity, children's books, and other domains.

Multimedia

Getting Stuck in the Negatives (and How to Get Unstuck)
https://www.youtube.com/watch?v=7XFLTDQ4JMk
Alison Ledgerwood discusses how people think and how they can think better.

Indigenous Wisdom
https://www.ted.com/speakers/elizabeth_lindsey
Elizabeth Lindsey, a fellow of the National Geographic Society, discusses indigenous wisdom and traditions.

The Art of Thinking Clearly
https://youtu.be/vNOV4nlOHtQ
Author Rolf Dobelli explains how we all have cognitive biases and make simple errors in our day-to-day thinking. Being aware of them can build and broaden our perspective to resolve our problems adaptively.

Center for Practical Wisdom - University of Chicago
https://www.uchicago.edu/research/center/the_center_for_practical_wisdom/
The mission of the center is to expand the scientific understanding of wisdom and its role in everyday decisions and choices. Bringing multidisciplinary experts together, the center aims to support research and disseminate research about practical wisdom.

Real Wisdom - Lessons from 40 films in 7 minutes
https://youtu.be/G2wIuTdf5FQ
This compilation of clips from famous movies illustrates the wise use of strengths in challenging situations.

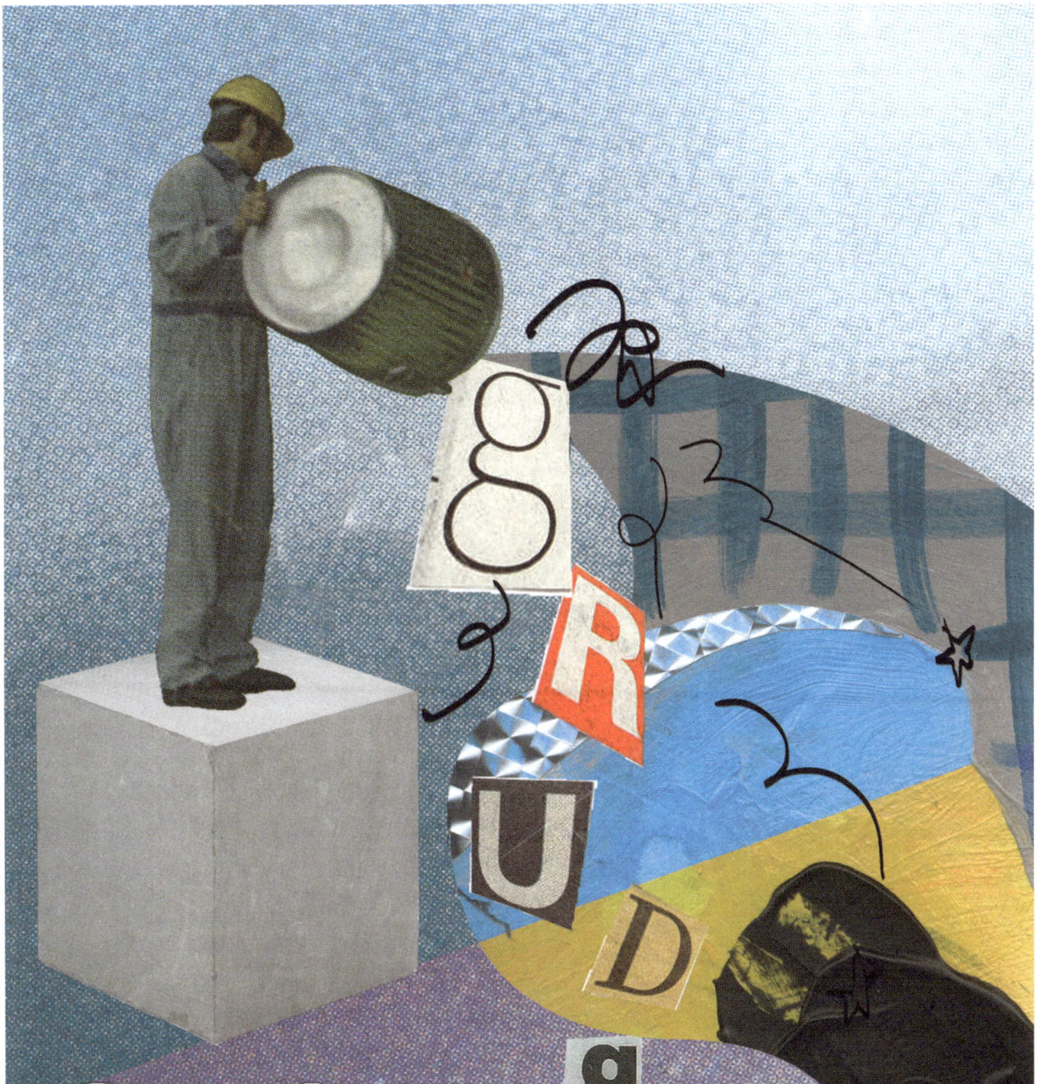
Grudge
& Gratitude

Module 8: Grudge and Gratitude

Module 8 explores negative and positive experiences related to interpersonal relationships. While holding on to grudges can lead to resentment and relationship stress, expressing gratitude builds positive emotions and healthy relationships. Participants learn that relationships can be strengthened by both releasing negative emotions and expressing positive ones.

Module Topic	Minutes to Allot	
Learning Outcomes Grudge: By reflecting on the impact of holding resentment, participants: • Gain access to and awareness of the consequences of holding a grudge • Learn the value of forgiveness for enhancing well-being and resilience Gratitude: By delivering in person a letter of gratitude, participants: • Attune their awareness toward the goodness of others • Build gratitude skills and positive emotions through concrete actions	5	5
Opening Activities Start the module with a relaxation or mindfulness practice Invite participants to share a few events from their gratitude journal that have occurred since the last session Invite questions about the previous module and practice(s)	10	15
Illustration of Core Concepts Review core concepts and show video illustrations Facilitate reflection and discussion: • *What are the key messages in the video(s) you just watched?* • *How might these concepts be relevant in your life?*	15	15
Practice 1: Let Go of Grudge Have participants complete *Worksheet: Holding a Grudge* Debrief learning from practice(s) using questions: • *How does this grudge affect your behaviors, relationships, and feelings?* • *In what way would your life be different if you let go of this grudge?* **Practice 2: Express Gratitude** Step 1: Introduce sample gratitude letter and have participants write their own letter of gratitude Debrief learning from letter-writing practice using questions: • *How did you feel as you wrote the letter?* • *What was the easiest part to write? The toughest?* • *Are there others for whom you are grateful? How might you express it?* Step 2: After a few days of reflection, rewrite the letter Step 3: Deliver letter in person and read it out loud (homework).	20	30
Closing Activities Invite discussion of everyday applications Remind participants of relevant resources at the end of the module Guide participants in a 3-minute closing relaxation or mindfulness practice	10	10
Total	60 minutes	75 minutes

Core Concepts of Grudge

Many of the themes here are also presented in the Core Concepts section of the Workbook (p. 103):

Grudge

- Life is often an unexpected blend of moments filled with joys and woes, delights and despairs, fulfillment and deprivation. Our brains retrieve information from these moments, process and encode it, and store it for later. This information creates the memories that play an important role in influencing our immediate and long-term well-being (Hupbach et al., 2008).
- Human evolution has seen to it that we remember failures more readily than successes. Our minds are naturally wired to focus more on negative events and experiences than those that are positive. This is called the *negativity bias*. Most people spend far more time thinking about how they can correct something that has gone wrong (or is about to go wrong) than they do basking in what has gone right. For example, we remember criticism, traumas, and other negative feedback in much greater detail than positive events (Baumeister et al., 2001; Ito et al., 1998; Rozin & Royzman, 2001; Williams et al., 2009).
- A *grudge* is a stubborn resentment that one holds against another person or group. This resentment can be for things that have actually occurred or for imagined reasons (Persoon-Gundy, 2014; Struthers et al., 2017). "Grudge" is usually associated with negative connotations such as malevolence, enmity, hatred, malice, rancor, and ill-will. However, it is important to understand that when someone is hurt, has been harmed or offended, the victim is likely to feel emotional pain, anger, or the urge to take revenge. This is a grudge (Rapske et al., 2010).
- As we saw in Module 2, holding onto a grudge can be a sign of a fixed mindset, often accompanied by thinking tendencies such as jumping to conclusions, tunnel vision, magnifying or maximizing, or overgeneralizing (see Module 2: Fixed and Growth Mindsets, Module 3: Cognitive Accuracy, and Module 4: Cognitive Flexibility). When we experience a grudge, our appraisal of the situation is neither accurate nor flexible.
- We feel bitter toward the other person when we hold on to a grudge. This can cloud our perception of the other person and lead us to question even their most well-intentioned actions. Studies indicate that clinging to resentments depletes our resilience, isolates us socially, and increases our risk for health problems. People who tend to hold grudges are also more likely to have heart disease, chronic pain, and high blood pressure (Blumenthal et al., 2018; Hupbach et al., 2008; van Monsjou et al., 2023; Zheng et al., 2015).

Illustrations of Grudge

Play at least one of the three videos below to illustrate the core concepts of grudge and encourage discussion.

The Power of Forgiveness
https://www.youtube.com/watch?v=8o9_TlZyB_Y
(Duration: 7:18 minutes)
A social experiment about the process of forgiveness, this video tests the theory that by exercising forgiveness, we can experience greater happiness.

Why Is It So Hard to Let Go of Grudges?
https://youtu.be/PrsRtKYsQhc
(Duration: 5:46 minutes)
This video clip explains why our brain harbors grudges and why it is difficult to let go, even though it is good for our physical and psychological health.

Can you Erase Bad Memories?
https://youtu.be/89shevn24L8
(Duration: 3:32 minutes)
This video explains how every time we recall a memory, our brain alters its details and over time our recall becomes less accurate.

Reflection and Discussion

Invite participants to complete the Reflection and Discussion section of their Workbook (p. 104) regarding the video(s) they have watched. Discuss the questions:

What are the key messages in the video(s) you just watched?

How might these concepts be relevant in your life?

Practice 1: Let Go of the Grudge

The goal of this practice is to increase participants' awareness about the impact of carrying grudges. When negative experiences occur, we cope with them in various ways. However, some of us carry them as "baggage" for a long time and are not aware of the burden that this creates in our lives. The practice is not about off-loading this baggage or resolving the conflict with the person who hurt or offended us. Nor does the practice involve simply venting about the negative experience. The goal of the practice is to help participants evaluate the impact the grudge might have on their well-being and provide them with some options for dealing with or minimizing its impact.

Much like other practices, a brief relaxation and mindfulness practice will likely help participants to ground themselves. Here are instructions to guide the practice:

- Instruct participants to think about a friend or a family member toward whom they are holding a grudge.
- Instruct participants to use the worksheet to describe the grudge and its effects (Workbook, Practice 1: Let Go of Grudge, p. 105). In the larger circle, have them describe the grudge that they are holding against this individual. In the smaller three circles, describe the effects this grudge has had on them.
- Inform participants that possible effects might relate to their feelings or emotions, level of energy, thoughts, behavior, or relationships. Sometimes, it can be helpful to think about what life would be like (how it might be different) if they did not hold this grudge.
- Invite participants to review the optional reading on dealing with grudges to learn about different strategies (p. 107 in Workbook).

Worksheet: Holding a Grudge (from Workbook, p. 105)

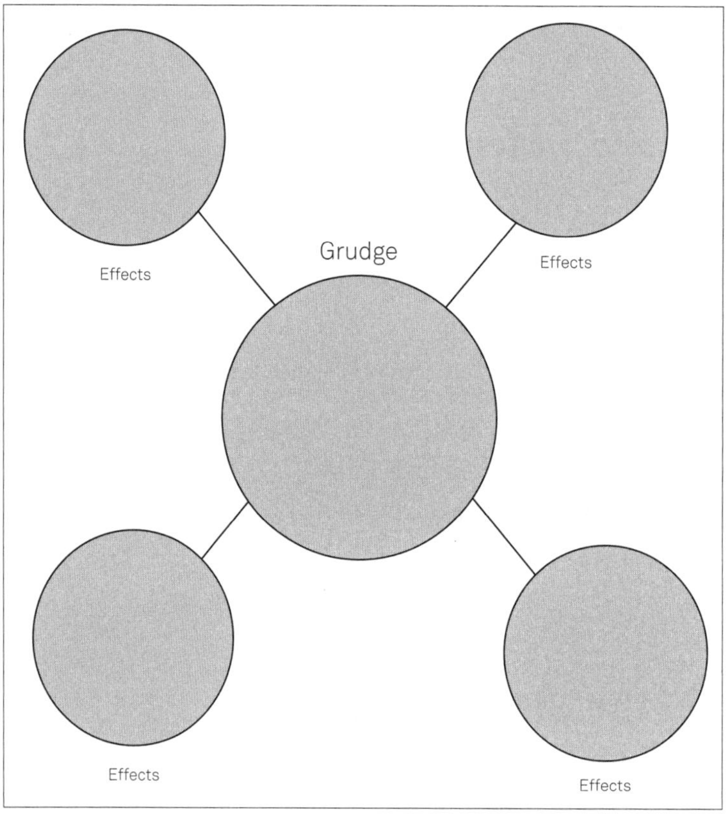

Practice Debrief

Refer participants to the Practice Debrief section in their Workbook (p. 106), which instructs them to write a few reflections or insights about themselves regarding the grudge they described using the following questions:

- *How does holding this grudge affect your behaviors, relationships, and feelings?*
- *Imagine letting go of this grudge or letting it fade away. In what ways would your life be different?*

Optional Reading: Dealing With Grudges (also on p. 107 in Workbook)

Sophie Hannah in her 2019 book How to Hold a Grudge distinguishes forgiveness from letting go of a grudge. She conceptualizes grudge as an awareness that others have harmed us. According to Hannah, a grudge does not necessarily involve strong feelings of anger and resentment. Hannah states that one can hold a grudge without strong emotions and that, in some cases, it can protect us against future harm. Hence, asking someone to let go of their grudges and move on could be perceived as dismissing or trivializing the pain, hurt, or injury that motivated the grudge. Hannah offers five alternative options to deal with grudges, leading with either forgiving or holding onto the grudge:

- Forgive willingly, let go of negative feelings. Hold no grudges. Maintain the same behavior with the person.
- Forgive willingly, let go of negative feelings toward the person, yet still hold on to some resentment, although you don't show it in your behavior with the person.
- Forgive willingly, let go of negative feelings toward the person, yet still hold the grudge. Change your behavior with the person. For example, in their presence, you are cautious in what you say to them and you don't go out of your way to be with them.
- Decide not to forgive, hold on to negative feelings toward the person and hold a grudge. Maintain the same behavior with the person. Essentially, you pretend to have the same relationship with them.
- Decide not to forgive and hold on to the negative feelings toward the person. Hold a grudge. Change your behavior with the person in the future. For example, you stop all contact with them.

Forgiving

If you choose to forgive willingly, reassure yourself that you are using and building strengths. For example, kindness and social intelligence can help you to reframe the hurt. Gratitude may help you to consider the person's positive aspects, which you may have overlooked previously or which remain hidden from you due to negativity bias. In deciding to forgive, make sure you are not absolving, avoiding, or ignoring the impact of the hurt which engendered the grudge in the first place. If you choose to forgive, please do so because handling the negative emotions associated with the offense or offender is difficult. Forgiveness typically does not follow a prescribed timeframe. Strive earnestly toward it, as research links letting go and forgiveness to improved psychological and physical health (Struthers et al., 2017).

Working Through Grudges

Awareness is the first step in letting go of grudges. Reflect on the cost of holding on to the grudge. Periodically appraise how holding that grudge is impacting you. Does holding it make you angry, anxious, ambivalent, or jealous? Reflect on how these disruptive emotions affect you. Also, try to foresee your emotional state; if you hold onto the grudge, what might be the emotional cost you will need to pay in the long run?

If you decide to hold a grudge against a person or situation, consider how much time, effort, and emotional energy you spend on it. Try to create some distance (e.g., unfollow them on a shared social media platform) so that you do not have readily available access to information about or contacts with the person or situation.

Think of some adaptive action you can readily engage in when you start to brood about the person or situation. Commit to starting a creative and adaptive activity that expresses your grudge. When doing these creative activities, remember that this is your way of harnessing negative feelings and redirecting them toward a positive and creative output.

Core Concepts of Gratitude

The themes here are also presented in the Core Concepts section of the Workbook (p. 108):

- *Gratitude* is an experience of thankfulness, which entails noticing and appreciating the positive things in life. In doing so, we acknowledge the value and meaning of positives. These positives could be an experience, an event, people, or an emotional state. To practice gratitude is to acknowledge the value and meaning of positive things.
- How do we benefit from gratitude? Sonja Lyubomirsky (Lyubomirsky, 2007), in her book *The How to Happiness*, mentions eight distinct benefits, which are:
  1. **Positive Experience.** Gratitude allows us to more fully enjoy the benefits of positive experiences.
  2. **Self-Worth and Self-Esteem.** Gratitude supports and increases our self-worth and self-esteem. It helps us realize how much we and others have accomplished, which in turn makes us more confident and capable. Thus, gratitude can help us unlearn negative habits such as self-pity, which is the tendency to dwell on negative experiences or feel victimized.
  3. **Improved Ability to Cope With Stress.** Gratitude can help us cope with stress and adversity. After a shocking experience, gratitude can help us evaluate what is most important in our lives.
  4. **Willingness to Help Others.** Grateful people are more likely to help others. They become more aware of the kind and caring acts others have done for them and feel a desire to do kind acts in return. They are less likely to be materialistic and more likely to appreciate what they have.
  5. **Better Relationships.** Gratitude can strengthen our relationships. When we become truly aware of the value of our friends and family members, we are likely to treat them better. When we treat them well, they treat us well.
  6. **Fewer Negative Comparisons.** Expressing gratitude decreases our tendency to compare ourselves with others. We become thankful and content with what we have (e.g., friends, family, home, and health) and are less likely to feel bad for what we may not have.
  7. **Less Time for Negatives.** When we express gratitude, we are likely to spend less time dwelling on negative emotions. For example, when we feel grateful, it is less likely that we will feel guilty, greedy, or angry.
  8. **Fuller and Deeper Appreciation.** The joy of a positive experience or a new possession generally does not last. Initially, we feel happy, but often the joy diminishes over time. By appreciating the meaning and value of the experience or object, we can enjoy our positive experiences for a longer period of time.
- Robert Emmons, one of the pioneers of gratitude research, explains the importance of gratitude in the context of resilience. Emmons argues that we have the most to gain through gratitude when faced with difficulties. "In the face of demoralization, gratitude has the power to energize. In the face of brokenness, gratitude has the power to heal. In the face of despair, gratitude has the power to bring hope. In other words, gratitude can help us cope with hard times." (Emmons, 2013). In addition, despite the ubiquity of adversities, challenges, and setbacks, we need to remember that human beings are remarkably adaptive creatures who can transform adverse circumstances into opportunities for personal growth. Recognizing how we have made it through difficult times can foster gratitude, just as we appreciate a mild spring after a harsh winter (Emmons, 2008).

Illustrations of Gratitude

Play at least one of the three videos below to illustrate the core concepts of gratitude and encourage discussion.

An Experiment in Gratitude
https://youtu.be/oHv6vTKD6lg
(Duration: 7:13 minutes)
This video illustrates the power of writing and reading a gratitude letter.

The Gratitude Letter Project
https://youtu.be/VLCQ_VomKLM
(Duration: 5:01 minutes)
Students at Lake Shore Public Schools joined up with Make a Wish, Macy's, and the Believe Campaign to write letters of gratitude to those they wanted to thank.

Say "Thank You" – A Motivational Video on the Importance of Gratitude
https://youtu.be/7uzynHWxn5Q
(Duration 5:10 minutes)
This video clip, with an opening speech from the actor Denzel Washington, underscores the important of gratitude and saying thank you for what is already yours.

Reflection and Discussion

Invite participants to complete the Reflection and Discussion section of their Workbook (p. 109) regarding the video(s) they have watched. Discuss the questions:

What are the key messages in the video(s) you just watched?

How might these concepts be relevant in your life?

Practice 2: Express Gratitude

As discussed in the Core Concepts section, gratitude is associated with a number of benefits, including better relationships, better psychological health, and enhanced life satisfaction. This practice aims to help participants experience some of these benefits in their own lives.

Discuss with participants that research demonstrates many benefits of interventions that help participants practice gratitude. In addition, practicing gratitude could be especially helpful for those who are experiencing symptoms of depression or who may not express gratitude much in their lives.

Help participants to contextualize this practice of gratitude with the gratitude journal, which is a regular practice. While the regular practice of gratitude helps to increase our awareness of everyday positive events and experiences, this practice introduces participants to the practice of expressing heartfelt, genuine gratitude to someone who has had a positive impact on them.

The gratitude letter is a powerful exercise that most people find moving. Encourage participants to take their time. However, it is critical to emphasize to participants to choose one individual to whom they will draft, rewrite, and deliver a gratitude letter.

This practice has two parts: Part A is writing the letter (Step 1 in the Workbook), and Part B is rewriting the letter (Step 2) and delivering it in person (Step 3). Instructions for facilitating and debriefing both parts of the practice are below.

Step 1: Writing the Letter

- Invite participants to sit in a relaxed position, with eyes closed or gaze lowered and fixed on a spot near the floor.
- Once participants settle down, read the following script, preferably verbatim, from Seligman's book *Flourish* (2011) to begin this practice:

  Close your eyes. Call up the face of someone still alive who, years ago did something or said something that changed your life for the better. Someone who you never properly thanked, someone you could meet face-to-face next week. (Seligman, 2011, p. 30).
- With their eyes still closed or gazing downwards, encourage participants to think of the people – parents, friends, teachers, coaches, teammates, or employers – who have been especially kind to them but who have never heard participants express their gratitude. Remind participants that gratitude may be long overdue, but it is not too late.
- With eyes still closed, encourage participants to focus on one such person and to start a letter to that person. What would they say? Encourage participants to describe specific details of the other person's kind act (or actions), how this helped them, including how the kindness may still be affecting participants' lives to this day.
- Ask participants to open their eyes and immediately, without any delay, begin writing the first draft of the gratitude letter to this person. Participants use the section in their Workbook, Step 1: Draft a Gratitude Letter (p. 111)
- Instruct participants to describe in concrete terms why they are grateful. Instruct participants to keep the letter short and concise, but also detailed. Recommend that participants name specific things the other person did for them and write out exactly how it affected their life. Recommend that they tell the recipient what they are doing now and how they often remember the other person's efforts. The following sample letter was written by a high school student to his teacher.

Sample Letter

Dear Ms. Robinson,

This letter is to thank you, with genuine gratitude, for the loving acts you bestowed upon me during my high school years. At a time when I felt misunderstood, angry, and lonely you offered me your compassionate ear and voice. The time you devoted to helping me, though it may seem small in your eyes, has had a big effect on the person I am constantly becoming. When others were trying to preach with words and advice, you taught me through action and care.

Do you remember the time when you picked me up with your van and talked to me for over an hour while we sat on the side of the road? It may seem like a little gesture, but the words I am using to describe your actions here are hopelessly inadequate to explain the effect you had on me. You made me feel wanted and worth caring about, and this is the greatest gift you ever gave me.

This letter is as much for me as it is for you. I truly am thankful for all you have done, and I hope you can now appreciate how much it meant to me.

Sincerely,
Nathanial

Homework

Step 2 Debrief

Ask participants to complete the Practice Debrief section in the Workbook (p. 112) Ask them to reflect on the following questions:

- *How did you feel as you wrote your letter?*
- *What was the easiest part to write, and what was the toughest?*
- *Have you thought of others with whom you wish to share your gratitude? Record some initial thoughts about how you might express your gratitude to them.*

Step 3: Polishing the Gratitude Letter and Delivering It

- Have the participants rewrite their gratitude letter (see the Workbook section Step 2: Rewrite Your Gratitude Letter) and then have them deliver it as homework (Workbook section Step 3: Deliver Your Gratitude Letter)
- Instruct participants to handwrite the version they will deliver and to call the person in advance to arrange a time to deliver the letter in person. Tell them not to reveal to the person the purpose of their visit. Invite them to deliver the letter personally and read it aloud to the recipient. Encourage them to discuss how they both feel about the experience of sharing gratitude.

Step 3 Debrief

Participants may have different timelines for completing the gratitude letter practice. Whenever they are able to complete this exercise, follow up with a debrief discussion. This can be woven into a future module. The following questions will help participants to reflect about the practice:

1. *What specific emotions did you experience while reading the letter?*
2. *What was the reaction of the person to whom you wrote the gratitude letter?*
3. *Would you repeat this experience with someone else? If so, what would you change to make the practice more effective?*

Learning and Cultural Fit

Adapt this practice to the learning and cultural needs of your participants, including its unique values and demographics. Possible adaptations include:

- The expression of gratitude can be different across cultures. For example, in some cultures, it is customary to express gratitude frequently. Consider discussing with participants how their cultural or family background might influence expressions of gratitude.
- Some participants may be going through life circumstances that make it very difficult for them to find something worth being grateful for in their everyday life. Gently encourage these participants to consider whether there are people who are helpful in providing support during this difficult time. If not, you might invite them to think of past accomplishments for which they are grateful and remember those who helped them succeed. If they simply cannot do this exercise authentically, then do not force them.
- Encourage participants to use different approaches and strategies to express gratitude toward diverse things. For example, participants can be grateful for things in the classroom, at their home, in their family, in their social circle, or in nature more broadly. Participants can be grateful for experiences and for people in their lives.

Closing Activities

The goal of closing this module is to help participants consolidate their understanding of grudge and gratitude and to take their new learning into everyday life.

Discuss with participants the Everyday Applications section, also found on p. 115 in their Workbook. Invite participants to be mindful in their day-to-day lives by noticing their own and others' actions in relation to grudge and gratitude. Encourage them to use relevant resources found at the end of this module and included in their Workbook starting on p. 115.

Choose a 3-minute activity from Regular Practice 1: Mindfulness and Relaxation to close the module.

Everyday Applications

Letting Go of Grudges

- Make grudge a choice. If you decide to let go of the grudge, you will choose to drop the emotional burden that you might have been carrying. If you feel hurt and the offender has not apologized, your anger or upset feelings may be justified. However, if you decide to let go of this negative feeling, it will free you emotionally. It will create fresh emotional space that had previously been occupied by the grudge.
- Letting go of a grudge can be gradual. If you feel strong negative emotions and cannot let go of the grudge, don't force yourself. Understand that it is a gradual process, and taking one small step a day can eventually move you toward complete resolution.
- Express your feelings in writing about the grudge, the impact on you of holding this grudge, and the process of letting go. You can also decide to write down your deepest feelings without worrying about structure, spelling, or fear of disclosure – that is, this writing is for your eyes only. Set aside your write-up for a couple of days and then write another page. Set it aside and repeat again after few days. With a calm mood and clear head, slowly read your three write-ups and see what patterns emerge. At the very least, the writing process can help you to see your grudge on a tangible piece of paper.
- Letting go of a grudge is a gift. Understand that letting go is a gift that you will give to the other person and yourself. However, some resentments are based on chronic abuse, ongoing discrimination, or exploitation. So letting go of such wrongdoings might be unfair and harmful. Therefore, remind yourself that forgiveness and letting go are personal decisions, not requirements. By forgiving someone, we are not necessarily condoning their behavior.

Cultivating Gratitude

- Use gratitude to overcome the hardwiring of negativity bias. Our daily living presents both positive and negative events and experiences that make us sad, happy, or sometimes a mix of both.
- Gratitude can be expressed to more than just people; one can be grateful toward an object, idea, event, or experience.
- Every day select one small yet important thing that you take for granted. Work on being mindful of this thing in the future.
- Notice negative mood swings that make you feel grouchy, tired, or irritable. Choose to think of one thing you are grateful for and see if this has a positive impact on your mood.
- Express thanks to all who contributed to your success, no matter how small their contribution might have been. Be aware of the degree to which other people help you in pursuing your goals or solving problems, in addition to your own hard work. When expressing thanks, do not just say "thanks" – be more descriptive and specific – for example, "I appreciate your prudent advice on how to write a better essay." Observe how people respond differently to more detailed thankfulness.
- Begin each day thinking about the people you are grateful to have in your life.
- Employ systematic approaches such as the gratitude journal and gratitude letter. They can be particularly helpful as they provide a new perspective on the day.

References

Baumeister, R. F., Bratslavsky, E., Finkenauer, C., & Vohs, K. D. (2001). Bad is stronger than good. *Review of General Psychology, 5*(4), 323–370. https://doi.org/10.1037/1089-2680.5.4.323

Blumenthal-Barby, J., & Opel, D. J. (2018). Nudge or grudge? Choice architecture and parental decision-making. *The Hastings Center Report, 48*(2), 33–39. https://doi.org/10.1002/hast.837

Emmons, R. (2008). *Thanks: How practicing gratitude can make you happy*. Houghton-Mifflin.

Emmons, R. (2013). *How gratitude can help you through hard times*. https://greatergood.berkeley.edu/article/item/how_gratitude_can_help_you_through_hard_times

Hannah, S. (2019). *How to hold onto a grudge: From resentment to content – the power of grudge to transform your life*. Simon & Schuster.

Hupbach, A., Hardt, O., Gomez, R., & Nadel, L. (2008). The dynamics of memory: Context-dependent updating. *Learning & Memory, 15*(8), 574–579. https://doi.org/10.1101/lm.1022308

Ito, T. A., Larsen, J. T., Smith, N. K., & Cacioppo, J. T. (1998). Negative information weighs more heavily on the brain: The negativity bias in evaluative categorizations. *Journal of Personality and Social Psychology, 75*(4), 887–900. https://doi.org/10.1037/0022-3514.75.4.887

Lyubomirsky, S. (2007). *The how of happiness: A scientific approach to getting the life you want*. Penguin Press.

Persoon-Gundy, J. (2014). The grudge. *Annals of Internal Medicine, 160*(12), 846. https://doi.org/10.7326/M14-0113

Rapske, D. L., Boon, S. D., Alibhai, A. M., & Kheong, M. J. (2010). Not forgiven, not forgotten: An investigation of unforgiven interpersonal offenses. *Journal of Social Clinical Psychology, 29*, 1100–1130. https://doi.org/10.1521/jscp.2010.29.10.1100

Rozin, P., & Royzman, E. (2001). Negativity bias, negativity dominance, and contagion. *Personality and Social Psychology Review, 5*, 296–320. https://doi.org/10.1207/S15327957PSPR0504_2

Seligman, M. E. P. (2011). *Flourish: A visionary new understanding of happiness and well-being*. Simon & Schuster.

Struthers, C. W., van Monsjou, E., Ayoub, M., & Guilfoyle, J. R. (2017). Fit to forgive: Effect of mode of exercise on capacity to override grudges and forgiveness. *Frontiers in Psychology, 8*, Article 538. https://doi.org/10.3389/fpsyg.2017.00538

van Monsjou, E., Struthers, C. W., Fergus, K., & Muise, A. (2023). Examining the lived experience of holding grudges. *Qualitative Psychology, 10*(1), 60–78. https://doi.org/10.1037/qup0000205

Williams, L. M., Gatt, J. M., Schofield, P. R., Olivieri, G., Peduto, A., & Gordon, E. (2009). "Negativity bias" in risk for depression and anxiety: Brain-body fear circuitry correlates, 5-HTT-LPR and early life stress. *NeuroImage, 47*(3), 804–814. https://doi.org/10.1016/j.neuroimage.2009.05.009

Zheng, X., Fehr, R., Tai, K., Narayanan, J., & Gelfand, M. J. (2015). The unburdening effects of forgiveness: Effects on slant Perception and jumping height. *Social Psychological and Personality Science, 6*(4), 431–438. https://doi.org/10.1177/1948550614564222

Resources

Literature

Andreassen, T. W. (2001). From disgust to delight: Do customers hold a grudge? *Journal of Service Research, 4*(1), 39–49. https://doi.org/10.1177/109467050141004

Brooks, V. A. (2005). No hard feelings: Finding the focus in a teacher-student function. *The High School Journal, 89*(1), 54–56. https://doi.org/10.1353/hsj.2005.0012

Froh, J., & Bono, G. (2014). *Making grateful kids: The science of building character.* Templeton Press.

Froh, J. J., Bono, G., & Emmons, R. A. (2010). Being grateful is beyond good manners: Gratitude and motivation to contribute to society among early adolescents. *Motivation and Emotion, 34*, 144–157. https://doi.org/10.1007/s11031-010-9163-z

Gilpin, T. (2020). *The long deep grudge: A story of big capital, radical labor, and class war in the American heartland.* Haymarket Books.
Messias, E., Saini, A., Sinato, P., & Welch, S. (2010). Bearing grudges and physical health: Relationship to smoking, cardiovascular health and ulcers. *Social Psychiatry and Psychiatric Epidemiology, 45*(2), 183–187. https://doi.org/10.1007/s00127-009-0054-0
Persampiere, J., Poole, G., & Murphy, C. M. (2014). Neuropsychological correlates of anger, hostility, and relationship-relevant distortions in thinking among partner-violent men. *Journal of Family Violence, 29*(6), 625–641. https://doi.org/10.1007/s10896-014-9614-5
Schwarzenegger, K. P. (2020). *The gift of forgiveness: Inspiring stories from those who have overcome the unforgivable.* Viking.
Toepfer, S. M., Cichy, K., & Peters, P. (2012). Letters of gratitude: Further evidence for author benefits. *Journal of Happiness Studies, 13*(1), 187–201. https://doi.org/10.1007/s10902-011-9257-7

Gratitude Letter

Kaczmarek, L. D., Kashdan, T. B., Drążkowski, D., & Enko, J. (2015). Why do people prefer gratitude journaling over gratitude letters? The influence of individual differences in motivation and personality on web-based interventions. *Personality and Individual Differences, 75,* 1–6. https://doi.org/10.1016/j.paid.2014.11.004
Kini, P., Wong, J., McInnis, S., Gabana, N., & Brown, J. W. (2016). The effects of gratitude expression on neural activity. *Neuroimage, 128*(1), 1–10. https://doi.org/10.1016/j.neuroimage.2015.12.040
Toepfer, S. (2009). Letters of gratitude: Improving well-being through expressive writing. *Journal of Writing Research, 1*(3), 181–198. https://doi.org/10.17239/jowr-2009.01.03.1
Toepfer, S. M., Cichy, K., & Peters, P. (2012). Letters of gratitude: Further evidence for author benefits. *Journal of Happiness Studies, 13*(1), 187–201. https://doi.org/10.1007/s10902-011-9257-7
Waters, L., & Stokes, H. (2015). Positive education for school leaders: Exploring the effects of emotion-gratitude and action-gratitude. *Australian Educational and Developmental Psychologist, 32*(1), 1–22. https://doi.org/10.1017/edp.2015.1

Additional Readings

Eight Keys to Forgiveness
https://greatergood.berkeley.edu/article/item/eight_keys_to_forgiveness
Forgiveness can be very challenging. Robert Enright, an eminent scholar and practitioner of forgiveness, explains where to begin.

Altering Traumatic Memories
https://www.sciencedaily.com/releases/2021/04/210408152250.htm
Researchers have discovered that traumatic memories can indirectly be altered and weakened.

Painful Memories Could Be Erased
https://www.cbc.ca/news/health/erase-memories-1.4186191
Research might one day lead to treatment of people with PTSD or anxiety disorders.

Websites

The Forgiveness Project
https://www.theforgivenessproject.com/
The Forgiveness Project collects and shares stories from both victims/survivors and perpetrators of crime and conflict who have rebuilt their lives following hurt and trauma.

Worthington Model of Forgiveness
http://www.evworthington-forgiveness.com/
One of the most distinguished scholars and practitioners of forgiveness, Evert Worthington offers a number of free resources.

Multimedia

Grudge and Forgiveness

How Holding a Grudge Can Be a Shortcut to Forgiveness
https://www.cbc.ca/player/play/1454576707958
This podcast discusses how holding a grudge can be a shortcut to forgiveness – it deepens our understanding of the hurt so that when we let it go, we experience even greater contentment.

When Hope Is 'Punk' and Grudges Are Forgiveness
https://www.cbc.ca/radio/tapestry/when-hope-is-punk-and-grudges-are-forgiveness-1.5046927
This podcast suggests that we replace the adage "forgive and forget" with "forgive and remember," as it helps us to build coping skills for future life challenges.

Mothers Who Found Forgiveness & Friendship
https://www.ted.com/talks/aicha_el_wafi_phyllis_rodriguez_the_mothers_who_found_forgiveness_friendship
Phyllis Rodriguez and Aicha el-Wafi have a powerful friendship born of unthinkable loss.

How to Forgive
https://www.youtube.com/watch?v=d-K5btaxEFY
This video describes why we need to flex our forgiveness muscles more regularly, yet mindfully.

Gratitude

This Film Shaped Everyone Matters: Gratitude
https://youtu.be/4115qFsdWKQ
This short video encourages us to open our hearts, feel grateful for everyday, for the beauty of this planet, and the people we meet.

Want to Be Happy? Be Grateful
https://www.ted.com/talks/david_steindl_rast_want_to_be_happy_be_grateful?referrer=playlist-give_thanks
David Steindl-Rast, a Benedictine monk, meditates and writes on "the gentle power" of gratefulness.

Gratitude Letter
https://www.youtube.com/watch?v=W1GrLfmbiPE
Tal Ben-Shahar explains in this clip the exercise of writing and delivering a gratitude letter.

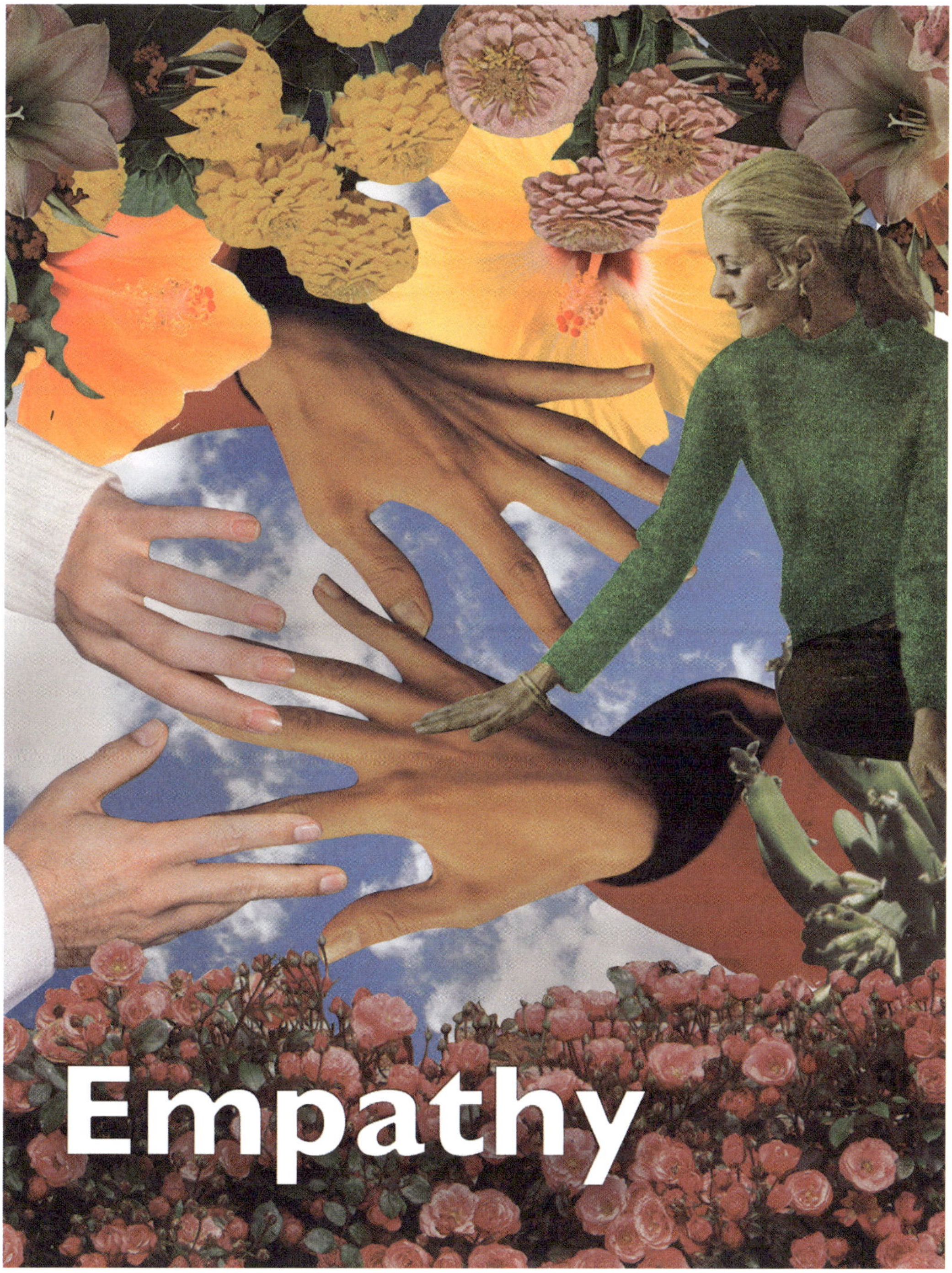
Empathy

Module 9: Empathy

The ability to put oneself in another's shoes is the focus of Module 9. The module encourages participants to identify thoughts, beliefs, and actions that foster healthy relationships. Participants learn about the power of empathy to understand others' challenges.

Module Topic	Minutes to Allot	
Learning Outcomes By reading a story of how one teen empathized with and acted on behalf of homeless people, participants: • Take the perspective of others who face challenging circumstances • Increase awareness of others' challenging experiences without feeling overwhelmed by negative thoughts and emotions	5	5
Opening Activities Start the module with a relaxation or mindfulness practice Invite participants to share a few events from their gratitude journal that have occurred since the last session Debrief participants' delivery of the letter of gratitude, if completed Invite questions about the previous module and practice(s)	10	15
Illustration of Core Concepts Review core concepts and show video illustrations Facilitate reflection and discussion: • *What are the key messages in the video(s) you just watched?* • *How might these concepts be relevant in your life?*	15	15
Practice: Build Empathy Read aloud *Kids Can Make a Difference: A Teen Story* Debrief learning from practice(s) using questions: • *How did perspective taking help Trevor?* • *How did Trevor's feelings, beliefs and behaviors change as a result?* • *What difficulties do you see in developing empathy?* • *How are flexible thinking and awareness of emotions important?* • *Do you see problems with perspective taking and too much empathy?* • *Are there any situations where empathy is not possible?*	20	30
Closing Activities Invite discussion of everyday applications Remind participants of relevant resources at the end of the module Guide participants in a 3-minute closing relaxation or mindfulness practice	10	10
Total	60 minutes	75 minutes

Core Concepts of Empathy

Many of the themes here are also presented in the Core Concepts section of the Workbook (p. 117):

- What is *empathy*? Empathy is putting ourselves in other people's shoes, in order to feel and understand their emotions, thoughts, actions, and motives. Empathy is an ability to imagine what others might be feeling or thinking (Gerdes et al., 2010). Generally, empathy can be (a) imagining what another person is feeling and thinking; (b) a wide range of perceptual, cognitive, and affective responses to events in the lives of others; or (c) both. To make sense of the term "empathy" and the role it plays in human behavior, it is useful to differentiate the many ways that psychologists have used the term (Stocksa & Lishnerb, 2009).
- Empathy is akin to perspective taking in the sense that it entails at least two processes. First, imagining what the other person is feeling, and second, imagining oneself in that specific situation. As a result of these two processes, the information empathy provides is something no other situation or mechanism can provide (Stocksa & Lishnerb, 2009). Empathy is distinct from mindfulness, which often entails nonjudgmental awareness of emotions and experiences. Mindfulness cultivates empathy, which in turn facilitates mindfulness.
- Empathy most often evokes an altruistic motive with the ultimate goal of supporting someone for whom one feels empathy and advocating for their welfare.
- Empathy can be of two types. Cognitive empathy is the ability to understand another person's perspective, whereas emotional empathy is the ability to share another person's thoughts and feelings.
- Whenever we hold on to any belief, view, or position too tightly, we undermine our ability to take others' perspectives. This also limits other strengths such as curiosity, open-mindedness, social intelligence, and kindness. Being empathic facilitates the growth of those other important strengths (Kostic et al., 2016).
- Empathy motivates prosocial behavior. The empathy-altruism hypothesis suggests that those with higher levels of empathy are more likely to want to help others (Andreoni & Miller, 2002; Eisenberg & Miller, 1987) Empathy predicts supportive bystander behavior such as helping victims, a core goal of antibullying interventions (Garandeau & Salmivalli, 2018). In a study of 900 children (aged 11–13 years), those with high empathy were more likely to stand up for their peers, when their peers were bullied (Abbott & Cameron, 2014). Healthy empathy development is associated with lower levels of aggression, being more inclusive of others, and increased perspective taking among children (Thompson & Melchior, 2019). Meta-analytic research (Imuta et al., 2022) has shown that children and adolescents who bully their peers are capable of taking other people's perspective, but engage in bullying and other antisocial behavior due to deficits in empathy. Children and adolescents who defend the victims of bullying have insights into other people's perspective as well as feelings of empathy to others in need.

Illustrations of Empathy

Play at least one of the three videos below to illustrate the core concepts of empathy and encourage discussion.

Wonder (2017) – There Are No Nice People Scene
https://youtu.be/C0KLb_v50-k
(Duration: 2:55 minutes)
In this short scene from Wonder, Auggie, born with facial differences, is comforted by love and empathy from his sister, Via.

Brené Brown on Empathy
https://youtu.be/1Evwgu369Jw?list=PL373A068F767AD185
(Duration: 2:53 minutes)
This animated clip discusses the ingredients of empathy and how it differs from sympathy. It explains how empathy builds meaningful connections to others and is important to living a fulfilling life.

Patch Adams (8/10) Movie Clip – You Treat a Person (1998)
https://youtu.be/Pr9ruvxA3K4
(Duration: 3:41 minutes)
For Patch Adams, masterfully played by Robin Williams in this clip, every human being has an impact on others. The greatest disease to be treated is indifference.

Reflection and Discussion

Invite participants to complete the Reflection and Discussion section of their Workbook (p. 118) regarding the video(s) they have watched. Discuss the questions:

What are the key messages in the video(s) you just watched?

How might these concepts be relevant in your life?

Practice: Build Empathy

Building empathy is important in today's world in which technological advances have connected people around the world instantly and constantly, yet many of us spend much of our lives in front of screens. As a result, we interact less in person. We lack time to listen and understand others. Research shows that the stock of social capital (the very fabric of our connections with each other) has plummeted, impoverishing our social and communal lives (Putnam, 2000).

This practice shares the story of a young boy who felt for others whom he did not know, showing perspective taking, followed by prosocial behavior. It helps participants sharpen their empathy skills and incorporate their understanding of concepts from previous modules such as fixed and growth mindset, cognitive accuracy, and cognitive flexibility.

Here are suggested steps to implement this activity:

- If it is helpful for your group, begin by asking participants to reflect on and share experiences that involved empathy, i.e., times when they showed empathy toward another person or another person showed empathy toward them.
- Discuss some of the common attitudes and behaviors that can interfere with empathy, such as diving into problem-solving mode or focusing on finding silver linings.
- Have participants read the story below "Kids Can Make a Difference: A Teen Story" from Burns, 2005 (Workbook, p. 119).
- Begin the discussion of the story by inviting their general reactions.
- Remind participants about the skills of cognitive flexibility and accuracy they learned in Modules 3 and 4. For example, you could ask them to complete the statement "Homeless people are always . . ." and ask them if they made any thinking shortcuts (i.e., jumping to conclusions) about homeless people.
- Draw their attention as well as to the negativity bias, which may have influenced their answers. Remind them that empathy can help counter the tendency toward negativity bias while spotting the strengths of others can also help us to build empathy.

Kids Can Make a Difference: A Teen Story

You know, sometimes when you are a kid, it is easy to feel pretty helpless or powerless. Indeed, if you stop and think about it, there are so many things that you can't do. You can't stay up as late as your bigger brother or sister. You can't play sports as well as your football or basketball heroes. You can't do some of the stunts that other kids do at the skate park. You can't get the results at school that your parents seem to expect that you should. Sometimes it is hard to see that you even have the potential to develop any of these abilities. How could you ever get to be a league football player when you fumble every time you try to pick up the ball? What you want to achieve may seem so far off in the future that it feels [like] you will never reach it.

Well, I once heard an inspiring story – a true story, I believe – about a boy named Trevor. It shows there are little things kids can do that make a big difference. One night Trevor was doing what a lot of other 13-year-old kids would be doing: He was watching TV. On the news he saw a story about some homeless people who were sleeping out in the cold on the streets in a downtown area of Philadelphia where he lived. Trevor had never really stopped to think how fortunate he was to live in a fairly well-to-do suburb of the same city. The story of the homeless people touched his heart, and he began to wonder what he could do to help these people.

It might have been easy for Trevor to forget about it. There are so many sad stories that you see on TV at times. This could have been just another that he ignored. Trevor also might have thought, "Well, what can I do about it? I'm just a kid," but he didn't. Instead he began to wonder how he might help and that led him to remember there were some spare, unused blankets in their garage. So, he went to his father and asked if he could take them to the people downtown who had no homes to go to for the night.

Trevor's father might have thought the request a bit strange. It is easy for us to want to hang onto the things that we have. It is easy for adults to think that they've worked hard to get what they own, so why should they give it away? It is much the same as a kid thinking, "It took a long time to save up my pocket money to help buy this new bike, so why should I lend it to a friend who needs to get home in a hurry?"

Now, Trevor's dad was a kind-hearted guy. He drove Trevor downtown to hand out their few surplus blankets to some of the people on the streets. I guess when it came time to curl up and sleep that night, the people were pretty happy for the added warmth of the new blankets. Trevor was happy too. He felt good about giving out the blankets. He felt inner warmth, almost like he had been wrapped up in an emotional blanket himself. But he realized there was a risk – it might feel so good that you'd want to do it again.

The next day Trevor went to his local grocery store and other public places in his neighborhood where there were notice boards. He put up signs asking for people to donate any spare blankets or food they didn't need. The result was surprising. Kindness was contagious. Trevor found so many people were willing to help that within a week he had filled his dad's garage with food and blankets. What Trevor had started with his kindness grew and spread throughout the community. It wasn't long before people's generosity overflowed from his dad's garage, and Trevor and his dad had to look for a bigger building to house all the gifts being donated. Would you believe there are now a number of special warehouses throughout Philadelphia that stock food and blankets to feed and warm the homeless? They are all called "Trevor's Place."

Practice Debrief

Ask participants to complete the Practice Debrief section in their Workbook (p. 120) and discuss their answers to the questions:

- *How did perspective taking help Trevor?*
- *How did Trevor's feelings, beliefs, and behaviors change as a result of developing empathy?*
- *What difficulties do you see in developing empathy?*
- *How are flexible thinking and awareness of emotions important for developing empathy?*
- *How might this be challenging for some people?*
- *Do you see any problems with perspective taking and too much empathy?*
- *Are there any situations where empathy is not possible?*

Learning and Cultural Fit

Adapt this practice to the learning and cultural needs of your participants, including their unique values and demographics. Possible adaptations include:

- It is important for us to empathize with emotional or painful experiences but not necessarily with the behavioral consequences of those feelings. For example, one can empathize with a participant's pain without condoning their drug use or aggression. Similarly, one can affirm another person's pain but not the thoughts that result, such as suicidal ideation or self-hatred.
- Conflicts, arguments, and even fights are inevitable and bullying is now a common experience in the social media landscape. Invite participants to appraise conflicts from all perspectives, even though sometimes they may find it difficult to put themselves in the shoes of a perpetrator or transgressor. Remind them they do not have to agree with a particular perspective; however, it will help them to understand emotional and cognitive states from different perspectives.
- Emphasize that having empathy for another person does not mean approval for their actions, forgiveness, or absolution.

Closing Activities

The goal of closing this module is to help participants consolidate their understanding of empathy and to take their new learning into everyday life.

Discuss with participants the Everyday Applications section, also found on p. 122 in the Workbook. Invite participants to be mindful in their day-to-day lives by noticing their own and others' actions and habits which show the use of empathy. Encourage them to use relevant resources found at the end of this module and included in their Workbook starting on p. 123.

Choose a 3-minute activity from Regular Practice 1: Mindfulness and Relaxation to close the module.

Everyday Applications

- Take time to understand at least one person who is different from you and who you would typically either avoid or dismiss. Take time to understand what might be their perspective.
- Appraise your circle of relationships. For whom is it easy to feel empathy? For whom is it difficult to feel empathy? Challenge yourself by putting yourself in the shoes of those in your circle for whom you feel less empathy. Then expand this practice to those outside your circle of relationships.
- When having a difficult conversation with a loved one, stop and ask yourself: Am I speaking to this person in a way that I would want to be addressed?
- When having a difficult conversation with a loved one, stop and notice what emotions are influencing your response and possibly distorting your message.
- When in a heated discussion with someone about politically or morally charged topics, ask the other person to share what's behind their perspective - why is it so important to them? This question can reveal their values and enable you to empathize with their perspective, whether you agree or disagree with their belief.
- Enhance empathy through lovingkindness meditation as discussed in Regular Practice 1 section of the Workbook (pp. 22–24). This practice invites you to express a wish for happiness, well-being, safety, and peace for yourself and for others.

The Everyday Applications for this module are adapted from "Building Social and Emotional Skills in Elementary Students: Empathy" by Randy Taran, https://www.edutopia.org/blog/project-happiness-empathy-randy-taran

References

Abbott, N., & Cameron, L. (2014). What makes a young assertive bystander? The effect of intergroup contact, empathy, cultural openness, and in-group bias on assertive bystander intervention intentions. *Journal of Social Issues, 70*(1), 167–182.

Andreoni, J., & Miller, J. H. (2002). Giving according to GARP: An experimental test of the consistency of preferences for altruism. *Econometrica, 70*, 737–753. https://doi.org/10.1111/1468-0262.00302

Eisenberg, N., & Miller, P. A. (1987). The relation of empathy to prosocial and related behaviors. *Psychological Bulletin, 101*(1), 91–119. https://doi.org/10.1037/0033-2909.101.1.91

Garandeau, C. F., & Salmivalli, C. (2018). Le programme anti-harcèlement Kiva [The anti bullying program Kiva]. *Enfance, 3*(3), 491–501. https://doi.org/10.3917/enf2.183.0491

Gerdes, K. E., Segal, E. A., & Lietz, C. A. (2010). Conceptualising and measuring empathy. *British Journal of Social Work, 40*(7), 2326–2343. https://doi.org/10.1093/bjsw/bcq048

Imuta, K., Song, S., Henry, J. D., Ruffman, T., Peterson, C., & Slaughter, V. (2022). A meta-analytic review on the social-emotional intelligence correlates of the six bullying roles: Bullies, followers, victims, bully-victims, defenders, and outsiders. *Psychological Bulletin, 148*(3-4), 199–226. https://doi.org/10.1037/bul0000364

Kostic, J., Nesic, M., Stankovic, M., Zikic, O., & Markovic, J. (2016). Evaluating empathy in adolescents with conduct disorders. *Vojnosanitetski Pregled, 73*(5), 429–434. https://doi.org/10.2298/VSP150121031K

Putnam, R. D. (2000). *Bowling alone: The collapse and revival of American community*. Touchstone/Simon & Schuster. https://doi.org/10.1145/358916.361990

Stocksa, E. L., & Lishnerb, D. A. (2009). Empathy. In S. J. Lopez (Ed.), *The encyclopedia of positive psychology* (pp. 320–326). Blackwell.

Thompson, E., & Melchior, S. (2019). Improving empathy in children: Interactive read-aloud as a counseling intervention. *Journal of Creativity in Mental Health, 15*(2), 199–211. https://doi.org/10.1080/15401383.2019.1676857

Resources

Literature

Abbott, N., & Cameron, L. (2014). What makes a young assertive bystander? The effect of intergroup contact, empathy, cultural openness, and in-group bias on assertive bystander intervention intentions. *Journal of Social Issues, 70,* 167–182. https://doi.org/10.1111/josi.12053

Bernard, M. E. (2006). It's time we teach social-emotional competence as well as we teach academic competence. *Reading & Writing Quarterly, 22*(2), 103–119. https://doi.org/10.1080/10573560500242184

Brackett, M. (2019). *Permission to feel: Unlocking the power of emotions to help our kids, ourselves, and our society thrive.* Celadon Books.

Burns, G. W. (2005). *Healing stories for kids and teens: Using metaphors in therapy.* Wiley.

Goleman, D., Bennett, L., & Barlow, Z. (2012). *Ecoliterate: How educators are cultivating emotional, social, and ecological intelligence.* Jossey-Bass.

Grant, L. (2014). Hearts and minds: Aspects of empathy and wellbeing in social work participants. *Social Work Education, 33*(3), 338–352. https://doi.org/10.1080/02615479.2013.805191

Maynard, N., & Weinstein, B. (2019). *Hacking school discipline: 9 ways to create a culture of empathy and responsibility using restorative justice.* Times 10 Publications.

Renati, R., Berrone, C., & Zanetti, M. A. (2012). Morally disengaged and unempathic: Do cyberbullies fit these definitions? An exploratory study. *Cyberpsychology, Behavior, and Social Networking, 15*(8), 391–398. https://doi.org/10.1089/cyber.2012.0046

Stepien, K. A., & Baernstein, A. (2006). Educating for empathy: A review. *Journal of General Internal Medicine, 21*(5), 524–530. https://doi.org/10.1111/j.1525-1497.2006.00443.x

Van Cuylenburg, H. (2019). *The resilience project: Finding happiness through gratitude, empathy and mindfulness* (H. Van Cuylenburg, Narr.) [Audiobook]. Random House Australia.

Zaki, J. (2019). *The war for kindness: Building empathy in a fractured world.* Broadway Books.

Additional Readings

The Difference Between Empathy and Sympathy
https://www.psychologytoday.com/intl/blog/hide-and-seek/201505/the-difference-between-empathy-and-sympathy
This Psychology Today article describe the difference between empathy and sympathy.

Websites

Roots of Empathy
https://rootsofempathy.org/
The program Roots of Empathy develops empathy in children today so they can build the world they deserve.

Center for Building a Culture of Empathy
http://cultureofempathy.com/
The Center for Building a Culture of Empathy is a leader of the global empathy movement. The aim of this center is to build a global culture of empathy and care.

Center for Empathy in International Affairs
https://www.centerforempathy.org/
The Center for Empathy in International Affairs provides a deeper understanding of others. It also informs foreign policymaking, strengthens diplomacy, and contributes to the prevention and resolution of violent conflict.

Multimedia

The Roots of Empathy and Compassion
https://youtu.be/3AgvKJK-nrk
Paul Ekman is a respected author and researcher on emotion. He discusses different levels of empathy from emotional recognition and resonance to compassion for our families, our global community, and all sentient beings.

Under the Surface. Empathy Film
https://www.youtube.com/watch?v=AZ-pU7ozt3g
This short video shows challenges people face in their daily lives without expressing or sharing them with anyone.

We're Experiencing an Empathy Shortage, but We Can Fix it Together
https://youtu.be/-DspKSYxYDM
Jamil Zaki from Standford University asks: "In a fractured world, can we hack our own sense of empathy and get others to become more empathic?"

Empathy Can Change the World
https://www.youtube.com/watch?v=aU3QfyqvHk8
This video was conceptualized, scripted, and acted out by 8th-grade students.

The Importance of Empathy
https://youtu.be/UzPMMSKfKZQ
This short film shows how different people experience the world and the benefits of perspective taking. It explains research in the field of brain science and the positive heath impacts of expressing empathy toward others.

Unsung Hero
https://www.youtube.com/watch?v=uaWA2GbcnJU
This commercial illustrates the priceless human emotions of kindness.

Slowness & Savoring

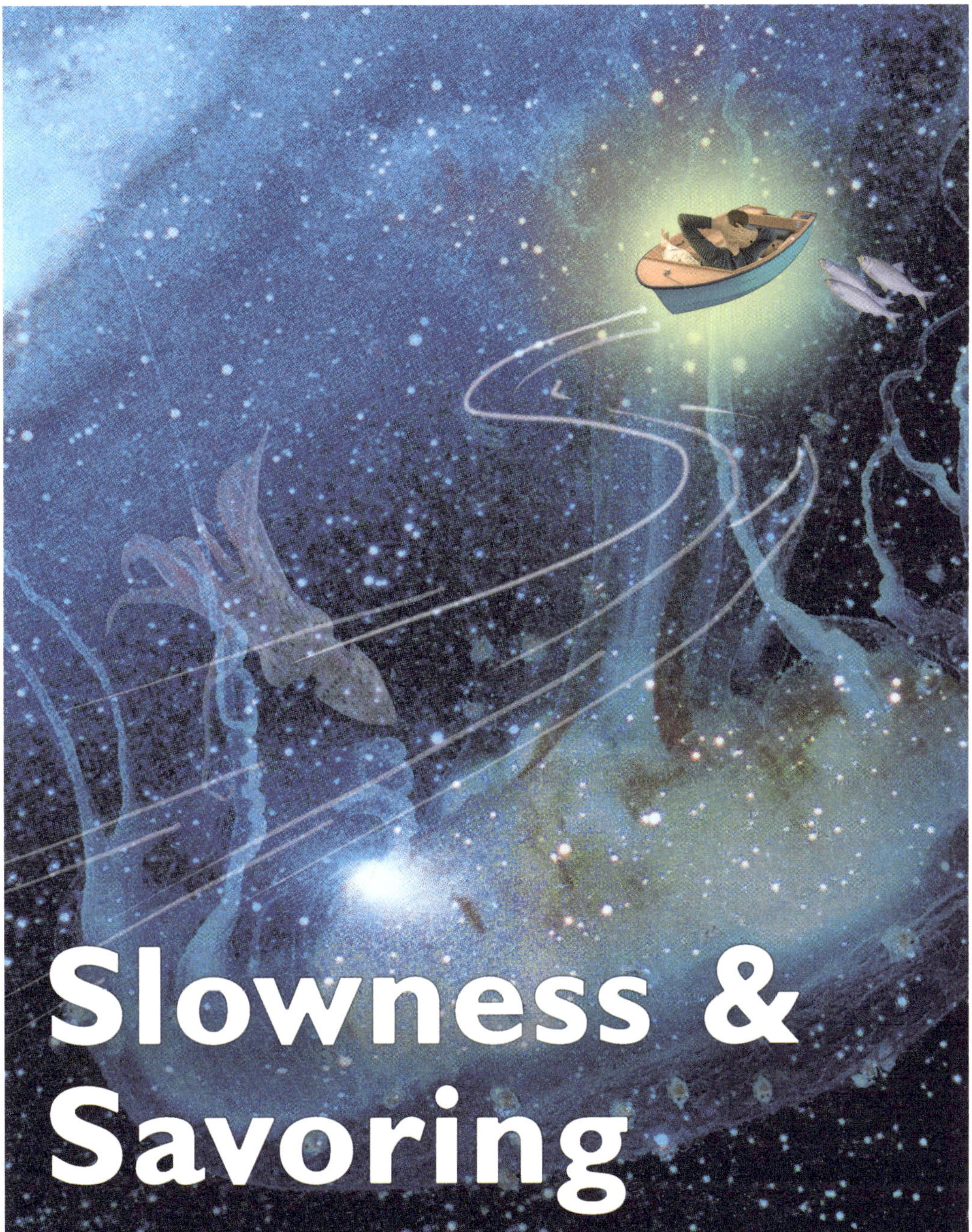

Module 10: Slowness and Savoring

This module invites participants to recognize the stressful impact of fast-paced, hectic lives with lengthy to-do lists and limited time. It debunks assumptions about the effectiveness of multitasking and elevates the power of slowing down and savoring the details of our daily experiences. Through a fun, engaging activity, participants learn how slowing down and savoring can generate positive emotions that carry over to our important relationships.

<table>
<tr><th>Module Topic</th><th colspan="2">Minutes to Allot</th></tr>
<tr><td>Learning Outcomes
By savoring a few chosen items and employing savoring types and techniques, participants:
• Recognize the pressure and cost of doing things faster
• Slow down to appreciate an experience in detail
• Experience how savoring amplifies positive emotions</td><td>5</td><td>5</td></tr>
<tr><td>Opening Activities
Start the module with a relaxation or mindfulness practice
Invite participants to share a few events from their gratitude journal that have occurred since the last session
Invite questions about the previous module and practice(s)</td><td>10</td><td>15</td></tr>
<tr><td>Illustration of Core Concepts
Review core concepts and show video illustrations
Facilitate reflection and discussion:
• What are the key messages in the video(s) you just watched?
• How might these concepts be relevant in your life?</td><td>15</td><td>15</td></tr>
<tr><td>Practice: Slow Down and Savor
Present your selection of savoring items that draw on five senses
Discuss savoring types and techniques with participants
Have participants individually or in small groups choose three items to savor and record their observations in the Practice Debrief worksheet
Debrief learning from practice(s) using questions:
• What savoring types did you use?
• What savoring techniques did you use to savor your item?
• What did you notice by slowing down to savor?</td><td>20</td><td>30</td></tr>
<tr><td>Closing Activities
Invite discussion of everyday applications
Remind participants of relevant resources at the end of the module
Guide participants in a 3-minute closing relaxation or mindfulness practice</td><td>10</td><td>10</td></tr>
<tr><td align="right">Total</td><td>60 minutes</td><td>75 minutes</td></tr>
</table>

Core Concepts of Slowness and Savoring

The themes here are also presented in the Core Concepts section of the Workbook (p. 125):

Slowness

- Why slow down? We live in an age of speed and anxiety. We fill up our time with more and more tasks at an increasing rate. It seems we are addicted to speed. Our desire for speed is also demonstrated by our tendency to multitask. Think of your daily life. How many apps and gadgets do you have turned on at the same time? (Facebook, Twitter/X, computer, smartphone, etc.). In his book *In Praise of Slowness*, journalist Carl Honoré (2005) describes how the current age is turbocharged, whereby every moment feels like a race against the clock. This attitude of impatience has, Honoré observes, infected every facet of our culture. Consider road rage, shopping rage, vacation rage, social-media rage. These exaggerated reactions have taken a toll on our health and turned our work into an undesired necessity. Research shows that people who are cognitively busy are also more likely to act selfishly, use sexist language, and make erroneous judgments in social situations (Kahneman, 2011).
- Multitasking has now become part of the job description as much as job performance. We value the ability to multitask, but, in fact, the human brain is not designed to multitask most higher order activities. We tend to confuse the act of switching between tasks with multitasking. What we actually do is go back and forth between activities. We have become quite good at this. However, research suggests that this kind of switching back and forth between activities is actually very unproductive. Tasks can take more than twice as long to complete when performed this way (Osward et al., 2007).
- Is speed bad? Speed is not always bad, of course, nor is slowness always good. Nobel Laureate and distinguished psychologist Daniel Kahneman (2011) posits that our minds have two systems. System 1 is fast, intuitive, and emotional. System 2 is slower, more deliberate, and more logical. System 1 is automatic, and System 2 is effortful. Each system is important: We need to respond quickly to accidents or dangerous events, but when people are in a relaxed state, their brain goes into a deeper, slower, more nuanced mode of thought. Artists have always known that you cannot hurry the act of creation. Businesses are beginning to realize the same thing.
- Workers need moments to relax, unplug, and be silent in order to be creative and productive. Let us clarify that slowness is not antispeed. High-speed internet is helpful. We would not enjoy ice hockey if it were slow. Similarly, although project deadlines force us to act more quickly than we might like, they also help to motivate us and increase our productivity.
- Slowness and savoring work together. Slowing down allows you to savor, and you can rarely savor without slowing down.

Savoring

- What is *savoring*? Fred Bryant and Joseph Veroff (2007) define savoring as a total experience that includes appreciating all sensations, perceptions, thoughts, behaviors, and emotions when mindfully attending to positive events or experiences. Examples of savoring include a tourist viewing the Egyptian Pyramids from the back of a camel, a diner tasting an exotic

dish in a gourmet restaurant, and a hiker soaking in a hot tub under the stars after a long day of backpacking. Savoring is becoming absorbed in a chosen subjective experience.
- Savoring amplifies or prolongs positive aspects of experiences. By focusing our attention on the positive aspects of the present moment, we improve our overall mood and satisfaction (Hurley & Kwon, 2012). Research has shown that people who spend more time in nature report greater well-being. Meredith and colleagues (2020) found in a review of studies that 10–50 minutes of sitting or walking in a diverse array of natural settings is associated with lower levels of psychological and physical indicators of stress when contrasted with equal durations spent in urbanized settings.
- When savoring objects or experiences with friends and family, we can deepen our connections to the meaningful people in our life. Savoring requires effort: We have to work against the pressures of a turbocharged culture that constantly asks us to multitask and do more at a rapid speed.

Illustrations of Slowness and Savoring

Play at least one of the three videos below to illustrate the core concepts of slowness and savoring and encourage discussion.

Carl Honoré – Author of "In Praise of Slow"
https://youtu.be/RvOUH5dIU24
(Duration: 4:46 minutes)
The author of *In Praise of Slowness* examines our compulsion to hurry and chronicles the global trend in slowing down our experiences (originally published as *In Praise of Slowness*).

Forget Multitasking, Try Monotasking
https://youtu.be/0YNeyBANrTI
(Duration: 2:52 minutes)
This TED talk by Designer Paolo Cardini questions the efficiency of multitasking and makes the case for monotasking.

Where Good Ideas Come From
https://youtu.be/gy09lzLfhgA
(Duration: 4:06 minutes)
This clip talks about spaces where good ideas lead to breakthroughs. They require collaboration, slowness, and the need for hunches to collide.

Reflection and Discussion

Invite participants to complete the Reflection and Discussion section of their Workbook (p. 127) regarding the video(s) they have watched. Discuss the questions:

What are the key messages in the video(s) you just watched?

How might these concepts be relevant in your life?

Practice: Slow Down and Savor

The purpose of this practice is to help participants develop skills of noticing, experiencing, prolonging, and generating positive emotions from a variety of objects. This practice will increase their awareness and enhance their appreciation of positive emotions in daily life.

Participants will engage with objects mindfully for a few minutes. While likely familiar with these objects and accompanying positive emotions, participants are encouraged to pay attention to some unique features of these objects, including features they might not have noticed previously.

This practice requires some preparation. Plan ahead by gathering a variety of savoring items. Listed in Table 9 are examples of items from different categories (also provided in the Workbook, Table WB3, p. 128).

- Assemble all items selected from Table 9 on a table and let participants pick one or two.
- Ask participants (individually, in pairs, or in small groups) to savor their items, slowly and deliberately experiencing the objects.
- Allow sufficient time (5–15 minutes) for them to savor their items. If working in pairs or in small groups, invite them to share a description of their experience using the language of savoring types (Table 10) and techniques (Table 11). These same tables can be found in the Workbook on p. 128.
- Remind participants that savoring requires effort and consistent practice.

Table 9. Savoring items (Table WB3 in the Workbook)

Items	Description
Food	Chocolate, pineapple, strawberry, orange, coffee grains, loose tea
Objects from nature	Smooth rocks, sea shells, flowers, pine cones, honey suckle
Materials	Cotton, sand paper, gauze
Sound	Wind chimes, music, nature sounds (birds, ocean waves)
Written words	Poem, story, reflection, quotation
Other	Kaleidoscopes, any object of sensory interest such as bubbles

Table 10. Savoring types (Table WB4 in the Workbook)

Types	Description
Basking	Taking great pleasure in one's accomplishments
Thanksgiving	Giving thanks, expressing gratitude
Luxuriating	Enjoying physical comforts and sensations
Marveling	Being filled with wonder and awe at great art, a performance, or action
Mindfulness	Being aware, attentive, and observant

Table 11. Savoring techniques (Table WB5 in the Workbook)

Techniques	Description
Sharing with others	Sharing with others the value of a moment, recapturing the details
Memory building	Taking mental or physical pictures
Self-praising	Using self-affirmative statements to congratulate oneself
Sharpening perceptions	Focusing on certain elements and blocking others
Getting deeply absorbed	Being emotionally absorbed in an object or experience
Behavioral savoring	Enjoying celebratory experiences such as laughing, cheering, clapping, moving
Exercising curiosity	Actively being open to exploring unique, new, and undiscovered aspects of an experience
Avoiding kill-joy thinking	Focusing on the present moment of an experience without dwelling on thoughts that an experience will eventually end, or that someone might be having a better experience

Practice Debrief

Invite participants to fill in descriptions of their own experiences in the Practice Debrief worksheet in their Workbook (p. 129). Read aloud the instructions on their Practice Debrief worksheet:

> *Describe your savoring experience. For example, for chocolate, one participant described their experience:*
>
> *"I noticed the slightly bitter smell of the dark brown chocolate before I put it in my mouth. It quickly began to melt, and I was absorbed by the strong, sweet flavor. I wanted to swallow almost right away, but I just let it melt in my mouth until the chocolatey liquid had spread all over my mouth."*

Facilitate a discussion of participants' observations with the group as a whole.

Learning and Cultural Fit

Adapt this practice to the learning and cultural needs of your participants, including their unique values and demographics. Possible adaptations include:

- Many of today's participants have been surrounded by fast-paced technology for their entire lives. It may be difficult for them to understand the value of slowing down when a person's success seems to be defined and determined by their ability to work at a rapid pace. It is important for participants to understand that one can be fast-paced at times when productivity is necessary, but that they also need to find time to slow down to take care of themselves and enjoy their activities and experiences.

- Encourage participants to savor through engaging multiple senses. For visual savoring, participants can take pictures of moments when they are in awe of what is going on and put them in their scrapbook or on an *awe wall*. For auditory savoring, participants can record their feelings while listening to music. They could record details, such as highs and lows of the song, the singer's facial expressions, the quality of the melody, and the depth of the voice.
- Some participants may have underlying difficulties with attention and self-regulation. Encourage these participants to proceed slowly through a concrete and time-limited task. For example, they could begin by slowing down for 5 minutes in a day. They can broaden this as they become better at slowing down.
- Not all cultures are as time-bound and fast-paced as many industrialized countries. Participants from diverse cultural backgrounds may already be accustomed to a slower pace at home. In group discussions, invite them to share their cultural perspectives. Assess and modify instructions accordingly.
- Participants should not confuse savoring adaptive activities with savoring maladaptive behaviors, such as smoking tobacco or marijuana, or engaging in other potentially harmful or dangerous activities.

Closing Activities

The goal of closing this module is to help participants consolidate their understanding of slowness and savoring and to take their new learning into everyday life.

Discuss with participants the Everyday Applications section (p. 130 in their Workbook). Invite participants to be mindful in their day-to-day lives by noticing their own and others' actions and habits related to slowness and savoring. Encourage them to use relevant resources found at the end of this module and included in their Workbook starting on p. 131.

Choose a 3-minute activity from Regular Practice 1: Mindfulness and Relaxation to close the module.

Everyday Applications

Ways to Slow Down

Making small but steady changes to slow down are better than following an ambitious plan to be serene and tranquil all of the time. In his book *In Praise of Slowness*, Carl Honoré (2005) recommends using the following everyday strategies to slow down:

- Pick one or two areas of your life that you usually hurry through. Slow down your pace. Options could be eating at least three meals slowly for one week, walking or talking slowly at least once a week.
- Deliberately focus on peaceful experiences, such as following floating clouds with your eyes, watching the sunset, feeling the breeze blow, or hearing and enjoying wind chimes. You may find that the rhythms of nature are slow but deeply satisfying.
- Talk to friends and family about the negative effects of speed (e.g., accidents, injuries, stress, anxiety). Think about starting a club in your school that sets examples of slowing down in different domains of school life. Involve school administration, teachers, and parents.
- Learn to say no to avoid overscheduling.
- Create gadget-free times or zones – for example, no social media after 10 p.m., no gadgets during homework, vacations.
- Technology can speed up the demands on our life and increase distraction. However, it can also help you slow down. Make use of the many apps on your phone or computer such as *Screen Time* to be more mindful of your technology usage or *Calm* to meditate.

Ways to Savor

Consider the following techniques to deepen your savoring.

- Have a relatively quiet and distraction-free dinner. Set for yourself a beautiful formal table with full cutlery, plates, and glassware. If you like, listen to background music of your choice. Take a bite and try to chew every bite at least 10 to 15 times. Savor the texture, taste, and smell of the food. Instead of rushing through the food, relish the flavor, paying attention to different ingredients and specific details. Try to lose yourself during that time.
- Spend quality time with one of your favorite family members or friends. Pick an activity that both of you enjoy. It could be as simple as having a conversation in a distraction-free environment, watching a movie together, or going for a walk. Try to be in the *here and now* with that person without worrying about the past or the future.
- Spend some time by yourself. It could be for half an hour or an entire day. You could choose to listen to favorite songs, explore a park, go to a favorite restaurant, or simply read a book of your choice. Pay close attention to your senses while you are engaged in the activity. What do you see, smell, and hear around you?

References

Bryant, F. B., & Veroff, J. (2007). *Savoring: A new model of positive experience.* Lawrence Erlbaum Associates Publishers.

Honoré, C. (2005). *In praise of slowness: Challenging the cult of speed.* HarperSanFrancisco.

Hurley, D. B., & Kwon, P. (2012). Results of a study to increase savoring the moment: Differential impact on positive and negative outcomes. *Journal of Happiness Studies, 13*(4), 579–588. https://doi.org/10.1007/s10902-011-9280-8

Kahneman, D. (2011). *Thinking, fast and slow.* Doubleday Canada.

Meredith, G. R., Rakow, D. A., Eldermire, E. R. B., Madsen, C. G., Shelley, S. P., & Sachs, N. A. (2020). Minimum time dose in nature to positively impact the mental health of college-aged students, and how to measure it: A scoping review. *Frontiers in Psychology, 10*, Article 2942. https://doi.org/10.3389/fpsyg.2019.02942

Oswald, F. L., Hambrick, D. Z., & Jones, L. A. (2007). Keeping all the plates spinning: Understanding and predicting multitasking performance. In D. H. Jonassen (Ed.), *Learning to solve complex scientific problems.* Lawrence Erlbaum Associates Publishers.

Resources

Literature

Bryant, F. B., & Veroff, J. (1984). Dimensions of subjective mental health in American men and women. *Journal of Health and Social Behavior, 25*, 116–135. https://doi.org/10.2307/2136664

Bryant, F. B., & Veroff, J. (2007). *Savoring: A new model of positive experience.* Lawrence Erlbaum Associates Publishers.

Honoré, C. (2005). *In praise of slowness: Challenging the cult of speed.* HarperSanFrancisco.

Kahneman, D. (2011). *Thinking, fast and slow.* Allen Lane.

Kasser, T. (2003). *The high price of materialism.* MIT Press.

McAlary, B. (2017). *Destination simple: Everyday rituals for a slower life.* Source Books.

McAlary, B. (2018). *Slow: Simple living for a frantic world.* Sourcebooks.

Osbaldiston, N., & Palgrave, M. (2013). *Culture of the slow: Social deceleration in an accelerated world.* Palgrave Macmillan.

Quoidbach, J., Berry, E., Hansenne, M., & Mikolajczak, M. (2010). Positive emotion regulation and well-being: Comparing the impact of eight savoring and dampening strategies. *Personality and Individual Differences, 49*(5), 368–373. https://doi.org/10.1016/j.paid.2010.03.048

Sunim, H. (2012). *The things you can see only when you slow down: How to be calm and mindful in a fast-paced world.* Penguin.

Websites

Slow Living LDN
https://slowlivingldn.com/what-is-slow-living/
This website aims to help people live better not faster, through carefully crafted content that promotes a meaningful and conscious lifestyle.

Slow Living 101
https://www.sloww.co/slow-living-101/
This website offers (for a subscription fee) book summaries, blogs, infographics, and practical ideas about slowing down.

Be More With Less
https://bemorewithless.com/artofslow/
Courtney Carver's website suggests that living in a new, smaller space allows for spending more time together and enjoying a new life in the city. Removing things like a big house, yard, shed, mortgage, high utility bills, property taxes, car, and a host of other items frees one to appreciate life's true value.

The Free Mindfulness Project
http://www.freemindfulness.org/welcome
This is a website that shares free resources on mindfulness and engages the community through its blog and discussion forums.

Multimedia

Savoring – The Science of Well-Being
https://youtu.be/AEY8vjAhQ6Y
This video is part of the Yale University online course, The Science of Well-Being.

Be Mindful and Savor, with Barbara Fredrickson
https://youtu.be/HMb2VyIeEZo
In this brief interview, Barbara Fredrickson, distinguished scholar and scientist of positive emotions, explains how savoring can amplify mindfulness.

National Geographic YouTube channel
https://www.youtube.com/@NatGeo/featured
National Geographic's YouTube channel NatGeo takes you up close to the stories about our planet.

Gratitude | Louie Schwartzberg | TEDxSF
https://www.youtube.com/watch?v=gXDMoiEkyuQ
Louie Schwartzberg's stunning time-lapse photography provides a visual meditation to be grateful every day.

Thinking, Fast and Slow by Daniel Kahneman | Animated book summary
https://youtu.be/uqXVAo7dVRU
This video clip summarizes Nobel laureate Daniel Kahneman's book *Thinking, Fast and Slow*. Learn how two systems of thinking can help you to make better decisions.

Tips for Savoring Life's Precious Moment
https://youtu.be/Ff4BuYDMC48
This short clip describes savoring as a sense of gladness, being real, and being present with eyes and ears in the moment.

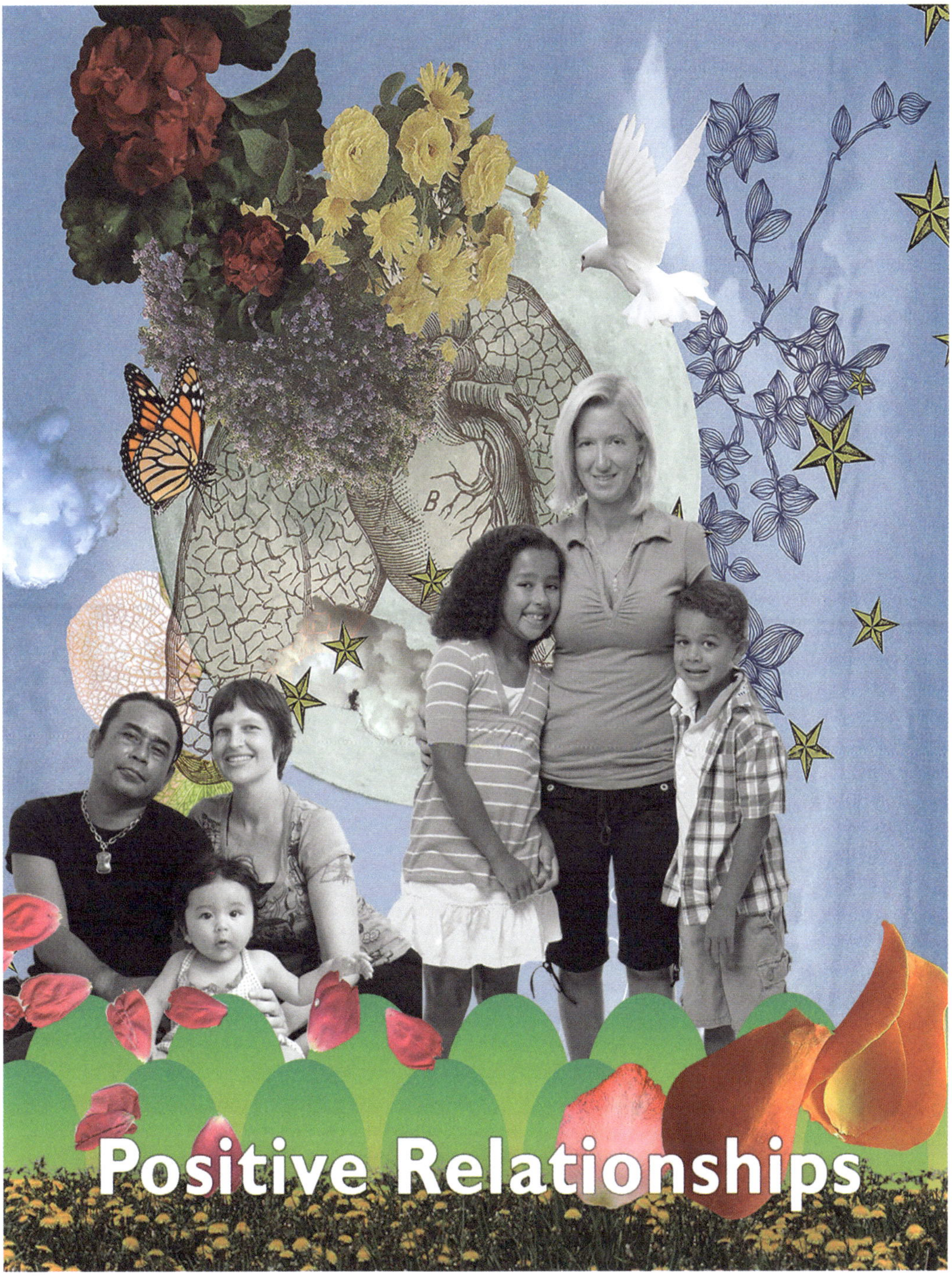
Positive Relationships

Module 11: Positive Relationships

Module 11 builds on participants' understanding that our signature character strengths can be a source of resilience and well-being. In relationships, this insight can be a powerful accelerator of community wellness and resilience, whereby valuing the strengths of those in our circle can be a source of shared positive emotion.

Module Topic	Minutes to Allot	
Learning Outcomes By creating a tree of positive relationships, participants: • Spot strengths of significant people in their lives • Plan ways to cultivate their relationships by engaging in activities with those who share similar strengths • Explore possibilities to discover the uniqueness of their closest relationships from a strengths perspective	5	5
Opening Activities Start the module with a relaxation or mindfulness practice Invite participants to share a few events from their gratitude journal that have occurred since the last session Invite questions about the previous module and practice(s)	10	15
Illustration of Core Concepts Review core concepts and show video illustrations Facilitate reflection and discussion: • *What are the key messages in the video(s) you just watched?* • *How might these concepts be relevant in your life?*	15	15
Practice: Celebrate Collective Strengths Have participants identify people in their circle with whom they have a positive relationship and list their top strengths by completing *My Tree of Positive Relationships* Debrief learning from practice using questions: • *Can you recall specific events that exemplify their strengths?* • *Have any of them helped you develop your strengths?* • *Do you share strengths with any and can you develop your relationship with them as a result?* • *Whose strengths differ from yours? Can you learn from them as a result?*	20	30
Closing Activities Invite discussion of everyday applications Remind participants of relevant resources at the end of the module Guide participants in a 3-minute closing relaxation or mindfulness practice	10	10
Total	60 minutes	75 minutes

Core Concepts of Positive Relationships

Many of the themes here are also presented in the Core Concepts section of the Workbook (p. 133):

- Positive relationships include family, but extend to other important relationships such as friends, colleagues, and the community at large. Learning ways to acknowledge the strengths of those in our circle can counter negativity bias and improve the quality of our interactions.
- Susan Sheridan and colleagues (2004) define "positive family" as a unit that is able to access and mobilize strengths and resources to acquire and build skills and competencies, through specific behaviors, to meet the needs and challenges of family members. More recently, Waters and colleagues have found that strengths-based parenting (SBP) predicts student well-being and academic achievement (Waters et al., 2019)
- One way to build positive relationships is by acknowledging the highest strengths of family members. Similarly, one way to build positive relationships with others in your network is by acknowledging their highest strengths. When you recognize the strengths of your important relationships, you are more likely to appreciate one another and build stronger connections.
- Learning about the strengths of important people in your life may also help you gain new insights into their behaviors that you may previously have misunderstood. This will enable you to know, acknowledge, and celebrate their strengths and promote interactions and family-centered activities. For instance, if you learn that one of your brother's top strengths is love of learning, then a trip to a museum would be a great place to visit when your family is on vacation.
- Learning about each other's strengths promotes empathy and fosters greater appreciation for each other's actions and intentions. For example, when a mother discovers that some of her son's top strengths are honesty, fairness, and bravery, she is better able to understand why he drives all the way across town to return an extra dollar he was accidentally given when checking out at a grocery store, even though he will spend over a dollar on gas in the process of driving back to the store. Rather than seeing this as illogical behavior, she can see that he is simply acting according to one of his defining character strengths.

Illustrations of Positive Relationships

Play at least one of the three videos below to illustrate the core concepts of positive relationships and encourage discussion.

How to Build Trust and Relationships
https://www.youtube.com/watch?v=wtNOq1Bwtt4
(Duration: 3:08 minutes)
This short video provides relationship-building insights from Dale Carnegie's 1936 classic *How to Win Friends and Influence People*, still used today for leadership and team training.

Healthy vs. Unhealthy Relationships
https://www.youtube.com/watch?v=Gn7ZQ2x0cOE
(Duration: 2:16 minutes)
This cartoon illustrates the difference between a healthy relationship and an unhealthy relationship with a friend or romantic partner.

A Touching Story of An Old Man, His Son, and a Sparrow
https://youtu.be/Ql5odcCvrbg?list=PL373A068F767AD185
(Duration: 4:12 minutes)
This touching story depicts the power of family relationships and connecting with the world in a positive way (in Greek with English subtitles).

Reflection and Discussion

Invite participants to complete the Reflection and Discussion section of their Workbook (p. 134) regarding the video(s) they have watched. Discuss the questions:

What are the key messages in the video(s) you just watched?

How might these concepts be relevant in your life?

Practice: Celebrate Collective Strengths

This practice is similar to creating a family genogram. A genogram is a graphic representation of a family tree. It maps out family and other close relationships. Often used in family therapy, the genogram helps to identify tensions and conflicts. In SBR, the worksheet My Tree of Positive Relationships helps participants map out at a glance the salient strengths of their closest relationships. The goal of this practice is to help participants explore patterns of strengths and imagine how awareness of these strengths can be used to deepen relationships.

This practice draws on the foundation built in Modules 5–7 that focus on strengths. It aims to sharpen the skills of spotting, labeling, acknowledging, and celebrating the strengths of loved ones. The practice can help increase participants' understanding of their loved ones, from a place of dignity, pride, and admiration which may reduce conflict and criticism.

- Briefly review the 24 strengths from Module 5.
- Review with participants Figure 6 below, the sample tree of positive relationships (Figure WB5 in the Workbook p. 135).
- Ask participants to use the worksheet My Tree of Positive Relationships on p. 136 of the Workbook to complete their tree by using each box to list a close connection (family, friend, other loved one) and what they guess might be that person's signature character strengths. Alternatively, they can invite their loved ones to complete the online VIA survey (www.viacharacter.org).

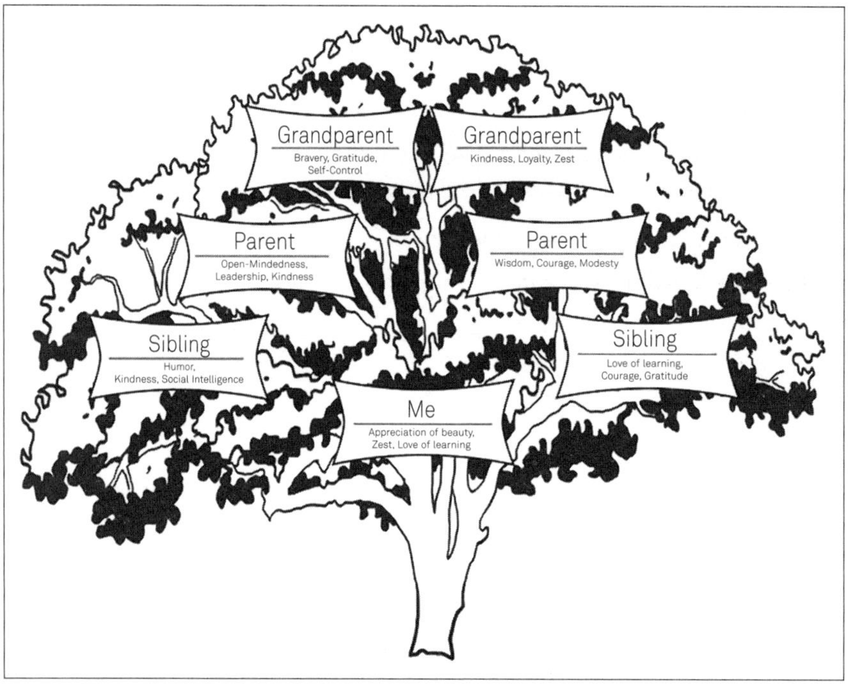

Figure 6. Sample tree of positive relationships (Figure WB5 in the Workbook)

Worksheet: My Tree of Positive Relationships (p. 136 in the Workbook)

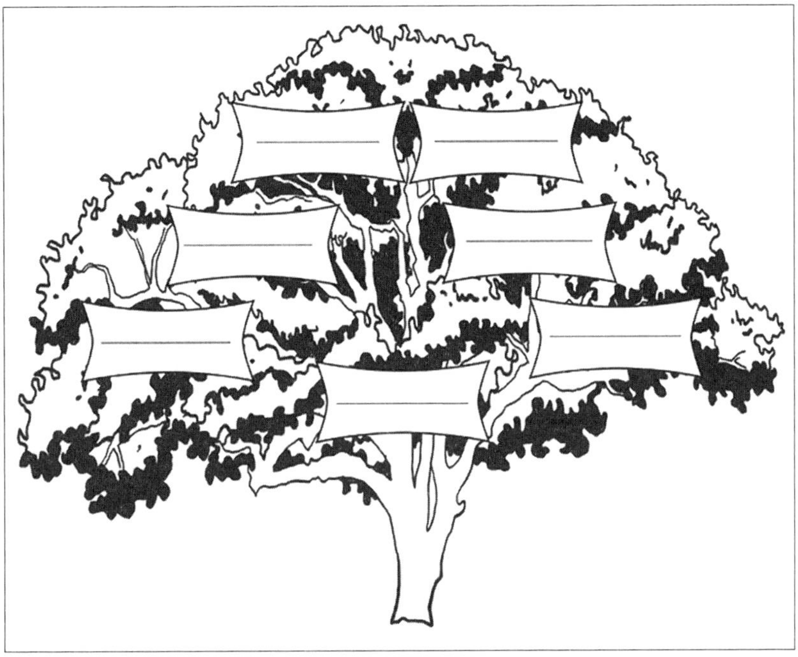

Practice Debrief

Ask participants to complete the Practice Debrief exercise in their Workbook on p. 137 that asks the questions:

- *Can you recall any specific events that exemplify the strengths of your loved ones (e.g., parents, siblings, romantic partners)?*
  - *Example 1: My mother is kind because she always tries to do nice things for me, without me even asking for them.*
  - *Example 2: My best friend is brave because she stands up for others when people say mean things.*
- *Can you identify the people in your tree who have helped you to develop your strengths?*
- *Do you share any strengths with those on your tree? Are there opportunities for you to further develop your relationship with them?*
- *What strengths do others have that are different from your strengths? Are there opportunities for you to learn strengths from others?*
- *Do you think some members on your tree overuse or underuse their strengths? Does any of this underusing or overusing cause difficulties for them or conflicts with you or others?*
- *Looking at the collective strengths on your worksheet: My Tree of Positive Relationships, how do they support your resilience and well-being?*

Learning and Cultural Fit

Adapt this practice to the learning and cultural needs of your participants, including their unique values and demographics. Possible adaptations include:

- Some family members and friends may find it easier to engage in this practice if their strengths are identified through stories or narratives related to important life events, such as migration from one country to another, death of a loved one, completing a degree or important project, or coping with challenges of adjusting to a new place or role. Paying close attention to these narratives will enable facilitators to identify strengths. Also, inquire if participants cultivated certain strengths as they negotiated with life's challenges.
- Assembling family members or loved ones might be challenging. This practice can also be done during family gatherings, for example, celebrating birthdays or other milestones, or during religious or cultural festivities such as Christmas, Easter, Passover, Diwali, Eid, Chinese New Year, or Kwanzaa, when family members often spend time together.
- When working with participants from different cultural backgrounds, facilitators should be mindful of the context in which strengths are perceived and valued. In cultures which value interdependent and collectivist norms, strengths which maintain interpersonal harmony are desired and hence easily spotted, acknowledged, and appreciated. For example, an immigrant mother from a collectivist cultural background may not appreciate strengths such as courage or creativity as these are not valued by the culture in which she was raised. Instead, she may perceive courage as a weakness if it risks rupturing relationships. Conversely, her daughter, if born and raised in the Western culture, may value courage as one of her core elements of personality and obedience as her weakness.

Closing Activities

The goal of closing this module is to help participants consolidate their understanding of positive relationships and to take their new learning into everyday life.

Discuss with participants the Everyday Applications section (p. 139 in their Workbook). Invite participants to be mindful in their day-to-day lives by noticing their own and others' actions and habits related to strengths, including those that promote positive relationships. Encourage them to use relevant resources found at the end of this module and included in their Workbook starting on p. 140.

Choose a 3-minute activity from Regular Practice 1: Mindfulness and Relaxation to close the module.

Everyday Applications

- Invite people who are close to you to talk with you about their strengths. Ask them what strengths are central to who they are.
- If you want, share information with them about the 24 character strengths discussed in Module 5. Share one or more of the strengths assessments with them. Invite them to think about important events or experiences in their lives that have brought them happiness or joy, and to consider the strengths that might have played a role.
- Once you have collected all of the strengths for people who are important to you, reflect again on specific events that exemplify your own strengths.
- Consider what activities you and your loved ones can do together that will allow you all to use your strengths. Arrange to meet (in person, online, or hybrid) with others in your tree (Worksheet: My Tree of Positive Relationships) who identified their strengths, and brainstorm how you can use your strengths together. Make a point of following through on doing these activities.
- Notice how your loved ones use their strengths in the roles they occupy and the activities they do every day.
- Discuss with family members and loved ones which specific strength stands out for each family member and why they admire this strength. Also connect your loved ones with someone within the family or extended family who they admire due to a specific skill, talent, or ability.

References

Sheridan, S. M., Warnes, E. D., Cowan, R. J., Schemm, A. V., & Clarke, B. L. (2004). Family-centered positive psychology: Focusing on strengths to build student success. *Psychology in the Schools, 41*(1), 7–17. https://doi.org/10.1002/pits.10134

Waters, L. E., Loton, D., & Jach, H. K. (2019). Does strength-based parenting predict academic achievement? The mediating effects of perseverance and engagement. *Journal of Happiness Studies, 20*(4), 1121–1140. https://doi.org/10.1007/s10902-018-9983-1

Resources

Literature

Amatea, E. S., Smith-Adcock, S., & Villares, E. (2006). From family deficit to family strength: Viewing families' contributions to children's learning from a family resilience perspective. *Professional School Counseling, 9*(3), 177–189. https://doi.org/10.5330/prsc.9.3.43751461038m4m68

Christie, D., & Barnard, K. D. (2012). *Supporting resilience and positive outcomes in families, children, and adolescents.* Springer. https://doi.org/10.1007/978-0-85729-573-6_3

Evans, J., & Kelsey, A. (2016). *Strengths based marriage: Build a stronger relationship by understanding each other's gifts.* Gallup Press.

Flouri E. (2004). Psychological outcomes in mid adulthood associated with mother's child-rearing attitudes in early childhood: Evidence from the 1970 British birth cohort. *European Child & Adolescent Psychiatry, 13*(1), 35–41. https://doi.org/10.1007/s00787-004-0355-5

Gronhoj, A., & Thogersen, J. (2012). Action speaks louder than words: The effect of personal attitudes and family norms on adolescents' pro-environmental behaviour. *Journal of Economic Psychology, 33*(1), 292–302. https://doi.org/10.1016/j.joep.2011.10.001

Houltberg, B. J., Henry, C. S., Merten, M. J., & Robinson, L. (2011). Adolescents' perceptions of family connectedness, intrinsic religiosity, and depressed mood. *Journal of Child and Family Studies, 20*(1), 111–119. https://doi.org/10.1007/s10826-010-9384-5

Korkeila, K., Kivelä, S. L., Vahtera, J., Kivimaki, M., Sundell, J., Helenius, H., & Koskenvuo, M. (2004). Childhood adversities, parent-child relationships and dispositional optimism in adulthood. *Social Psychiatry and Psychiatric Epidemiology, 39*(4), 286–292.

Reckmeyer, M., & Robison, J. (2016). *Strengths based parenting: Developing your children's innate talents.* Gallup Press.

Waters, L. (2017). *The strength switch: How the new science of strength-based parenting can help your child and your teen to flourish.* Penguin Random House.

Additional Readings

Maintaining Healthy Relationships and Mental Wellbeing
https://www.nhs.uk/every-mind-matters/lifes-challenges/maintaining-healthy-relationships-and-mental-wellbeing/
This web article from the National Health Service (NHS), UK, outlines some practical steps to improve our relationships.

Building Positive Relationships with Students: What Brain Science Says
https://www.understood.org/en/school-learning/for-educators/empathy/brain-science-says-4-reasons-to-build-positive-relationships-with-students
This web article shares insights from neuroscience about what happens to students' brains when they feel safe and understood.

Why Teacher-Student Relationships Matter?
https://www.edweek.org/ew/articles/2019/03/13/why-teacher-student-relationships-matter.html
This web article shares ideas about how to build a relationship that could ignite a student's lifetime love of learning.

Websites

Strongest Families Institute
https://strongestfamilies.com/
The Strongest Families Institute is a not-for-profit corporation providing evidence-based services to children and families seeking help for mental health and other issues impacting health and well-being.

How to Stop Taking Your Partner for Granted
https://greatergood.berkeley.edu/relationships
Sara Algoe explains a practice to help you feel more appreciation for your partner.

Centre for Family Research, University of Cambridge
https://www.cfr.cam.ac.uk/
The Centre for Family Research is one of the foremost centers in the world exploring familial relationships.

Strengths Switch
https://www.leawaters.com/
Lea Water's website offers free resources for strengths-based parenting.

Relationships – Greater Good Magazine
https://greatergood.berkeley.edu/relationships
Find articles on relationships, from the Greater Good Center.

Multimedia

Love No Matter What | Andrew Solomon | TEDMED 2013
https://www.ted.com/talks/andrew_solomon_love_no_matter_what?referrer=playlist-what_does_family_mean&language=en
Writer Andrew Solomon discusses what it is like to raise a child who is different and what he learned about unconventional love and unconditional acceptance as a result.

The Sibling Bond | Jeffrey Kluger | TEDxAsheville
https://www.ted.com/talks/jeffrey_kluger_the_sibling_bond?referrer=playlist-what_does_family_mean
Jeffery Kluger discusses the life-long bonds between siblings and the effects of birth order.

Positive Parenting: Lea Waters on Strength Based Parenting:
https://youtu.be/RMhVopiQYzM
Lea Waters, a distinguished expert in positive psychology, discusses strengths-based parenting.

Let's Eat Rice Daddy
https://youtu.be/LzP8E8KSgPc
A Chinese New Year commercial depicts the unconditional love between a father and son.

Unsung Hero
https://youtu.be/uaWA2GbcnJU?si=pi7ZPBPlLOZTwLaR
This video is a poignant illustration of positive relationships kindled by kindness.

The Attachment Theory: How Childhood Affects Life
https://www.youtube.com/watch?v=WjOowWxOXCg
Attachment theory examines the emotional and physical bonds between children and their caregivers and how these early bonds play an important role in psychological development.

How Children and Adults Can Build Core Capabilities for Life
https://youtu.be/6NehuwDA45Q
This animation from the Center on the Developing Child at Harvard University explains how we develop and use core capabilities, also known as executive functions.

The Secret of Successful Relationships: Rupture and Repair
https://youtu.be/rgQvqi6aYD8
This video clip describes how two key concepts "rupture" and "repair" can help us to foster healthy, loving and trusting relationships.

The Color of Paradise
https://youtu.be/nZyrQGrWaA8?si=J4FrATTxLirk5Oak
This clip is a collage of scenes from the Persian Movie, Color of Paradise (1999), showing how a gifted blind young boy, Mohammed, experiences the world with his senses, with the exception of sight.

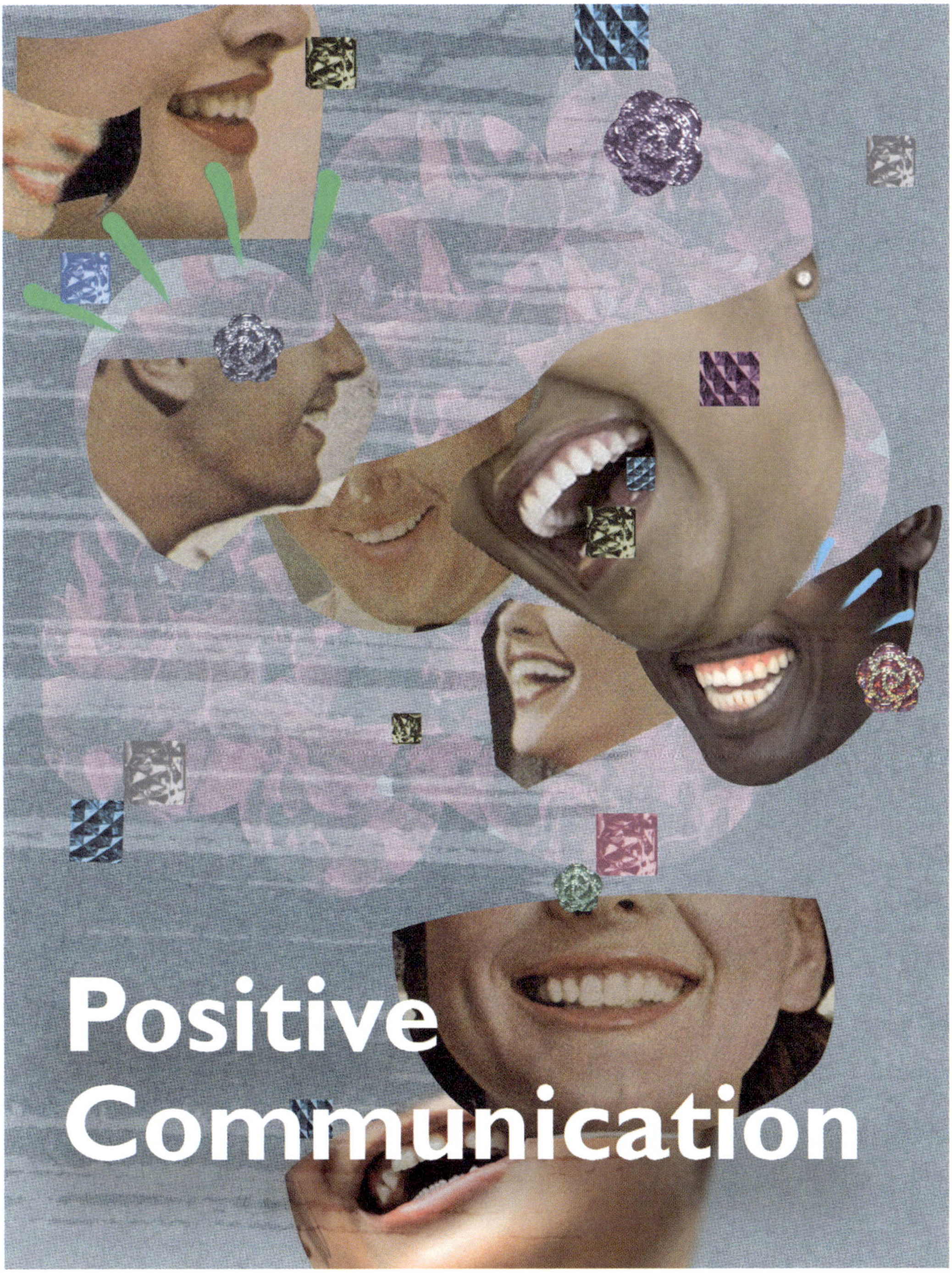
Positive
Communication

Module 12: Positive Communication

Module 12 looks closely at a common verbal communication situation – the sharing of good news – to identify four distinct communication responses, only one of which is ideal. This module examines the emotional experience of receiving feedback through not just words but also tone and body language.

Module Topic	Minutes to Allot	
Learning Outcomes Through an exercise that illustrates four different ways to respond to positive news shared by a loved one, participants: • Discover the emotional impact of communication that is active or passive, constructive or destructive • Engage in active constructive responding, which can help others to feel seen and valued, especially when sharing positive news	5	5
Opening Activities Start the module with a relaxation or mindfulness practice Invite participants to share a few events from their gratitude journal that have occurred since the last session Invite questions about the previous module and practice(s)	10	15
Illustration of Core Concepts Review core concepts and show video illustrations Facilitate reflection and discussion: • *What are the key messages in the video(s) you just watched?* • *How might these concepts be relevant in your life?*	15	15
Practice: Communicate Actively and Constructively Referring to the four styles of responding to positive news, have participants rate the style of a significant person in their life using scaled questions Debrief learning from practice(s) using questions: • *If the person's response is not active constructive, what might be going on (e.g., timing, mixed feelings, stress, or pre-occupation)?* • *How might the person be influenced by family and cultural factors?* • *How does this practice offer you insights about your own style of responding when others share positive news with you?*	20	30
Closing Activities Invite discussion of everyday applications Remind participants of relevant resources at the end of the module Guide participants in a 3-minute closing relaxation or mindfulness practice	10	10
Total	60 minutes	75 minutes

Core Concepts of Positive Communication

Many of the themes here are also presented in the Core Concepts section of the Workbook (p. 143):

- Good things happen. In fact, positive events generally outnumber negative ones in our daily lives (Gable & Haidt, 2005). When people experience positive events, one of the most common reactions is to share them with their loved ones (Pagani et al., 2019). Gable and colleagues refer to the social sharing process of positive events as "capitalization" (Gable et al., 2004). It is the process of taking advantage of, or capitalizing on, positive events, with an assumption that expressive displays (e.g., communicating about the event with others, celebrating, etc.) augment the benefits of the event, improve mood in the moment, and add to longer-term well-being (Langston, 1994). Research has identified sharing good news with a close friend as one of the most important rules of friendship (Argyle & Henderson, 1984). The capitalization process encompasses both the capitalization attempt, i.e., the act of relating the positive event to another person, and the perceived responses to these capitalization attempts, i.e., the perceived responses of the individual with whom the event is shared (Gable & Reis, 2010).
- Gable and colleagues (2004) posit that when people share positive events, responses from others can vary along two important dimensions: active-passive and constructive-destructive. On the active-passive continuum, the partner shows involvement, interest, attention (active) OR they can be disengaged, inattentive, and quiet (passive). On the constructive-deconstructive continuum, the partner can be supportive or unsupportive. Four types of responses emerge from the intersection of these two orthogonal dimensions: active-constructive (AC), passive-constructive (PC), active-destructive (AD), and passive-destructive (PD):
  - Active-constructive: Is a response in which the responder expresses excitement or enthusiasm about the event. The responder asks questions, seeks additional details about the event, elaborates on possible implications and benefits of the event for the discloser, and comments on why the event is meaningful to the person who shared. Over all, the AC response includes interest, shared happiness, and pride.
  - Passive-constructive: Is a response in which the responder expresses some positive attitude toward the event, but does not ask for details and is mostly silent about the event. Hence, the interaction is short.
  - Active-destructive: An AD response is one in which the responder is involved and attentive. However, the tone of the response is largely negative. Negative or adverse implications of the shared event are highlighted and its significance minimized. The sharer is left deflated and dejected.
  - Passive-destructive: A PD response acknowledges the event minimally, if at all. Interest in the event is not shown or minimized. More importantly the responder quickly shifts the topic, discusses something unrelated, and keeps the conversation focused on this irrelevant topic.

  An example of these four types of responses can be found in Table 12.
- Research has shown that AC responding has personal and relational benefits. The personal benefits include increased positive emotions, subjective well-being and self-esteem, and decreased loneliness. Relational outcomes linked with capitalization include increased relationship satisfaction, intimacy, commitment, trust, liking, closeness, and stability (Gable & Reis, 2010; Otto et al., 2015; Paek et al., 2022; Woods et al., 2014).

- Maintaining relationships requires effort, just like taking good care of your car or your room. In most relationships, people experience conflicts, but it makes a big difference if they put effort into learning how to manage them. Most relationships go through very difficult phases, but we can manage them peacefully if we make the effort to develop effective communication skills (Kelly, 1997).
- Positive communication and conflict management are key building blocks to any relationship. Awareness that comes from recognizing the strengths of our loved ones can significantly improve our relationships.

Table 12. Four styles of responding to positive news of partner (Adapted from Gable et al., 2004; see Table WB6 in the Workbook)

Style	Constructive	Destructive
Active	Sharer: *I got the promotion.* Responder maintains eye contact, smiles, shows positive emotions, says: *That is wonderful! I'm so happy for you. You will be excellent in that role. Let me know if there is anything I can do to support you in your transition.* Sharer feels validated and understood.	Sharer: *I got the promotion.* Responder brings conversation to an end, points out downside, displays negative emotions through grimace, tense forehead, says: *If you take this role, you will have to do additional work in the evenings, we will have less time together.* Sharer feels ashamed, embarrassed, doubtful, or angry.
Passive	Sharer: *I got the promotion.* Responder says: *That's nice.* Is subdued and lacks enthusiasm. Conversation fizzles out. Sharer feels unimportant, misunderstood, guilty, or negated.	Sharer: *I got the promotion.* Responder displays little or no eye contact, lacks interest, turns away or leaves the room after saying: *Another role, huh? Well, hurry up and get changed so that we can get lunch. I'm starving.* Sharer feels confused, disappointed, let down, or angry.

Note. Table is based on the scenario: A friend responds to her friend's good news that she was chosen for the lead role in the school play. For illustrations of the four styles, watch YouTube video on Active Constructive Responding (see details in the Illustrations of Positive Communication).

Illustrations of Positive Communication

Play at least one of the three videos below to illustrate the core concepts of positive communication and encourage discussion.

Active-Constructive Responding
https://youtu.be/qRORihbXMnA
(Duration: 5:34 minutes)
This educational video illustrates the four main responding styles of people.

How Miscommunication Happens (and how to avoid it)
https://www.youtube.com/watch?v=gCfzeONu3Mo
(Duration: 4:32 minutes)
Sharing the dangers of miscommunication, Katherine Hampsten provides useful strategies for effective communication.

Empathy: The Heart of Difficult Conversations
https://youtu.be/2UvDMQyBVLs
(Duration: 8:21 minutes)
Michelle Stowe, a trainer and consultant, discusses how instead of blaming and shaming others, we can communicate with them in authentic manner.

Reflection and Discussion

Invite participants to complete the Reflection and Discussion section of their Workbook (p. 145) regarding the video(s) they have watched. Discuss the questions:

What are the key messages in the video(s) you just watched?

How might these concepts be relevant in your life?

Practice: Communicate Actively and Constructively

Participants may be more knowledgeable about how to respond when loved ones share negative news or experiences. Typically, it would be to sympathize with them and offer support, suggestions, or advice if the situation is ongoing. When loved ones share sad news with us, we console them.

However, what do we do when our loved ones share positive news? Do we do the opposite, that is, offer them our support with enthusiasm? This exercise is about practicing how to respond when loved ones share good news with us.

The goal of this module's practice is to help participants engage in active-constructive responding (ACR) and discover how this process can strengthen relationships. Providing ACR demonstrates to the partner that they are heard and understood, both in times of stress and also in joy. Furthermore, sharing a partner's initial positive emotions creates an upward spiral of positive interpersonal interaction and has been linked to relationship satisfaction. Sharing positive events improves an individual's feelings about these events, including positive affect and meaningfulness (Algoe et al., 2010; Gable & Reis, 2010).

Ask participants to think about situations in which they share positive news or experiences with someone who is close to them and how this person generally responds (see Workbook, Practice: Communicate Actively and Constructively, p. 146).

1. *When I share my good news, most of the time the person understands, validates my joy, and asks me a few questions about the good news. I feel connected.*

   Rarely .... *Sometimes* .... *Almost Always*

2. *When I share my good news, most of time the person does not make a big deal. Although I know they are supportive, they do not show this support through words or other ways. I feel somewhat embarrassed, disappointed, and guilty.*

   Rarely .... *Sometimes* .... *Almost Always*

3. *When I share my good news, the person's first response is typically to spot the negative aspects of it. I feel angry and upset.*

   Rarely .... *Sometimes* .... *Almost Always*

4. *When I share my good news, the person changes the conversation to other unimportant things. I feel dismissed and ignored.*

   Rarely .... *Sometimes* .... *Almost Always*

Instruct participants to rate the frequency of this person's use of four response styles: (1) active-constructive, (2) passive-constructive, (3) active-destructive, (4) passive-destructive.

Practice Debrief

After the activity, ask the participants to refer to Table WB6. Four styles of responding to positive news of partner (see Table 12 here) to complete this Practice Debrief section in their Workbook (p. 146) and to address the following reflection questions:

- *If the person's response is not active and constructive, consider what might be going on. For example, is your timing off, for example, are they preoccupied with another task? Is the person experiencing stress unrelated to your good news or mixed feelings about your good news?*
- *How might this person's response be influenced by family or cultural factors? For example, some families and cultures are less verbal, explicit, and expressive than others.*
- *How does this practice offer you insights about your style of responding when others share positive news with you?*
- *How can you respond more actively and constructively to others?*

Optional Practice: Active-Constructive Responding (ACR)

This activity is not in the Workbook and is provided as an optional activity if time allows. We recommend you do this activity after the opening activities but before reviewing the core concepts, as it is a powerful experiential illustration of ACR. Participants can engage in this activity without knowing the core concepts, which will become much clearer after they have done the activity.

People experience more positive events than negative ones. We often put energy and thought into how to respond when our loved ones share negative, sad, or distressing events with us. However, we may not think as deeply about our response when our loved ones share positive events. This practice will engage participants in a paired role-play activity, enabling them to experience four different types of responses that may occur when someone shares a positive event.

This activity has been adapted from Gable (2013). Below are directions for the ACR practice.

In this role-play activity, anticipate grouping participants into pairs. One member of the pair is a Sharer. The other is a Responder. There is only one Sharer role – i.e., someone who will share a positive experience. There are four Responder roles:

- Active-Constructive Responder (ACR)
- Passive-Constructive Responder (PCR)
- Active-Destructive Responder (ADR)
- Passive-Destructive Responder (PDR)

Prior to your session, print out a sufficient quantity of handouts – one role per handout described on the following page. To illustrate, for a group of 24 participants, you will need 12 sharer role handouts, and 12 responder role handouts (3 copies respectively of ACR, PCR, ADR and PDR roles).

> CAUTION: The Active Destructive Response (ADR) role can be stressful for both sharer and the responder. Facilitators should judge whether group cohesion and support are strong enough to have participants engage in this particular role. If not, use only the three other response roles and calculate your numbers accordingly, i.e., 3 sharers, 3 responders.

- During the session, distribute a single role to each participant. Instruct participants to place them blank side up so they can only read them once you provide additional instructions. When you've handed out all the roles, have participants read their roles quietly. Instruct them to NOT show or reveal their assigned role to their neighbors.
- Ask participants to make pairs, ensuring that each pair has a sharer and a responder. If there are odd numbers, have the remaining participant join a pair as a responder, but ensure that the responder role differs from the other participant.
- Once everyone is ready, ask them to complete the activity with their partner without showing their role to their partner. Instruct the sharers to begin and responders to engage according to their role. All pairs work on the activity at the same time.
- Allow 3 to 5 minutes for the role-play activity.
- After the time expires, ask participants to stop and stay in their pairs.
- Facilitate debriefing by asking how sharers and responders felt during the practice.
- Discuss the four styles with the help of Table 12, p. 255 (also in their Workbook on p. 144, Table WB6.)

Roles

Sharer Role

Your role in this practice is to share a positive event with the person you will be paired with. Please recall a recent positive event you feel comfortable sharing. Select an event that made you very happy. Share the details of the event with your partner. For example, when and where did the event happen? And what made you excited about it? Your partner will ask you some questions about the event. They may or may not choose to ask follow-up questions.

During this interaction, try to remember how you felt while you described the event and how you felt about the interaction with your partner.

Active-Constructive Responding (ACR) Role

In this activity, you will be paired with a partner who plays the role of sharer. Your partner will share a recent positive event they experienced. Your task is to offer an active-constructive response (ACR). AC responders convey interest and enthusiasm regarding the event and positive regard towards the person. ACRs often include questions about the event, elaboration of its positive aspects, and comments on its positive implications for the sharer of the event. The AC responder is often enthusiastic, excited, or happy. To convey this during the practice, make good eye contact, show positive emotion, and make enthusiastic comments such as "that sounds great" and "you must be/have been so excited." Ask open-ended questions, showing genuine curiosity about the event. Ask what they did to help make the event happen, which aspects they feel most excited about, and how this event contributes to their overall well-being. Point out potential benefits of the event. Try your best to convey your genuine interest and avoid coming across as scripted or superficial.

During this interaction, try to remember how you felt while you responded to the event and how you felt about the interaction with your partner.

Passive-Constructive Responding (PCR) Role

In this practice, you will be paired with a partner who plays the role of sharer. Your partner will share a recent positive event they experienced. Your task is to offer a passive-constructive response (PCR). PC responders may appear positive or supportive on the surface, but the responses are reserved and subtle. These responses are often quiet exchanges that involve few, if any, questions about the positive event shared. Do not elaborate or discuss the implications of the positive event. To convey PCR during this practice, smile and make occasional eye contact as your partner shares their positive experience. Avoid asking questions about the event or inviting your partner to elaborate on their statements. When the sharer is finished speaking, ask them if they are done, smile at them, and say, "that sounds good." In short, try to be a pleasant but uninvolved responder when your partner shares a positive event with you.

During this interaction, remember how you felt while you responded to the event and how you felt about the interaction with your partner.

Active-Destructive Responding (ADR) Role

In this practice, you will be paired with a partner who plays the role of sharer. Your partner will share a recent positive event they experienced. Your task is to offer an active-destructive response (ADR). ADR responders are quite engaged but treat the positive event shared as having minimal or no importance. Your task is to list potential downsides and limitations of the event. Please be actively involved but focus on picking up all possible deficits or risks of the positive experience. To convey this during the one-to-one interaction with the sharer, list all possible negative consequences of this experience. Try to be active. To demonstrate that you are carefully listening, carefully ask questions. However, with each question, list potential risks or problems this positive event may pose for the sharer.

During this interaction, remember how you felt while you responded to the event and how you felt about the interaction with your partner.

Passive-Destructive Responding (PDR) Role

In this practice, you will be paired with a partner who plays the role of sharer. Your partner will share a recent positive event they experienced. Your task is to offer a passive-destructive response (PDR). PD responders show no interest in the positive event. Once your partner has shared the event, change the topic quickly and start discussing an irrelevant topic. When your partner is finished, do not ask questions about the positive event that was shared. The goal is to give the impression that you are not very interested in the positive event your partner shared. You can continue the conversation and talk about something different or start discussing mundane issues such as the weather, traffic, breakfast, or dinner. Avoid acknowledging the shared event, and do not validate any associated emotions. Your job is to be a detached and uninterested responder.

During this interaction, remember how you felt while you responded to the event and how you felt about the interaction with your partner.

Optional Practice Debrief

Discuss with participants their reactions and reflections on this role-play activity using the following questions:

- *What was your experience of sharing or responding to this activity?*
- *What was most comfortable and uncomfortable about this practice?*
- *Did you see yourself or others in any of the response styles?*

Learning and Cultural Fit

Adapt this practice to the learning and cultural needs of your participants, including their unique values and demographics. Possible adaptations include:

- ACR can be an effective and powerful skill for strengthening relationships. However, it is important to be mindful of cross-cultural differences in communicating and responding to events and associated emotions. Be mindful that there are cross-cultural differences in the expression of emotions and the degree to which positive events are attributed to individual accomplishments or to family, group, or context. Communication also varies according to the social standing of both the sharer and receiver (Hurn & Toalin, 2013).
- Some participants may find the ACR practice ostentatious, as being self-effacing and showing modesty are culturally desirable. For example, Australians are relatively more self-effacing than Americans. Likewise, some participants prefer not to talk about events and associated emotions directly, openly, and publicly. Facilitators need to consider cultural humility (Yeager & Bauer-Wu, 2013) – that is, the ongoing process of reflecting on and discovering what they know about a culture and what they don't, while remaining receptive to learning from others. Build an honest and trustworthy relationship with participants by asking about a culturally appropriate way of expressing and responding to positive emotions.
- Participants' personalities may also affect their preferences for sharing or responding to positive events. Participants with a more introverted or reserved personality may state that the ACR practice is not for them. Underscore that this practice is more about communicating authentically than the vociferous verbal display of positive emotions. Listening carefully to the details of the positive event, asking few but relevant questions authentically, and showing genuine interest in connecting with the sharer, are more important actions. Introverts can do better as responders as they can listen carefully to details without interrupting sharers.
- Remind participants that sharing and responding to positive experiences does not come easy to everyone, especially in light of the diversity of learning needs. For example, participants with limited communication skills may struggle to share and respond to positive experiences. Likewise, those with nonverbal learning challenges may have difficulty discerning nuanced responses and interpreting body language. Offer participants multiple ways of expressing and responding to positive events, e.g., verbal, written, through art or technology.
- Secrecy generally is not good for our well-being (Critcher & Ferguson, 2014). Most people, upon learning positive news, tend to share it with others. However, there are important variations in how and when we disclose positive events. Recent research indicates that keeping good news a secret before sharing it could make people feel more energized and alive. Slepian and colleagues (Slepian et al., 2023) conducted several studies examining people's experiences reflecting on positive events that they either shared or kept secret for some time. They found that some positive events in life begin as secrets, including marriage proposals, pregnancies, milestone surprise birthday parties, and surprise gifts. The authors posit that negative news often is not shared because of potential shame, embarrassment, or perceived failure. All of these are linked to external perception or reputation. On the other hand, when we choose not to share positive news, it is mostly due to internal or personal desires. For example, a person may want to share positive news only when they feel ready to share, such as in the case of a pregnancy or marriage proposal. People sometimes go to great lengths to orchestrate the revealing of a positive event to enhance excitement and enjoyment.

Closing Activities

The goal of closing this module is to help participants consolidate their understanding of positive communication and to take their new learning into everyday life.

Discuss with participants the Everyday Applications section (p. 148 in their Workbook). Invite participants to be mindful in their day-to-day lives by noticing their own and others' actions and habits related to positive communication. Encourage them to use relevant resources found at the end of this module and included in their Workbook starting on p. 148.

Choose a 3-minute activity from Regular Practice 1: Mindfulness and Relaxation to close the module.

Everyday Applications

- Positive communication, a hallmark of positive relationships, is not about volume – that is, you do not have to be loud, expressive, verbal, and extroverted. It is about being sincere, authentic, and willing to be with others, especially when they share good news. One can do so, by listening actively, asking a few focused questions, and validating emotions – attributes not dependent on an extroverted personality. In fact, an introvert is likely to listen and understand more and ask thoughtful questions.
- Building positive relationships, from the perspective of positive communication, does not require an active and constructive response to all minor good events shared in everyday life. Nor do all positive events shared need flamboyant celebration. Know your loved ones well and offer positive and active responses for triumphs and accomplishments which are meaningful to them.
- Active-constructive responding can help us to become better listeners and attend to the person's experience. By refraining from criticizing or interrupting, we learn how to modulate our own emotions, but we also encourage others to express themselves without fear of judgment. By asking the person questions to elaborate on their experience, we build their confidence and improve communication outcomes.
- Communicating with your loved ones is key, especially during challenging times. For example, when you are facing a dilemma, knowing who within your circle of relationships can offer wise counsel can help you resolve the situation. Consult them for their advice. They will appreciate that you reached out and value their opinion. Likewise, when you feel down, communicating with someone who can voice hope and optimism can be an effective antidote.

References

Algoe, S. B., Gable, S. L., & Maisel, N. C. (2010). It's the little things: Everyday gratitude as a booster shot for romantic relationships. *Personal Relationships, 17*(2), 217–233. https://doi.org/10.1111/j.1475-6811.2010.01273.x

Argyle, M., & Henderson, M. (1984). The rules of friendship. *Journal of Social and Personal Relationships, 1*(2), 211–237. https://doi.org/10.1177/0265407584012005

Critcher, C. R., & Ferguson, M. J. (2014). The cost of keeping it hidden: Decomposing concealment reveals what makes it depleting. *Journal of Experimental Psychology: General, 143*(2), 721–735. https://doi.org/10.1037/a0033468

Gable, S. L. (2013). Capitalizing on positive events. In J. Froh & A. C. Parks (Eds.), *Activities for teaching positive psychology: A guide for instructors* (pp. 71–75). American Psychological Association.

Gable, S. L., & Haidt, J. (2005). What (and why) is positive psychology? *Review of General Psychology, 9*(2), 103–110. https://doi.org/10.1037/1089-2680.9.2.103
Gable, S. L., & Reis, H. T. (2010). Good news! Capitalizing on positive events in an interpersonal context. In M.P. Zanna (Ed.), *Advances in experimental social psychology* (Vol. 42, pp. 195–257). Elsevier Academic Press. https://doi.org/10.1016/S0065-2601(10)42004-3
Gable, S. L., Reis, H. T., Impett, E. A., & Asher, E. R. (2004). What do you do when things go right? The intrapersonal and interpersonal benefits of sharing positive events. *Journal of Personality and Social Psychology, 87*(2), 228–245. https://doi.org/10.1037/0022-3514.87.2.228
Hurn, B. J., & Toalin, B. (2013). *Cross-cultural communication: Theory and practice*. Palgrave McMillan. https://doi.org/10.1057/9780230391147
Kelly, J. R. (1997). Changing issues in leisure-family research – again. *Journal of Leisure Research, 29*(1), 132–134. https://doi.org/10.1080/00222216.1997.11949787
Langston, C. A. (1994). Capitalizing on and coping with daily-life events: Expressive responses to positive events. *Journal of Personality and Social Psychology, 67*(6), 1112–1125. https://doi.org/10.1037/0022-3514.67.6.1112
Otto, A. K., Laurenceau, J. P., Siegel, S. D., & Belcher, A. J. (2015). Capitalizing on everyday positive events uniquely predicts daily intimacy and well-being in couples coping with breast cancer. *Journal of Family Psychology, 29*(1), 69–79. https://doi.org/10.1037/fam0000042
Paek, J. J. W., Zee, K. S., Fitzsimons, G. M., & Higgins, E. T. (2022). Congratulations, so happy for you! Promotion motivation predicts social support for positive events. *Motivation Science, 8*(4), 285–297. https://doi.org/10.1037/mot0000272
Pagani, A. F., Parise, M., Donato, S., Gable, S. L., & Schoebi, D. (2019). If you shared my happiness, you are part of me: Capitalization and the experience of couple identity. *Personality and Social Psychology Bulletin, 46*(2), 258–269. https://doi.org/10.1177/0146167219854449
Slepian, M. L., Greenaway, K. H., Camp, N. P., & Galinsky, A. D. (2023). The bright side of secrecy: The energizing effect of positive secrets. *Journal of Personality and Social Psychology, 125*(5), 1018–1035. https://doi.org/10.1037/pspa0000352
Woods, S., Lambert, N., Brown, P., Fincham, F., & May, R. (2014). 'I'm so excited for you!' How an enthusiastic responding intervention enhances close relationships. *Journal of Social and Personal Relationships, 32*(12), 24–40. https://doi.org/10.1177/0265407514523545
Yeager, K. A., & Bauer-Wu, S. (2013). Cultural humility: Essential foundation for clinical researchers. *Applied Nursing Research, 26*(4), 251–256. https://doi.org/10.1016/j.apnr.2013.06.008

Resources

Literature

Cooperidder, D. D., Jen Hetzel, S., & Jo Mann, A. (2008). *Positive family dynamics: Appreciative inquiry questions to bring out the best in families*. Taos Institute Publication.
Gable, S. L., & Reis, H. T. (2010). Good news! Capitalizing on positive events in an interpersonal context. In M. P. Zanna (Ed.), *Advances in experimental social psychology* (Vol. 42, pp. 195–257). Elsevier Academic Press. https://doi.org/10.1016/S0065-2601(10)42004-3
Gable, S. L., Reis, H. T., Impett, E. A., & Asher, E. R. (2004). What do you do when things go right? The intrapersonal and interpersonal benefits of sharing positive events. *Journal of Personality and Social Psychology, 87*, 228–245. https://doi.org/10.1037/0022-3514.87.2.228
Hughes, A. M., & Read, V. (2012). *Building positive relationships with parents of young children: A guide to effective communication*. Routledge.
Maisel, N. C., & Gable, S. L. (2009). The paradox of received support: The importance of responsiveness. *Psychological Science, 20*, 928–932. https://doi.org/10.1111/j.1467-9280.2009.02388.x
Pawelski, S. P., & Pawelski, J. (2018). *Happy together: Using the science of positive psychology to build love that lasts*. Penguin Random House.

Socha, T. J., & Yingling, J. (2010). *Families communicating with children: Building positive developmental foundations*. Polity.

Tuhovsky, I. (2018). *The science of effective communication: Improve your social skills and small talk, develop charisma and learn how to talk to anyone* (Positive Psychology Coaching Series: Vol. 15) (R. Streu, Narr.) [Audiobook].

Websites

The Seven Elements of Positive Communication – 20-Minute Guide
https://the20minuteguide.com/parents/helping-with-words/positive-communication/
This web resource offers 7 elements of positive communication, including being brief, specific, positive, authentic, understanding, and collaborative.

Effective Communication
https://www.helpguide.org/articles/relationships-communication/effective-communication.htm
Access tips that can help you avoid misunderstandings and improve your work and personal relationships.

The Power of Positive Communication
https://www.londonschool.com/nordic/blogg/power-positive-communication/
A language-learning school illustrates simple techniques to express oneself in a positive manner.

Benefits of Active Constructive Responding
https://vennleader.com/index.php/2017/01/22/benefits-of-active-constructive-responding/
This article describes the four response styles, factors that lead to ACR and non-ACR response, and tips for ACR.

Multimedia

A Study on Praise and Mindsets
https://www.youtube.com/watch?v=NWv1VdDeoRY
Carol Dweck describes a study on the effects of praising children involving a series of experiments on over 400 5th-grade students.

Instant Family (2018) – You Were What Was Missing
https://youtu.be/HceqAAw60vQ
A teenager learns about the value she has brought to the parents who adopted her.

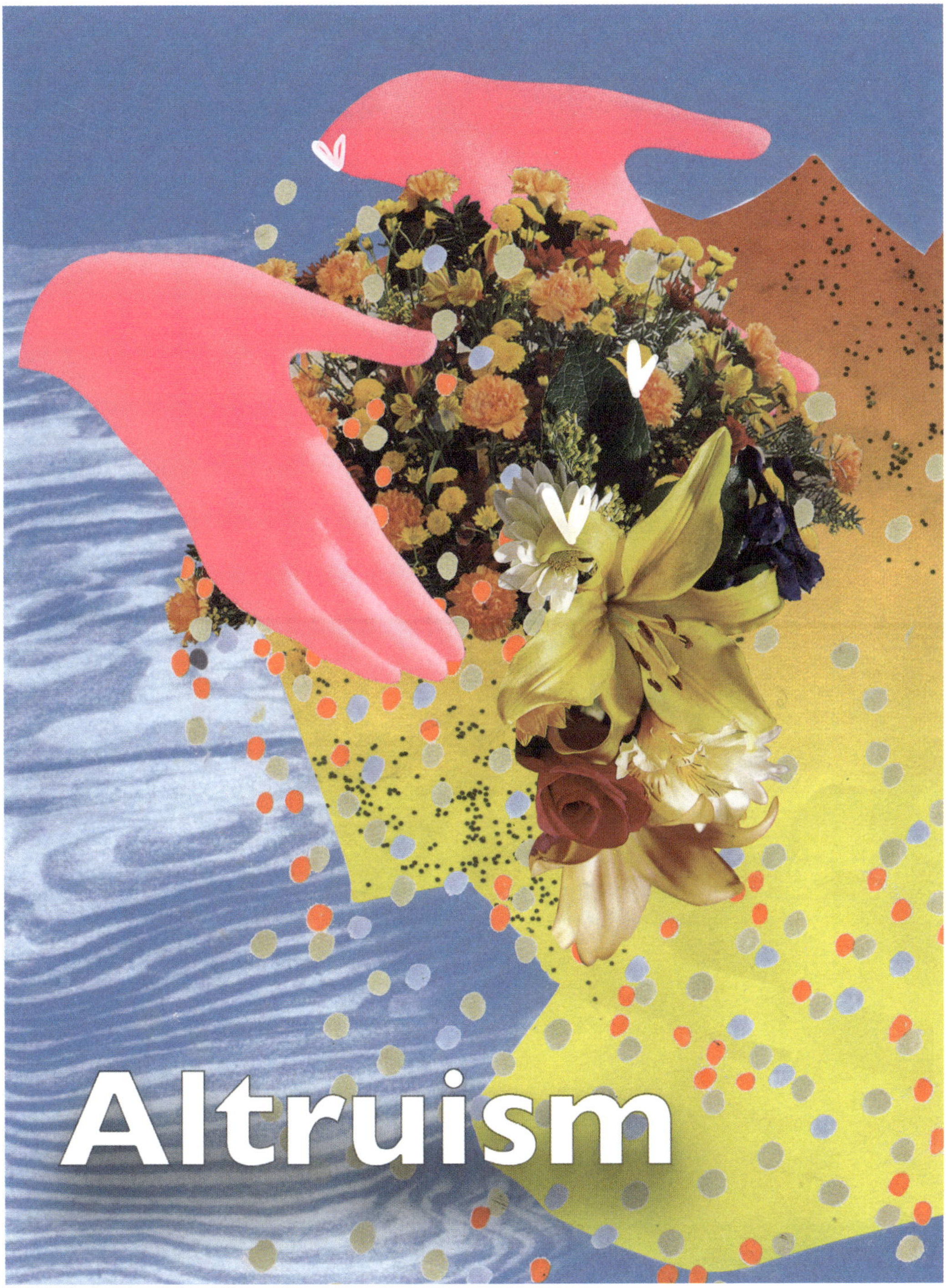
Altruism

Module 13: Altruism

This module on Altruism begins the shift toward engaging participants in reflections on life purpose and meaning. It encourages thinking beyond one's own individual well-being needs and those of immediate loved ones, toward considering the broader needs of the community and the importance of philanthropic endeavors.

Module Topic	Minutes to Allot	
Learning Outcomes By planning to give the gift of time while doing something helpful that also uses their strengths, participants: • Build a sense of connection • Experience positive emotions • Understand that altruism demands effort by the helper with no obvious benefit in return	5	5
Opening Activities Start the module with a relaxation or mindfulness practice Invite participants to share a few events from their gratitude journal that have occurred since the last session Invite questions about the previous module and practice(s)	10	15
Illustration of Core Concepts Review core concepts and show video illustrations Facilitate reflection and discussion: • *What are the key messages in the video(s) you just watched?* • *How might these concepts be relevant in your life?*	15	15
Practice: Give the Gift of Time Instruct participants to plan and carry out a "Gift of Time" using one of their signature strengths in the service of someone they care about After participants have completed the practice, have them write about their experience and schedule a later time to debrief learning using questions: • *In what ways has this experience encouraged you to extend similar gifts of time:* • *To other friends and family members?* • *To organizations involved in meaningful causes in your community?*	20	30
Closing Activities Invite discussion of everyday applications Remind participants of relevant resources at the end of the module Guide participants in a 3-minute closing relaxation or mindfulness practice	10	10
Total	60 minutes	75 minutes

Core Concepts of Altruism

Many of the themes here are also presented in the Core Concepts section of the Workbook (p. 151):

- Altruism refers to behaviors that people engage in to benefit another person or to alleviate another person's distress, without expecting any reward or benefit in return. Engaging in altruistic behavior includes a genuine desire to improve the well-being of others. There are many forms of altruism, including volunteering, giving money, donating blood, and any number of behaviors which benefit others (Pfattheicher et al., 2022). Research indicates that higher levels of altruism and prosocial behavior are associated with lower levels of depression and anxiety (Eli et al., 2021; Fujiwara, 2007). Altruism is closely related to the well-being of people of different genders and from different ethnocultural backgrounds (Giovanis & Ozdamar, 2022).
- One of the most important findings from the science of positive psychology and happiness is that altruism increases happiness (Aknin et al., 2013). Spending money on others makes us happier than spending it on ourselves. Some may think this is only true for affluent North Americans. However, the latest research shows that this finding holds up around the world, even in countries where sharing with others might threaten one's own livelihood. Findings from more than 200,000 people in 136 countries suggest that cross-culturally, people report greater happiness recalling a time when they spent money on others than when they spent their money on themselves (Aknin et al., 2015).
- An 18-year longitudinal study of nearly 70,000 participants in the United Kingdom found that people who volunteered in the past year were more satisfied with their lives and rated their health as better (Lawton et al., 2021). Other research indicates that individuals who spend more hours volunteering have higher levels of resilience and gratitude (Llenares et al., 2020).
- Practicing altruism is one way to find and pursue meaning in life (Smith, 2018). Social activism, social service, and international relief initiatives, as well as careers experienced as callings (missions) and interpersonal spiritual pursuits, are also forms of altruism. Sometimes, one altruistic act can encourage us to pursue further similar acts. For example, if you help a student who is bullied, this may motivate you to start an antibullying campaign. Similarly, if you received support during a crisis or challenging situation, you may want to support the cause by investing some of your time and resources.
- Altruistic acts are gifts that can be enjoyed and do not have to be a burden. Altruistic individuals do not sacrifice at every given moment. People are best able to help those around them when they have developed themselves and their abilities. Although it is important to act selflessly at times, we need to be sure to also take care of ourselves.
- Altruism is associated with character strengths such as love, social intelligence, kindness, gratitude, optimism, and zest. Likewise, using our character strengths can help us to become more altruistic.

Illustrations of Altruism

Play at least one of the three videos below to illustrate the core concepts of altruism and encourage discussion.

Pay it Forward
https://youtu.be/qfW0wCV9iFI
(Duration: 2:20 minutes)
A teacher challenges his students to think of an idea that could change our world, then put it into action.

Gift – Do Your Parents Embarrass You?
https://youtu.be/1DUYlHZsZfc?list=PL8m
(Duration: 7:30 minutes)
This short film depicts a son who discovers a big secret about his father, one that changes his understanding of him.

Life Vest Inside – Kindness Boomerang – "One Day"
https://www.youtube.com/watch?v=nwAYpLVyeFU
(Duration: 5:44 minutes)
Watch as a videographer tracks how an act of kindness passes around from person to person, spreading joy at every turn.

The Science of Kindness
https://www.youtube.com/watch?v=FA1qgXovaxU
(Duration: 2:00 minutes)
This animation summarizes scientific evidence on the benefits of kindness.

Reflection and Discussion

Invite participants to complete the Reflection and Discussion section of their Workbook (p. 152) regarding the video(s) they have watched. Discuss the questions:

What are the key messages in the video(s) you just watched?

How might these concepts be relevant in your life?

Practice: Give the Gift of Time

The aim of this practice is to help participants understand how they can use their signature strengths to help others. Through engaging in purposeful, helpful actions that make use of their strengths, participants can enhance relationships and meaning in their lives. When a person uses their signature strengths to help or serve others, they are more likely to be intrinsically motivated to engage in and sustain altruistic behaviors. They may also find that they are best able to help others through activities that call on their strengths.

This practice builds on Module 9: Empathy. It provides participants with another opportunity to feel empathic towards someone struggling or needing something. Participants can translate this empathy into a concrete plan of action for helping.

This is a homework practice. Its goal is to make participants aware of the fact that regardless of their financial circumstances, they have the power to give one of the greatest gifts of all, the gift of time. Suggested steps to implement this practice include:

- Refer participants to p. 153 of the Workbook Practice: Give the Gift of Time.
- Read aloud and discuss the preamble to the practice (see text in italics below).
- Give participants time to brainstorm possible people who could use their gifts of time and which of their strengths they can offer as a gift.
- Invite participants to share their ideas and clarify any questions or concerns.
- Ask that participants complete the Give the Gift of Time practice prior to the next session. Instruct them to complete the Worksheet reflection questions on p. 153 after they have given the gift of time to someone. Ask participants to write about their experience and to record what they did and how long it took.
- At the beginning of the next Module, invite participants to share their reflections and respond to the Practice Debrief questions below.

The purpose of this homework exercise is to make you aware of the fact that regardless of your financial circumstances, you have the power to give one of the greatest gifts of all, the gift of time.

This exercise contrasts with pursuits that provide immediate gratification. You may perceive that the time you spend giving this gift might be boring, tedious, or even exhausting. However, many people find that the sustained gratification that comes with giving the gift of time is more rewarding than time spent pursuing the pleasurable life – for example, eating chocolate, watching a good movie, or getting a massage.

Your goal is to give someone you care about the gift of time by doing something for them that requires a fair amount of time and involves using one of your signature strengths to deliver the gift, which will make the exercise more gratifying for you. For example, someone who is creative might draw, design, or sketch for a best friend who could benefit from therapeutic art. Someone who is playful and humorous might cheer a friend who is feeling sad. Someone who is kind and can cook might prepare a four-course dinner for their sick roommate.

Write in your Workbook about your experience of giving the gift of time. Be sure to record exactly what you did and how long it took.

- *How did you decide to give this specific gift of time? Did anything about the recipient or their situation help you choose?*
- *In what ways does your gift of time (and effort) differ from a material gift?*
- *Beyond feeling good about yourself, in what ways can this practice and the process be beneficial for you, especially from the perspective of your interpersonal growth?*

Practice Debrief

Facilitators can encourage participants to discuss the following questions upon completion of homework:

How does giving the gift of time help you understand and appreciate the needs of others?

In what ways has this experience encouraged you to extend similar gifts of time to:

- *Other friends and family members?*
- *Organizations involved in causes in your community that are meaningful to you?*

After completing this exercise, encourage participants to consider offering additional gifts of time to those who would truly benefit from their efforts. Opportunities might include mentorship, providing pro bono services such as tutoring, offering rides, or performing specific tasks suited to your skills.

Learning and Cultural Fit

Adapt this practice to the learning and cultural needs of your participants, including their unique values and demographics. Possible adaptations include:

- Some participants who may have learning or mental health challenges (e.g., executive deficits, including difficulties starting and completing tasks, using equipment and resources efficiently and safely) may not be able to complete the task in this module as outlined. Some other participants may have logistical constraints (such as long work hours or dealing with a major life transition) that make it difficult to complete an altruistic endeavor. Offer them flexibility and multiple avenues commensurate with their circumstances to complete the task. Emphasize that altruism does not always have to involve a large amount of time or planning. Smaller, everyday acts of altruism can be meaningful as well.
- Some participants who are socially anxious or shy by disposition may have difficulty approaching other people, as fear of social judgment may get in the way. These participants can begin with tiny steps, such as opening a door for someone or simply asking a classmate how they are doing and helping them with a small problem.
- It is crucial to approach the concerns of other people wisely. We must never forget that what we believe to be a problem may not be a problem for others. Encourage participants to maintain an open and empathic perspective, allowing themselves to be guided by the other person's needs.
- Hands-on altruistic endeavors could offer diverse ways of helping the environment and others. Some illustrations include planting new trees or caring for existing ones, litter removal, mentoring youth, volunteering at a homeless shelter or food bank, and conversing with a lonely senior living in a nursing home.

Closing Activities

The goal of closing this module is to help participants consolidate their understanding of altruism and to take their new learning into everyday life.

Discuss with participants the Everyday Applications section (p. 155 in their Workbook). Invite participants to be mindful in their day-to-day lives by noticing their own and others' altruistic actions and habits. Encourage them to use relevant resources found at the end of this module and included in their Workbook starting on p. 155.

Choose a 3-minute activity from Regular Practice 1: Mindfulness and Relaxation to close the module.

Everyday Applications

- Imagine a world where young people are knowledgeable and equipped with skills for lifelong engagement in philanthropy as givers of time, talent, and treasure for the common good. In order to be altruistic, you do not have to give big things. Look for simple opportunities in everyday life to be generous with your time by helping someone out or supporting a communal cause.
- Learn more about important altruists such as Martin Luther King, Jr., Gandhi, Princess Diana, Greta Thunberg, Malala Yusufzai, Amanda Gorman, and Dan Levy. What prompted them to give to their causes? How did their actions change the world?
- When you watch TV, read the news, or listen to the radio, notice any issues that bother you or create concern for others. Notice stories about people who are working to improve the lives of others. For those issues that inspire you or motivate you to do something, find out more about organizations working actively to make things better. Then consider donating time, money, or skills.

References

Aknin, L. B., Barrington-Leigh, C. P., Dunn, E. W., Helliwell, J. F., Burns, J., Biswas-Diener, R., Kemeza, I., Nyende, P., Ashton-James, C., & Norton, M. I. (2013). Prosocial spending and well-being: Cross-cultural evidence for a psychological universal. *Journal of Personality and Social Psychology, 104*(4), 635–652. https://doi.org/10.1037/a0031578

Aknin, L. B., Broesch, T., Hamlin, J. K., & Van de Vondervoort, J. W. (2015). Prosocial behavior leads to happiness in a small-scale rural society. *Journal of Experimental Psychology: General, 144*(4), 788–795. https://doi.org/10.1037/xge0000082

Eli, B., Zhou, Y., Liang, Y., Cheng, J., Wang, J., Huang, C., Xuan, X., & Liu, Z. (2021). Depression in children and adolescents on the Qinghai-Tibet plateau: Associations with resilience and prosocial behavior. *International Journal of Environmental Research and Public Health, 18*(2), Article 440. https://doi.org/10.3390/ijerph18020440

Fujiwara, T. (2007). The role of altruistic behavior in generalized anxiety disorder and major depression among adults in the United States. *Journal of Affective Disorders, 101*(1), 219–225. ttps://doi.org/https://doi.org/10.1016/j.jad.2006.11.024

Giovanis, E., & Ozdamar, O. (2022). Who is left behind? Altruism of giving, happiness and mental health during the Covid-19 period in the UK. *Applied Research in Quality of Life, 17*(1), 251–276. https://doi.org/10.1007/s11482-020-09900-8.

Lawton, R. N., Gramatki, I., Watt, W., & Fujiwara, D. (2021). Does volunteering make us happier, or are happier people more likely to volunteer? Addressing the problem of reverse causality when estimating the wellbeing impacts of volunteering. *Journal of Happiness Studies, 22*(2), 599–624. https://doi.org/10.1007/s10902-020-00242-8

Llenares, I. I., Sario, J. A., Bialba, D., & Dela Cruz, J. M. (2020). Volunteerism influences on student resilience and gratitude. *Journal of Psychology in Africa, 30*(3), 211–216. https://doi.org/10.1080/14330237.2020.1777031

Pfattheicher, S., Nielsen, Y. A., & Thielmann, I. (2022). Prosocial behavior and altruism: A review of concepts and definitions. *Current Opinion in Psychology, 44*, 124–129. https://doi.org/10.1016/j.copsyc.2021.08.021

Smith, H. C. (2018). Finding purpose through altruism: The potential of 'doing for others' during asylum. *Journal of Occupational Science, 25*(1), 87–99. https://doi.org/10.1080/14427591.2017.1371633

Resources

Literature

Aknin, L. B., Barrington-Leigh, C. P., Dunn, E.W., Helliwell, J. F., Burns, J., Biswas-Diener, R., Kemeza, I., Nyende, P., Ashton-James, C., & Norton, M. I. (2013). Prosocial spending and well-being: Cross-cultural evidence for a psychological universal. *Journal of Personality and Social Psychology, 104*(4), 635–652. https://doi.org/10.1037/a0031578

Barr, J. J., & Higgins-D'Alessandro, A. (2009). How adolescent empathy and prosocial behavior change in the context of school culture: A two-year longitudinal study. *Adolescence, 44*(176), 751.

Cemalcilar, Z. (2009). Understanding individual characteristics of adolescents who volunteer. *Personality and Individual Differences, 46*(4), 432–436. https://doi.org/10.1016/j.paid.2008.11.009

Keltner, D. (2009). *Born to be good: The science of a meaningful life*. W.W. Norton.

Landis, S. K., Sherman, M. F., Piedmont, R. L., Kirkhart, M. W., Rapp, E. M., & Bike, D. H. (2009). The relation between elevation and self-reported prosocial behavior: Incremental validity over the five-factor model of personality. *Journal of Positive Psychology, 4*(1), 71–84. https://doi.org/10.1080/17439760802399208

Ludden, A. B. (2011). Engagement in school and community civic activities among rural adolescents. *Journal of Youth and Adolescence, 40*(9), 1254–70. https://doi.org/10.1007/s10964-010-9536-3

Otake, K., Shimai, S., Tanaka-Matsumi, J., Otsui, K., & Fredrickson, B. (2006). Happy people become happier through kindness: A counting kindness intervention. *Journal of Happiness Studies, 7*(3), 361–375. https://doi.org/10.1007/s10902-005-3650-z

Post, S., & Neimark, J. (2008). *Why good things happen to good people: How to live a longer, healthier, happier life by the simple act of giving.* Broadway Books.

Ricard, M. (2016). *Altruism: The power of compassion to change yourself and the world.* Hachette Books.

Singer, P. (2016). *The most good you can do: How effective altruism is changing ideas about living ethically.* Yale University Press.

Websites

Better Together
http://robertdputnam.com/better-together/
Better Together was an initiative of the author Robert Putnam. The website offers a variety of ways to participate in and strengthen community life.

Spread Kindness
https://www.spreadkindness.org/
SpreadKindness.org is a nonprofit organization dedicated to encouraging and empowering people to practice kindness in their everyday lives.

Think Kindness
https://thinkkindness.org/
The nonprofit organization Think Kindness attempts to promote kindness in schools and communities across the US.

Effective Altruism
https://www.effectivealtruism.org/
The website offers ideas on how we can use our strengths and resources to help others in a way that will have the greatest impact on the world's problems. It encourages being generous with your time and your money to do the most good you can.

Centre for Effective Altruism
https://www.centreforeffectivealtruism.org/
The Centre for Effective Altruism helps to grow and support the effective altruism community.

Random Acts of Kindness Foundation
https://www.randomactsofkindness.org/the-science-of-kindness
This website and blog share the science behind acts of kindness. They provide educational resources to encourage people to undertake random acts of kindness in their everyday lives.

80,000 Hours
https://80000hours.org/
This organization researches the world's most pressing problems and promotes "effective altruism." It provides career resources to encourage graduates aged 20–35 to focus their strengths and careers on socially beneficial outcomes.

Multimedia

The Altruism Revolution
https://www.youtube.com/watch?v=mRY8zbv2qYI
This trailer introduces The Altruism Revolution, a documentary that examines the scientific reasons behind the call for a more caring society.

Random Acts of Kindness - Faith In Humanity Restored - Good People 2019
https://www.youtube.com/watch?v=jadl5ZYtcPI
This 13-minute collage captures everyday occurrences of people helping people and other sentient beings through difficult times.

A Selfish Argument for Making the World a Better Place - Egoistic Altruism
https://youtu.be/rvskMHn0sqQ
Making an argument for a positive-sum world, this video states that no matter what the motivation may be, working for a better world for all will benefit everyone.

Simple Acts of Kindness
https://www.youtube.com/watch?v=_Nl2sT0rTDc
Watch how people of all ages offer strangers simple acts of kindness to brighten their day.

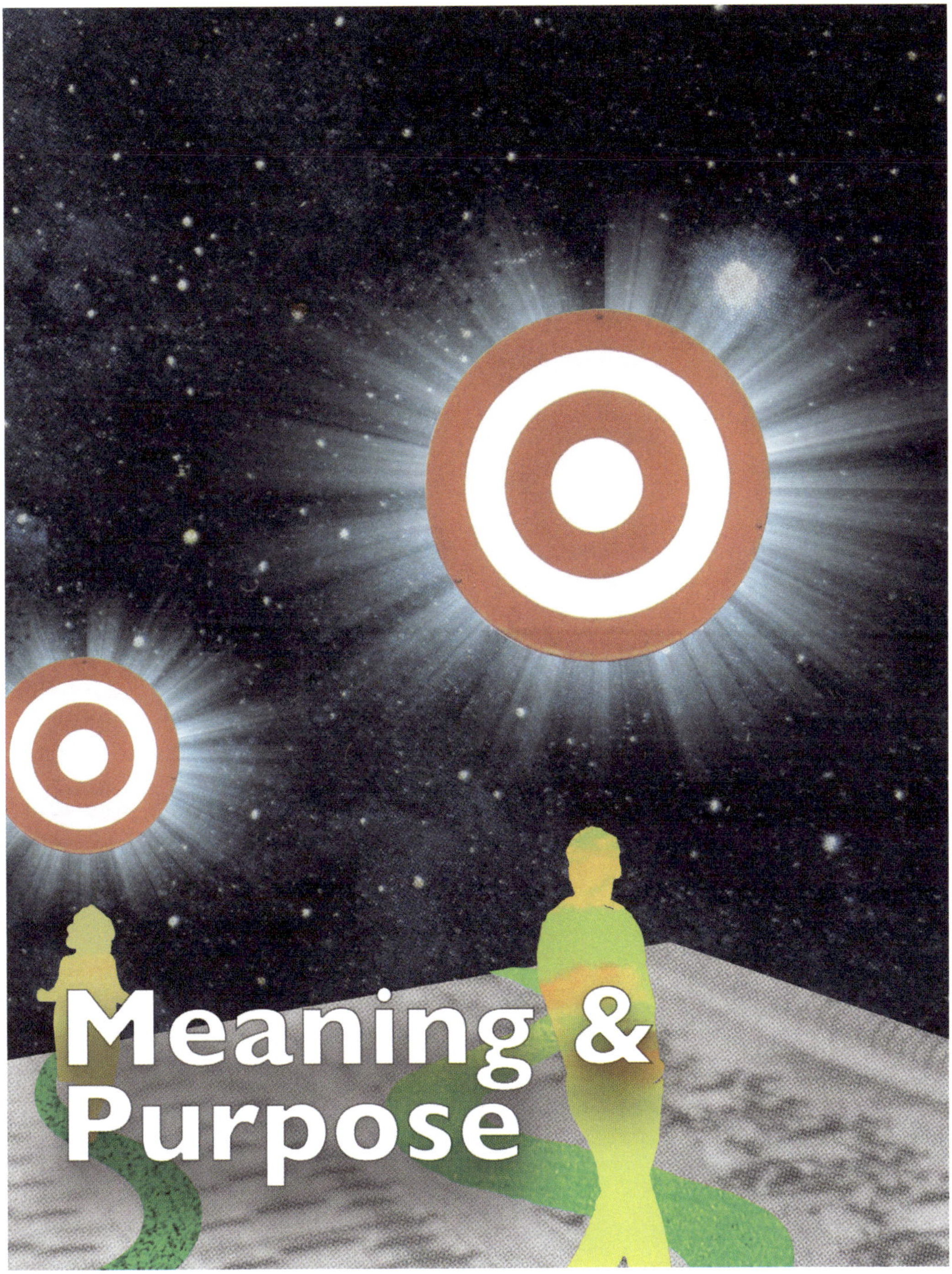
Meaning &
Purpose

Module 14: Meaning and Purpose

The closing module focuses directly on the value of living meaningful and purposeful lives. It comes full circle from Module 1 where participants shared a story of resilience from their past to an activity that invites them to imagine a meaningful, purpose-filled future.

Module Topic	Minutes to Allot	
Learning Outcomes By re-examining their initial story of resilience and by writing a story of how they would like to be remembered in the future, participants: • Reinterpret their story of resilience for clues to meaning and purpose • Envision a meaningful lifetime accomplishment • Envision a plan of action to achieve the vision within 10 years	5	5
Opening Activities Start the module with a relaxation or mindfulness practice Invite participants to share their experiences giving the gift of time. Invite questions about the previous module and practice(s)	10	15
Illustration of Core Concepts Review core concepts and show video illustrations Facilitate reflection and discussion: • *What are the key messages in the video(s) you just watched?* • *How might these concepts be relevant in your life?*	15	15
Practice 1: Reflect on your Story of Resilience Have participants complete Story of Resilience reflection to uncover aspects that hold meaning and purpose for them **Practice 2: Envision a Story of Your Future** Have participants complete long-term goal-setting questions Have participants imagine and write about their life 10 years from now, having accomplished these goals Debrief learning from practice(s) using questions: • *Does your story reveal themes about what has meaning in your life and your broader life purpose?* • *How can your strengths help you build into your life more of what matters most to you?* • *What actions or habits can you build into your future to maintain a sense of meaning and purpose?*	20	30
Closing Activities Invite discussion of everyday applications Remind participants of relevant resources at the end of the module Guide participants in a 3-minute closing relaxation or mindfulness practice Celebrate conclusion of the program	10	10
Total	60 minutes	75 minutes

Core Concepts of Meaning and Purpose

Many of the themes here are also presented in the Core Concepts section of the Workbook (p. 157):

- *Meaning* refers to a coherent understanding of the world that promotes the pursuit of long-term goals that provide a sense of purpose and fulfillment. Multiple lines of research (Lambert et al., 2013; Stillman & Baumeister, 2009) suggest that pursuit of meaning serves several purposes in our lives, for example:
  1. It helps us articulate life goals within the timeframe that includes our past, present, and future.
  2. It provides a sense of efficacy or control and allows us to believe that we are more than just pawns controlled by the events of the world.
  3. It guides our actions.
  4. Activities associated with meaning often bond people in a shared sense of community.
- Viktor Frankl, in his seminal works on meaning – for example, *The Will to Meaning* (Frankl, 1988), *Man's Searching for Meaning* (Frankl, 1963), and *The Doctor and the Soul* (Frankl, 1973) – argued that meaning is always possible and that it is a fundamental drive for people. No matter what the circumstances, individuals are always free to choose the perspective they will take on their experiences. Frankl posits that the pursuit of meaning must be included as one of the core human motivations alongside the pursuits of pleasure and power.
- Meaning does not need to be a grand, life-encompassing concept. Small scale events can also be a source of meaning. Examples might be picking up a used plastic bag and depositing it in the appropriate recycling bin, holding a door for others, buying a cup of coffee for the person next in line, or standing up for someone being verbally bullied. These small daily life events make a meaningful chain which is attached to a larger purpose or meaning such as serving others, spreading kindness, or being environmentally conscientious.
- Meaning tends to exist in interpersonal settings. Because humans are such social animals, people tend to have goals that promote their group (e.g., "I want to become a doctor to help my community") or goals that are derived from the values of their group (e.g., "I want to become a doctor because that is a valued profession").
- Meaning in life is primarily cognitive. Meaning involves having a firm belief that there is an overarching purpose to one's life. Secondly, a sense of meaning enhances self-control which guides one to transcend momentary urges and overrides more primitive and impulsive urges (Li et al., 2021; Martela & Steger, 2016)
- Steger (2012) posits that human beings have a strong desire to make sense of their experiences, gain some clarity about who they are, and identify the purpose of their lives. In other words, humans want to know what their lives are all about and how they fit in the grand scheme of things and the world around them. Steger contends that although meaning is part of our DNA, it is not fixed. Rather, we can choose some actions or activities to experience more meaning (Steger, 2012).
- There are many ways to achieve meaning. Committing to something larger than oneself – often through altruism and service to others – is important in the quest for meaning (Frankl, 1963; Kahana et al., 2013).
- A sense of meaning or purpose is linked to greater well-being and mental health. For example, meaning is associated with lower levels of depression and anxiety (e.g., Mascaro & Rosen, 2006, 2008). Research indicates that individuals who possess a clear sense of purpose tend to be more altruistic (Steger et al., 2006).

Illustrations of Meaning and Purpose

Play at least one of the three videos below to illustrate the core concepts of meaning and purpose and encourage discussion.

The Time You Have
https://www.youtube.com/watch?v=BOksW_NabEk
(Duration: 2:44 minutes)
A visual illustration of the time you have in your life, this video motivates viewers to start doing things that you love now.

Hugo – Purpose
https://www.youtube.com/watch?v=7jzLeNYe46g
(Duration: 2:33 minutes)
This short clip from the 2011 film *Hugo* illustrates the importance of finding purpose in our lives.

Peaceful Warrior – Everything Has a Purpose
https://youtu.be/w1jaPahTM4o?list=PL8m55lz0Oco4BRLkwj9KM9yxbCsLC5mjb
(Duration: 3:20 minutes)
Based on a true story and a book by Dan Millman, the story of a college gymnast illustrates the difference between mindless pursuit of a goal and connecting actions to serve a larger purpose.

Reflection and Discussion

Invite participants to complete the Reflection and Discussion section of their Workbook (p. 158) regarding the video(s) they have watched. Discuss the questions:

What are the key messages in the video(s) you just watched?

How might these concepts be relevant in your life?

Practice: Meaning and Purpose

The present is all we experience. In our minds, we recall our past and anticipate our future, reflecting on events and imagining possibilities for how things will work out in a certain way. These last two practices of SBR connect the past, present, and future into a narrative which is meant to provide coherence to our temporal self (Blouin-Hudon & Pychyl, 2017). With these concluding practices, we hope to provide participants with a feeling of continuity and belonging in their social networks as well as a greater sense of meaning and purpose in their lives.

Practice 1: Reflect on Your Story of Resilience

The goal of this practice is to review the Story of Resilience that participants wrote in Module 1 and to make meaning from it in light of the concepts and skills they have learned throughout the program.

Follow the steps below to guide this practice.

- Refer participants to the Story of Resilience they wrote in Module 1: Resilience.
- Have them read their story and encourage them to look for themes that might relate to their own sense of meaning and purpose.
- Encourage participants to look for dimensions of their story which are beyond themselves. That is, elements of their story that serve others, as serving others can be a source of meaning and purpose. Examples include pursuing causes to help others or the environment, safeguarding the rights of a vulnerable individual or community, raising awareness about sociocultural issues, or even engaging in creative activities.
- After participants have read and drawn insights from their story, invite them to pair up or form small groups of 3–4 participants and discuss what their story has revealed about themselves now that several weeks have passed since writing it.

Practice Debrief

Invite participants to discuss the following three questions:

- *What meaning can you derive from the experience in your resilience story?*
- *What does your story of resilience tell you about what is important to you?*
- *Does your story of resilience connect to your life purpose? How?*

Practice 2: Envision a Story of Your Future

The goal of this exercise for participants is to imagine their future self in 10 years' time and reflect on how they can use their strengths to be the person they would like to be.

Writing about our vision for the future is related to resilience. According to the expectancy-value model of motivation, progress toward a goal leads to positive emotions and confidence of a good outcome (Carver & Scheier, 2001). Mental simulation of this imagined future and its transfer onto paper through writing can help in planning and facilitate the actual behavior towards the goal.

Follow the steps below to implement this practice:

- Refer participants to the Worksheet on p. 160 of the Workbook that begins the practice with the prompt, "Imagine your life 10 years from now. You run into an old friend who asks what you have been up to since you left high school."
- Before having them write their story, have them brainstorm possible content. Ask them to write down a few realistic accomplishments they would like to achieve and how they would use their strengths in pursuing these accomplishments. Refer them to the examples in Table 13 (Table WB7 in Workbook on p. 160).

- Continue the brainstorming by inviting them to reflect on the questions following the table:
  - *What makes these achievements important to you and to others? Why?*
  - *What steps do you need to take to accomplish these goals in the next 10 years? What would you need to do, year-by-year?*
  - *What hurdles will you have to overcome to accomplish these achievements?*
  - *Which of your signature strengths will you use most often to accomplish your goals?*
- Once they have brainstormed their ideas, refer them to p. 162 of the Workbook to write their Story of My Future Self.
- Draw participants' attention to the instruction at the bottom of p. 162, inviting them to keep this story, read it at least once every 3 years and adjust their goals accordingly. Suggest that they can also share their story with a friend or loved one and update them on their progress.

Table 13. Some examples of significant achievements or accomplishments

• Reuse, repurpose, and recycle electronics	• Play a role in protecting the planet
• Explore and promote corporate social responsibility	• Be a transformative teacher in a classroom of special students
• Promote innovative ways to increase charitable giving	• Research a major disease in search of a treatment, cure, or intervention
• Invest talents in causes that bring about change for the better	• Develop art installations that contribute to your community
• Get involved politically to advocate for an important social issue	• Reduce crime or conflict in your neighborhood
• Volunteer your marketing skills to improve the image of an important cause	• Support parents to learn parenting or partnering skills
• Contribute to a cause that can comfort the needy	• Teach a skill that helps others to be more independent
• Become a mentor to disadvantaged people	• Be the best parent you can be
• Stand up for the rights of others	• Be the best partner you can be

Practice Debrief

Instruct the participants to reflect on and discuss what they wrote in Practice 2: Story of My Future Self (in their Workbook, p. 162) and then consider the following questions:

Does the Story of My Future Self reveal themes about what has meaning in your life and what your broader life purpose might be?

How can your strengths help you build into your life more of what matters most to you?

What actions or habits can you build into your life to create a sense of meaning and purpose?

Learning and Cultural Fit

Adapt this practice to the learning and cultural needs of your participants, including their unique values and demographics. Possible adaptations include:

- The search for meaning is highly culturally sensitive. For example, in Chinese Taoism, the meaning of life may be primarily based on living naturally instead of struggling against the Tao (Lin, 2001). Similarly, Buddhism advocates an attitude of acceptance, contentment, and non-attachment in relation to adverse situations, because suffering is inevitable (Lin, 2001). In other cultures, the meaning of life is closely tied with one's ability to forge close relationships with family and community.
- Some participants may find meaning a very abstract concept. They might have difficulty thinking about meaning in terms of specific goals. You can use the following questions to help participants develop a more concrete sense of the role of meaning in their lives:
  - Why are they in school? In this job? At this stage of their life?
  - How does being in school fit with their bigger purpose in life?
  - What are they learning and how will it help them later in life?
  - What do they need to learn in order to understand their purpose?
- Some participants may define meaning in spiritual contexts, such as being a good Buddhist, Christian, Hindu, Jew, or Muslim. The goal is to help participants find meaning through the sources that they deem most appropriate for them.
- What gives an event or experience meaning varies from person to person and across the lifespan. For example, what one finds meaningful at age 16 may change drastically at age 26. Help participants to understand that meaning and purpose do not need to be one well-defined, unchangeable, and grand cause. Our concept of meaning can be very personal and changeable.
- Participants who have experienced a significant loss or adversity may also find it difficult to find meaning. For such people, the process of finding meaning may be long, but it is never hopeless. Continue to gently encourage them.

Closing Activities

The goal of closing this module is to help participants consolidate their understanding of meaning and purpose and to take their new learning into everyday life.

Discuss with participants the Everyday Applications section (p. 164 in their Workbook). Invite participants to be mindful in their day-to-day lives by noticing their own and others' actions and habits which reveal purpose and meaning. Encourage them to use relevant resources found at the end of this module and included in their Workbook starting on p. 164.

Choose a 3-minute activity from Regular Practice 1: Mindfulness and Relaxation to close the module.

Everyday Applications

- Before going to bed, take 5 minutes to reflect on or write about what you did today that was meaningful for you. Does it in some way bring you closer to your goals?
- Before beginning an activity – for instance, doing a presentation, taking an exam, or even a simple thing such as making a comment to your friend – pause and take a few seconds to reflect on why you are doing what you are doing. Is it important to say what you are saying, and will it be helpful? When you spend time thinking about the "why?" of actions, you do them with more zest. Alternatively, you choose to avoid actions that are not important or meaningful to you.
- One at a time, try to reduce your activities or learn to say no to activities that do not feel purposeful to you. This is called decluttering your life. This could look like letting go of people, ideas, and things in your life which no longer make you happy. Look around your room. Are there clothes or books in your room, which you do not need anymore? Consider donating them. Are there unhelpful and self-defeating thoughts in your mind that visit you frequently? Consider replacing them with more helpful ones. Are there people in your life who bring you hurt and may be distracting you from your meaning in life? Can you think of ways to limit their importance in your life?
- With your life now decluttered, think about who in your life brings out your best and helps you live a purposeful, meaningful existence. Build time in your schedule to be with them and enjoy fulfilling activities.

Program Wrap-Up

Congratulations on facilitating this 14-module Strengths-Based Resilience program.

As you wrap up the program, make sure you build in sufficient time to celebrate participants' completion of the program. Encourage a conversation about their SBR journey, including questions that invite them to share their reflections about what they have learned. Examples include:

- What are the most valuable lessons or skills you have learned from SBR?
- What concrete changes, big or small, have you noticed in your behavior that you can attribute to SBR?
- What are helpful and practical things you learned during the SBR program which will enhance or maintain your resilience?
- What are you taking away from SBR that you can apply in the weeks, months, and years ahead?

If you are planning a formal evaluation, this is the time to have participants provide written feedback or to direct them to an online survey.

No matter where participants are in their journey toward experiencing greater resilience and well-being, they have taken a major step by completing this program. Remind them that building a repertoire of resilience skills is not an easy undertaking. It is a life-long process. Cultivating resilience means translating the SBR Program lessons into habits, thereby building strong character to surmount challenges and embrace opportunities.

References

Blouin-Hudon, E.-M. C., & Pychyl, T. A. (2017). A mental imagery intervention to increase future self-continuity and reduce procrastination. *Applied Psychology: An International Review, 66*(2), 326–352. https://psycnet.apa.org/doi/10.1111/apps.12088

Carver, C. S., & Scheier, M. F. (2001). Optimism, pessimism, and self-regulation. In E. C. Chang (Ed.), *Optimism & pessimism: Implications for theory, research, and practice* (pp. 31–51). American Psychological Association.

Frankl, V. E. (1963). *Man's search for meaning: An introduction to logotherapy*. Washington Square Press.

Frankl, V. E. (1973). *The doctor and the soul: From psychotherapy to logotherapy*. Penguin Books.

Frankl, V. E. (1988). *The will to meaning: Foundations and applications of logotherapy* (exp. ed.). Penguin Books.

Kahana, E., Bhatta, T., Lovegreen, L. D., Kahana, B., & Midlarsky, E. (2013). Altruism, helping, and volunteering: Pathways to well-being in late life. *Journal of Aging and Health, 25*(1), 159–187. https://doi.org/10.1177/0898264312469665

Lambert, N. M., Stillman, T. F., Hicks, J. A., Kamble, S., Baumeister, R. F., & Fincham, F. D. (2013). To belong is to matter: Sense of belonging enhances meaning in life. *Personality and Social Psychology Bulletin, 39*(11), 1418–1427. https://doi.org/10.1177/0146167213499186

Li, J.-B., Dou, K., & Liang, Y. (2021). The relationship between presence of meaning, search for meaning, and subjective well-being: A three-level meta-analysis based on the Meaning in Life Questionnaire. *Journal of Happiness Studies, 22*(1), 467–489. https://doi.org/10.1007/s10902-020-00230-y

Lin, A. (2001). *Exploring sources of life meaning among Chinese* [Unpublished master's thesis]. Trinity Western University.

Martela, F., & Steger, M. F. (2016). The three meanings of meaning in life: Distinguishing coherence, purpose, and significance. *The Journal of Positive Psychology, 11*(5), 531–545. https://doi.org/10.1080/17439760.2015.1137623

Mascaro, N., & Rosen, D. H. (2006). The role of existential meaning as a buffer against stress. *Journal of Humanistic Psychology, 46*(2), 168–190. https://psycnet.apa.org/doi/10.1177/0022167805283779

Mascaro, N., & Rosen, D. H. (2008). Assessment of existential meaning and its longitudinal relations with depressive symptoms. *Journal of Social and Clinical Psychology, 27*, 576–599. https://doi.org/10.1521/jscp.2008.27.6.576

Steger, M. F. (2012). Making meaning in life. *Psychological Inquiry, 23*, 381–385. https://doi.org/10.1080/1047840X.2012.720832

Steger, M. F., Frazier, P., Oishi, S., & Kaler, M. (2006). The Meaning in Life Questionnaire: Assessing the presence of and search for meaning in life. *Journal of Counseling Psychology, 53*(1), 80–93. https://doi.org/10.1037/0022-0167.53.1.80

Stillman, T. F., & Baumeister, R. F. (2009). Uncertainty, belongingness, and four needs for meaning. *Psychological Inquiry, 20*(4), 249–251. https://doi.org/10.1080/10478400903333544

Resources

Literature

Baumeister, R. F. (1991). *Meanings of life*. Guilford Press.

Emmons, R. A., Barrett, J. L., & Schnitker, S. A. (2008). Religion and personality. In R. Robins, O. P. John, & L. A. Pervin (Eds.), *Handbook of personality* (3rd ed., pp. 634–653). Guilford Press.

Esfahani Smith, E. (2017). *The power of meaning: Crafting a life that matters*. Broadway Books.

Kaukmann, S. B. (2020). *Transcend: The new science of self-actualization*. Penguin Random House.

Frankl, V. E. (1963). *Man's search for meaning: An introduction to logotherapy*. Washington Square Press.

Lightsey, O. (2006). Resilience, Meaning, and well-being. *Counseling Psychologist, 34*(1), 96–107. https://doi.org/10.1177/0011000005282369

Lin, A. (2001). *Exploring sources of life meaning among Chinese* [Unpublished master's thesis]. Trinity Western University.
Parks, S. D. (2019). *Big questions, worthy dreams: Mentoring emerging adults in their search for meaning, purpose, and faith*. Fortress Press.
Peterson. C., & Park, N. (2012). Character strengths and the life of meaning. In P. T. P. Wong (Ed.), *The human quest for meaning: Theories, research, and applications* (2nd ed., pp. 277–296). Routledge.
Peterson, J. B. (1999). *Maps of meaning: The architecture of belief.* Routledge.
Schnell, T., & Becker, P. (2006). Personality and meaning in life. *Personality and Individual Differences, 41*(1), 117–129. https://doi.org/10.1016/j.paid.2005.11.030
Stillman, T. F., & Baumeister, R. F. (2009). Uncertainty, belongingness, and four needs for meaning. *Psychological Inquiry, 20*(4), 249–251. https://doi.org/10.1080/10478400903333544
Wong, P. T. P. (2012). *The human quest for meaning: Theories, research, and applications*. Routledge.

Websites

John Templeton Foundation:
https:// www.templeton.org/about
The John Templeton Foundation serves as a philanthropic catalyst for discoveries relating to the deepest and most perplexing questions facing humankind. It supports research on subjects ranging from complexity, evolution, and emergence, to creativity, forgiveness, and free will.

Laboratory for the Study of Meaning and Quality of Life
http://www.michaelfsteger.com/
This is the website of Prof. Michael Steger, the founder and director of the Center for Meaning and Purpose, and professor of psychology at Colorado State University.

Meaning-Centered Counselling Institute: Home of Meaning Therapy
http://www.meaningtherapy.com/
Meaning Therapy is a website that offers counseling services, articles, and resources for people in search of discovering greater meaning in their lives.

Hold the Door for Others – Growth Through Adversity
https://holdthedoor.com/
This website offers resources for people to grow in the face of grief, trauma, and adversity.

Multimedia

Viktor Frankl: Our Need for Meaning and Purpose
https://youtu.be/lD09bOOHt0O
In a 1972 interview, the author of *Man's Search for Meaning* discusses his theory of logotherapy: how humans' search for meaning, especially in the face of crisis, enhances their chance of survival.

Can Science Explain Meaning and Purpose?
https://youtu.be/P07oEAlxkD8
Jay Lombard and Massimo Pigliucci discuss limits of science in explaining our beliefs.

The Theory of Everything
https://youtu.be/KLp6N46er6Y
In this movie clip, the distinguished scientist Stephen Hawking is shown explaining there should be no boundary to human endeavor. "While there is life, there is hope."

This Is How Terribly Short Your Life Is
https://youtu.be/LrRfjmv-5cQ
Your life is much shorter than you think. If you subtract essentials chores of life, including, sleeping, going to school, eating, and running errands, your remaining hours are precious and few. Make sure you use them wisely.

Artist's Notes on Illustrations

The notes below serve as captions to the artwork associated with each module in this Manual. Use these captions to guide your classroom discussion of the artwork.

Regular Practice 1: Mindfulness and Relaxation
Scaffolding the tumultuousness of the contemporary mind, the olive branches on the sides of the head remind us about our ability to cultivate tolerance for inevitable stressors and to cultivate a habit of calmness through sustained effort.

Regular Practice 2: Gratitude
The presenting gymnasts encourage us to recall the positive people, places, and things that are around us and the need to make an effort to acknowledge and appreciate them. The two hands represent the effort we need to make to focus on positive but genuine aspects of our lives and not slide into narrow and boxed negative thinking.

Module 1: Resilience
Nelson Mandela said, "The greatest glory in living lies not in never falling, but in rising every time we fall." The pole in this piece illustrates climbing up, falling, and then trying again.

Module 2: Fixed and Growth Mindsets
With a growth mindset, we can open up to possibilities and opportunities as illustrated by opening the net to a wider universe in this piece. With a fixed mindset, our view becomes narrow, within the bounds of this net, and we view problems and obstacles as unsolvable and ourselves as incapable.

Modules 3 and 4: Cognitive Accuracy and Flexibility
This piece captures self-growth and a change in perspective. As our thinking style becomes more flexible, we are able to become more advanced versions of ourselves. The abstract circles remind us to view challenging situations from all sides, open our thinking, and expand our viewpoint.

Modules 5: Character Strengths
This piece depicts core psychological assets — our character strengths. The diamond in the illustration symbolizes assets whereas the tree denotes growth that stems from these assets. Character strengths are traits that help us to grow as grateful, kind, curious, creative and cooperative individuals.

Module 6: Signature Strengths
This piece captures strengths that are central to one's existence. These are our unique character, represented through the orbits of ease, comfort, and originality we feel when we exercise our signature strengths.

Module 7: Problem-Solving and Strengths
The maze of life, illustrated here, presents challenges, stressors, and hassles. Our best option to try to overcome them lies not in focusing on our weaknesses but in using our strengths creatively and adaptively.

Module 8: Grudge and Gratitude
This piece depicts grudge as a dogged ill-feeling, which one can hold against a person or group. The illustration shows that one spends a lot of thinking and attentional resources on replaying this ill-feeling, hoping to gain insight, which often remains elusive, and one is left with brooding, shown as a black mass on the floor. Note: Gratitude is depicted in the Regular Practice: Gratitude.

Module 9: Empathy
This piece shows our ability to feel vicariously – putting ourselves in others' shoes. Hands touching symbolize care and concern for others while multicolored flowers show different perspectives. We can understand, at a deeper level, why people have scorn or a smile on their face.

Module 10: Slowness and Savoring
This piece reminds us to take a break from our busy lives to reconnect with ourselves. The individual returns to nature and rests peacefully in a boat. The limitless nature of the ocean and the cosmos represents the increased creativity and imagination we actually achieve when we work in a relaxed state.

Module 11: Positive Relationships
This piece illustrates that a significant part of our resilience and happiness is related to our close ties to our loved ones, especially our families. These relationships offer us opportunities to acknowledge, express, and enhance our strengths in a close interpersonal realm.

Module 12: Positive Communication
The smiling faces in the illustration depict the essence of this module – positive communication. These smiles are external display of feeling that we and our positive experiences are seen, understood, and valued by our friends and loved ones.

Module 13: Altruism
When we are altruistic, we give selflessly to others without expecting anything in return. In this image, two hands present a bouquet of flowers, symbolizing the gift of time, work, and energy. Multicolored circles spill out of the bouquet, symbolizing the rewarding feeling that results from helping others selflessly.

Module 14: Meaning and Purpose
The paths in this piece symbolize routes paved by actions taken in pursuit of a goal that is greater and beyond the self. This is depicted by red and white circles. These paths connect us with the universe, represented by space in the image.